Adam Arthur · Kevin Foley
C. Wayne Hamm
Editors

Perioperative Considerations and Positioning for Neurosurgical Procedures

A Clinical Guide

Springer

Editors
Adam Arthur
Semmes-Murphey Neurologic
and Spine Clinic
Memphis, TN, USA

Kevin Foley
Semmes-Murphey Neurologic
and Spine Clinic
Memphis, TN, USA

C. Wayne Hamm
Medical Anesthesia Group
Germantown, TN, USA

ISBN 978-3-030-10250-0 ISBN 978-3-319-72679-3 (eBook)
https://doi.org/10.1007/978-3-319-72679-3

Softcover re-print of the Hardcover 1st edition 2018

Printed on acid-free paper

This Springer imprint is published by the registered company Springer International Publishing AG part of Springer Nature
The registered company address is: Gewerbestrasse 11, 6330 Cham, Switzerland

Foreword

"It wasn't raining when Noah built the arc."

Howard Joseph Ruff *(December 27, 1930–November 12, 2016), financial adviser and author of the investing newsletter The Ruff Times*

The importance of preparation and attention to detail in the field of neurosurgery cannot be overemphasized. Perhaps in no other endeavor of surgery is there so little tolerance for error.

In the history of medicine, the chapter on neurosurgery is among the most interesting. Archaeological evidence proves that humans were performing trephinations since prehistoric times. Despite the early genesis of surgery on the human skull and brain, the specialty of neurosurgery is a relatively recent evolutionary product of the broader field of general surgery. The field made little progress until Harvey Cushing established neurosurgery as a unique discipline in the twentieth century. Our specialty was limited by a poor understanding of pathology, archaic imaging of that pathology, primitive anesthesiology, limited intraoperative visualization, and marginal postoperative care.

The past few decades have witnessed dramatic improvements in all of these important facets of neurosurgical care: introduction of the operating microscope, mind boggling advances in neuroimaging, development of the subspecialty of neuroanesthesiology, introduction of neurocritical care, neuroendovascular therapy, neuromodulation and molecular biology, to name a few. Despite these remarkable advances, the practicing neurosurgeon must never lose sight of the basic surgical principles and details that often determine the outcome for our patients.

The attention to detail required for success in neurosurgery begins with patient selection and continues throughout the patient's hospital course and postoperative care. Once the decision for surgery has been agreed upon, every detail matters and proper preparation will influence the outcome. The natural tendency to focus on high-tech issues may create complacency and neglect of the basics.

The editors have provided the first monograph dedicated to the important, but often trivialized, issue of surgical positioning in neurosurgical procedures. This seemingly routine issue may have a profound influence on the outcome of an otherwise well-planned procedure.

Although certain standard positions are typically used for most common neurosurgical procedures, the positioning must be tailored to the individual patient body habitus and comorbidities. Selection of the appropriate position must balance patient comfort, surgeon comfort, and a vast array of physiological issues and therefore must be tailored to the unique patient and their procedure.

The contributing authors have created an authoritative reference book that includes a balanced presentation of the positions commonly utilized in neurosurgery, alternative positions for unique situations, and a comprehensive discussion of the potential complications associated with all positioning options. This treatise should be read and studied by neurosurgeons of all levels of training and experience as well as those anesthesiologists who are so vitally important in determining the outcomes of our procedures.

Department of Neurosurgery
Emory University School of Medicine
Atlanta, GA, USA

Daniel L. Barrow
Pamela R. Rollins

Preface

"I would like to see the day when somebody would be appointed surgeon somewhere who had no hands, for the operative part is the least part of the work."

—Harvey Cushing

If a neurosurgical patient isn't positioned well, it can make operating with both hands unfeasible for the surgeon. Neurosurgical positioning errors can make surgery difficult or impossible in a myriad of ways. Aside from making the pathology inaccessible, improper positioning can result in increased blood loss, cardiopulmonary complications, and herniation.

Patients undergoing a procedure at the hands of any type of surgeon must be positioned properly to allow access to the surgical pathology and to keep the patient safe during the procedure. Most surgical specialties involve one or two "standard" and well-described positions that allow surgical access. In some surgical specialties, positioning requires consideration as a means of minimizing blood loss. Some surgical specialties must even give consideration to positioning with regard to using gravity as a means of minimizing retraction on eloquent tissues. Neurosurgery requires that we consider all of these factors and how they are impacted in a number of different positions.

The neurosurgeon is confronted with variations in pathology that are constantly requiring adjustments to "standard" positions. Thus, a full working knowledge of how to position patients to achieve the above desired goals, the expected results of the applied position, the complications of the applied position, and means of minimizing and/or avoiding those complications is necessary. This working knowledge must incorporate existing recommendations and guidelines and be applied with a reciprocal knowledge of the operating room nurses and anesthesia personnel for maximum surgical benefit with minimum surgical complications. As certain positions are infrequently used and operating room personnel and anesthesia providers are often changing, the neurosurgeon can sometimes find themselves the party most acquainted with the position and its attendant risks and benefits.

Our intent is that this work helps to advance the understanding of neurosurgical positioning and improve the safety of surgery for neurosurgical patients.

This book owes a great debt to Dr. John Martin and Dr. Mark Warner for their pioneering work in the three editions of *Positioning in Anesthesia and Surgery*.

Memphis, TN — Adam Arthur
Memphis, TN — Kevin Foley
Germantown, TN — C. Wayne Hamm

Contents

Contributors

Shaheryar F. Ansari Goodman Campbell Brain and Spine, Indianapolis, IN, USA

Department of Neurological Surgery, Indiana University School of Medicine, Indianapolis, IN, USA

Kenan I. Arnautović Department of Neurosurgery, Semmes-Murphey Clinic, University of Tennessee, Memphis, TN, USA

Adam Arthur Semmes-Murphey Neurological and Spine Clinic, University of Tennessee Health Sciences Center, Memphis, TN, USA

Jaafar Basma University of Tennessee Health Sciences Center, Memphis, TN, USA

Matthew T. Brown Department of Neurosurgery, University of Tennessee, Memphis, TN, USA

Raul Cardenas Department of Neurosurgery, University of Tennessee, Memphis, TN, USA

Department of Neurosurgery, Semmes-Murphey Clinic, University of Tennessee, Memphis, TN, USA

Michael DeCuypere Department of Neurosurgery, University of Tennessee Health Science Center, Memphis, TN, USA

LeBonheur Children's Hospital, Memphis, TN, USA

Semmes-Murphey Neurologic and Spine Institute, Memphis, Tennessee, USA

Lucas Elijovich Department of Neurology, University of Tennessee Health Sciences Center, Memphis, TN, USA

Semmes-Murphey Neurologic Institute, University of Tennessee Health Sciences Center, Memphis, TN, USA

Julius Fernandez (deceased) Department of Neurosurgery, University of Tennessee, Memphis, TN, USA

Department of Neurosurgery, Semmes-Murphey Clinic, University of Tennessee, Memphis, TN, USA

Kevin Foley Semmes-Murphey Clinic, University of Tennessee Health Science Center, Memphis, TN, USA

Thomas Scott Guyton Methodist Le Bonheur Healthcare, Memphis, TN, USA

C. Wayne Hamm Medical Anesthesia Group, Germantown, TN, USA

Daniel Hoit Department of Neurosurgery, Semmes-Murphey Brain and Spine Institute, University of Tennessee Health Sciences Center, Memphis, TN, USA

Emily Hamm Huseth Harris Shelton Hanover Walsh, PLLC, Memphis, TN, USA

Nickalus R. Khan Department of Neurosurgery, University of Tennessee Health Science Center, Memphis, TN, USA

L. Madison Michael II Semmes-Murphey Clinic, Memphis, TN, USA

Department of Neurosurgery, University of Tennessee Health Science Center, Memphis, TN, USA

Jean-Pierre Mobasser Goodman Campbell Brain and Spine, Indianapolis, IN, USA

Department of Neurological Surgery, Indiana University School of Medicine, Indianapolis, IN, USA

Michael S. Muhlbauer Department of Neurosurgery, University of Tennessee, Memphis, TN, USA

Vincent Nguyen University of Tennessee Health Sciences Center, Memphis, TN, USA

Christopher Nickele Department of Neurosurgery, Semmes-Murphey Clinic, University of the Tennessee Health Sciences, Memphis, TN, USA

Abhi Pandhi Department of Neurology, University of Tennessee Health Sciences Center, Memphis, TN, USA

Semmes-Murphey Neurologic Institute, University of Tennessee Health Sciences Center, Memphis, TN, USA

Prayash Patel Department of Neurosurgery, Semmes-Murphey Clinic, University of the Tennessee Health Sciences, Memphis, TN, USA

Mirza Pojskic Department of Neurosurgery, Philipps University Marburg, Marburg, Germany

Department of Neurosurgery, Semmes-Murphey Clinic, University of Tennessee, Memphis, TN, USA

Ganesh Rao Department of Neurosurgery, The University of Texas MD Anderson Cancer Center, Houston, TX, USA

Mallory Roberts Department of Neurosurgery, University of Tennessee, Memphis, TN, USA

Jon H. Robertson Department of Neurosurgery, University of Tennessee, Memphis, TN, USA

Emily P. Sieg Department of Neurosurgery, Milton S. Hershey Medical Center, Penn State University College of Medicine, Hershey, PA, USA

Jeffrey Sorenson University of Tennessee Health Sciences Center, Memphis, TN, USA

Semmes-Murphey Clinic, Memphis, TN, USA

Douglas R. Taylor Department of Neurosurgery, University of Tennessee Health Science Center, Memphis, TN, USA

Shelly D. Timmons Department of Neurosurgery, Milton S. Hershey Medical Center, Penn State University College of Medicine, Hershey, PA, USA

Jason A. Weaver Department of Neurosurgery, Semmes Murphey Clinic, University of Tennessee Health Sciences Center, Memphis, TN, USA

George F. Young Germantown, TN, USA

Pascal O. Zinn Baylor College of Medicine, and The University of Texas MD Anderson Cancer Center, Houston, TX, USA

Positioning Patients for Neurosurgical Procedures: A Historical Perspective

1

Mallory Roberts and Jon H. Robertson

History of Anesthesia in Neurological Surgery

Archaeological evidence exists of intracranial neurosurgical procedures being performed as early as during the Paleolithic period, but there is little known about what, if any, efforts were taken to anesthetize these subjects before extracting sections of their skulls (Fig. 1.1) [1]. There is speculation that coca leaves were chewed before procedures in areas where the plant grows naturally, but early neurosurgical patients likely found themselves having their heads drilled upon after a skull fracture or in order to release the supernatural elements thought to be causing convulsions or headaches (Figs. 1.2 and 1.3) [1].

Though the Egyptians recorded descriptions of spine pathology as early as 2900 BC, some of the first known spinal procedures were performed in the late fifth and early fourth centuries BC by Hippocrates, the father of spine surgery [2]. Hippocrates made note of the positions used to manipulate the spine and hips for his procedures (Figs. 1.4 and 1.5).

M. Roberts · J. H. Robertson (✉)
Department of Neurosurgery, University of Tennessee, Memphis, TN, USA
e-mail: Mrober41@uthsc.edu; jrobertson@semmes-murphey.com

In the first century AD, Dioscorides of Greece recorded the use of botanical substances for pain relief including mandrake, alcohol, and opium and he perhaps coined the term "anesthesia" [1]. Use of these substances during cranial procedures was not widespread at the time or for years to come, as some thought that the pain would "render [the patient] strong in endurance" and was considered "noble" even as late as the Middle Ages (Fig. 1.6).

Modern anesthesia was born in the mid-1800s with the advent of antiseptic technique and general anesthesia using ether. Dr. Morton in 1846 demonstrated the use of vaporized ether for surgical anesthetic (Fig. 1.7). Ether's widespread use was implemented within a year of its introduction and chloroform was used as an anesthetic agent just one year later; however, it took several decades for the use of these two agents to become prevalent in neurosurgical procedures [1, 3]. Once general anesthesia was broadly available, surgeons were able to perform longer and more complicated surgeries. With the utilization of this new technology came new hurdles concerning preoperative patient positioning by the surgeon and the anesthetist. Frequent patient complications and deaths were associated with the use of ether, and the rate of implementation of vital sign monitoring did not increase with the rapidity to parallel the drug's use. Once vital sign monitoring devices were widely used, accessing the patient's limbs or anterior chest again influenced preoperative positioning.

A. Arthur et al. (eds.), *Perioperative Considerations and Positioning for Neurosurgical Procedures*,
https://doi.org/10.1007/978-3-319-72679-3_1

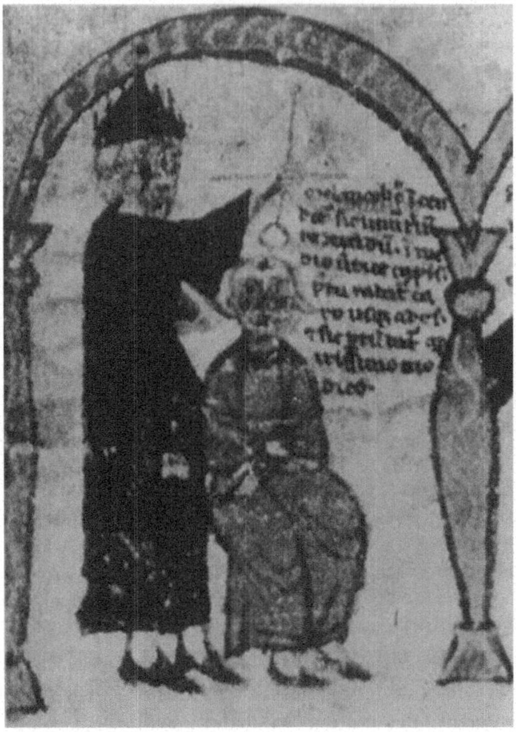

Fig. 1.1 Patients often received no anesthetics prior to "trephination," the drilling of holes in the skull [1]

Endotracheal tube placement for ventilation assistance in neurosurgical operations was first used with chloroform anesthesia soon after in the late 1870s by Sir William Macewen; oral intubation, too, took many years to be widely accepted [3]. The first general anesthesia department was not formed until the 1920s at the University of Wisconsin, headed by Ralph Waters, and anesthesia up until this point was performed by the surgical team [4].

In the early twentieth century neurosurgical operations, especially intracranial procedures, involved high morbidity rates. The importance of delivering intraoperative intravenous fluids, performing blood transfusions, maintaining adequate blood pressure, and understanding cerebrospinal fluid circulation were paramount to improving patient outcomes. This was especially important in the developing field of neurosurgery, as manipulation of the brainstem and spinal cord could cause rapid hemodynamic deterioration in addition to the risks of intraoperative blood loss and hypothermia that exist with all surgeries.

Many early developments in operative monitoring techniques, improving the safety of delivering anesthetic agents, and in defining neurological surgery as a specialized practice can be attributed to Harvey Cushing.

Harvey Cushing

Dr. Harvey Cushing is considered the father of neurosurgery in the United States. Cushing, who avidly journaled, described experiences while a student at Harvard Medical School where he was called to anesthetize patients who routinely suffered from the crude mechanisms used in the late 1800s [5].

> *Dr. Codman and I having entered the hospital together… we gave the anesthesia. I hesitate to recall what an awful business it was and how many fatalities there were. I was called down from the seats (of the surgical amphitheater) and told to put the patient to sleep. I proceeded as best I could under the orderly's directions. The operation was started… there was a sudden great gush of fluid from the patient's mouth, most of which he inhaled and he died… Codman and I resolved that we would improve our technique of giving ether.*

After witnessing many patients die due to ether administration during surgical procedures, Cushing and his classmate Earnest Codman began regularly recording pulse rate [5].

> *We made a wager of a dinner as to who could give the best anesthesia. We both became very much more skillful in our jobs than we otherwise would have become but it was particularly due to the detailed attention which we had to put upon the patient by the careful recording of the pulse rate throughout the operation* [5].

Co-residents E. A. Codman and Harvey Cushing are credited as the first to regularly record patient vital signs and interventions performed by those administering anesthesia. Codman was the first to record an anesthesia record in 1894 and Cushing improved upon it, with his earliest chart recorded in 1895 [5]. Pulse rate, respirations, pupillary size, mucus production, and drugs used were recorded. Though he often made notes of pulse quality in his anesthesia notes, Cushing did not begin recording blood pressure until 1901 upon his return from Europe [5].

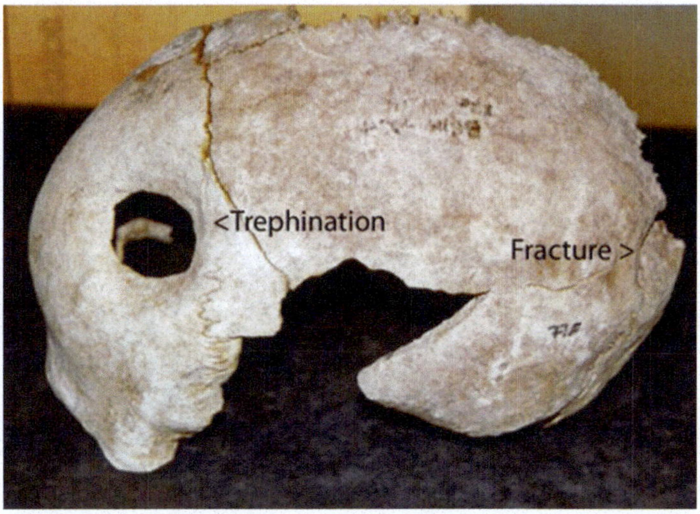

Fig. 1.2 Skull fragment carbon dated to the late Neolithic to early Bronze Age with evidence of frontal trephination found near Berlin. Posterior healed fractures extending over the lambdoid suture are also present. The trephination could have been employed as a treatment for the posterior fracture or perhaps for a separate anterior injury. (Reproduced from Piek J, Lidke G, Terberger T. The neolithic skull from Bölkendorf—evidence for Stone Age neurosurgery? Cent Eur Neurosurg. 2011;72(1). With permission from Thieme)

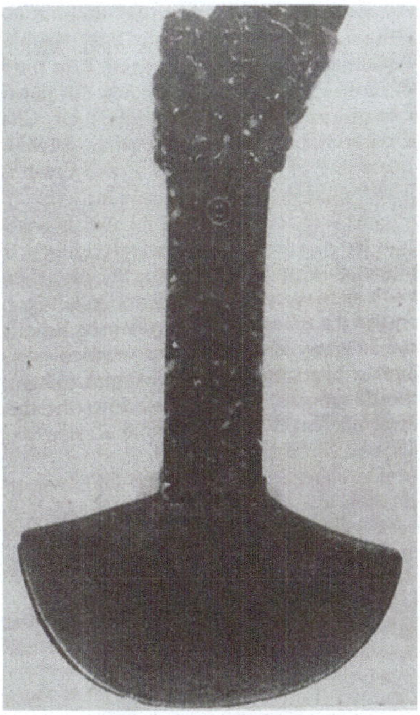

Fig. 1.3 Instrument used for trephination found in Peru as depicted by the handle's engraving. This was used around 1300–1500 BC. Coca leaves were perhaps chewed as a pain relief measure prior to cranial procedures [1]

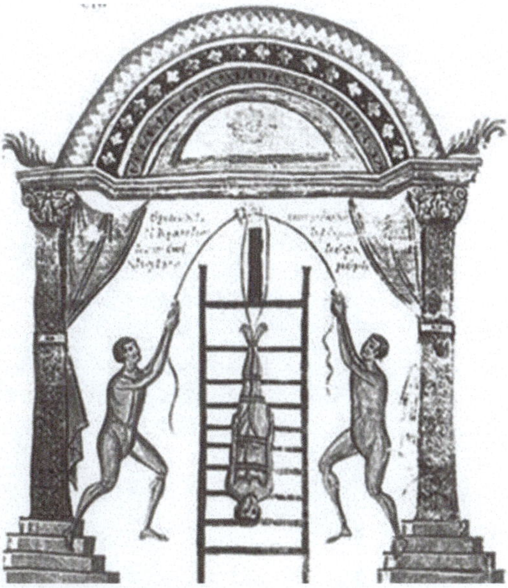

Figs. 1.4 and 1.5 Hippocrates used a platform or upright ladder and bound patients to physically reduce spinal curvature with external force. He has been called "the father of spine surgery" due to these techniques [3, 4]. (Reproduced from Marketos SG, Skiadas P. Hippocrates: the father of spine surgery. Spine. 1999;24(13). With permission from Wolters Kluwer Health, Inc.)

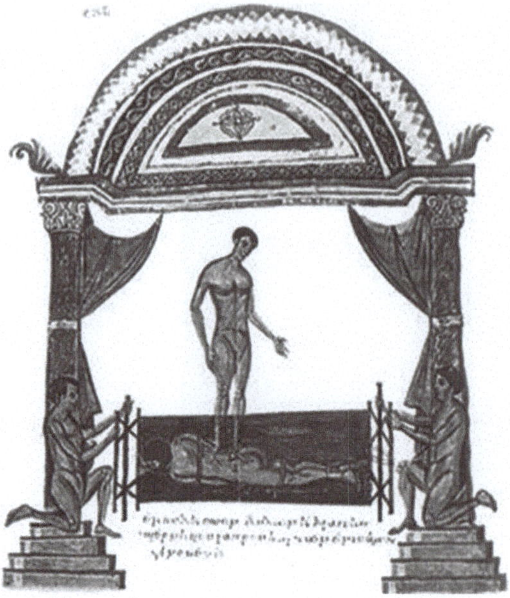

Figs. 1.4 and 1.5 (continued)

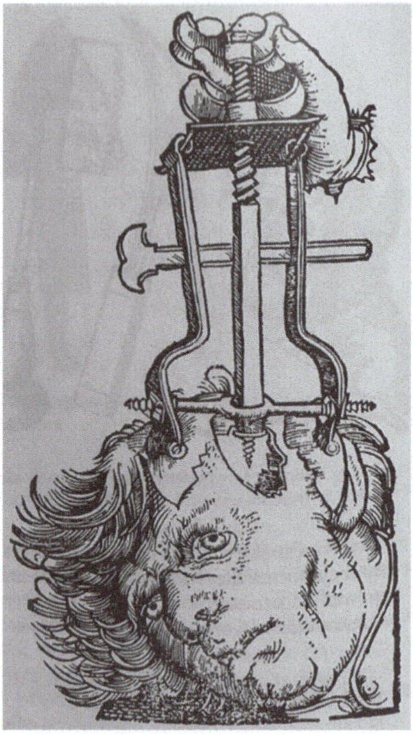

Fig. 1.6 Though anesthetic agents were available at the time (alcohol, opium, mandrake), pain was thought to be useful and its endurance noble—as such, their use was uncommon in the Middle Ages [1]

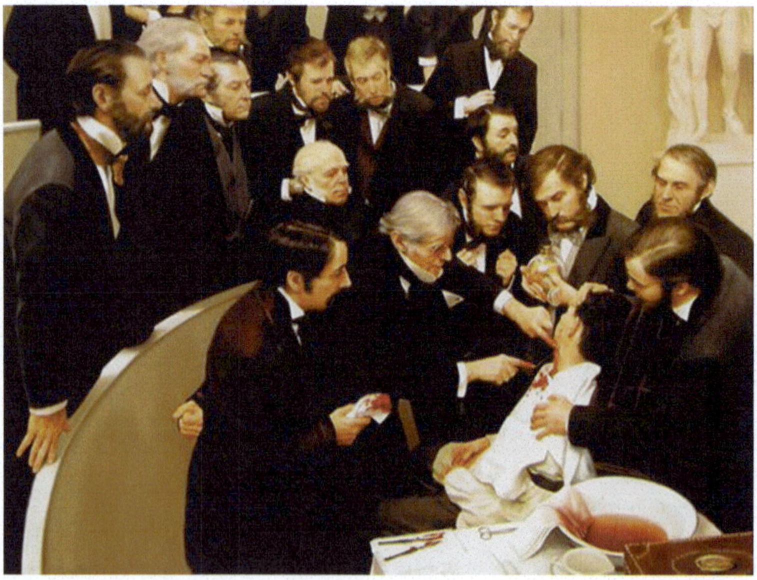

Fig. 1.7 "Ether Day 1846," a painting by Warren and Lucia Prosperi. A public demonstration of anesthesia using ether as administered by Dr. Morton (pictured holding anesthesia delivery device) in the amphitheater of Massachusetts General Hospital. (Reproduced from Desai SP, Desai MS. A tale of two paintings: depictions of the first public demonstration of ether anesthesia, Anesthesiology. 2007;106(5). With permission from Wolters Kluwer Health, Inc.)

On going abroad and getting interested in blood pressure I discovered in Padua a simple recording instrument in Riva-Rocci's clinic. On returning home I came to utilize this always during the course of my neurological operations… A much more elaborate ether chart was thereupon prepared, on which not only pulse rate and respiration but the systolic blood pressure was recorded [5].

Cushing's excitement for having found an objective measure of blood pressure is evident in his writings though he was met with considerable skepticism upon return to Boston [5–8]. Harvard Medical School went so far as suggesting "The adoption of blood-pressure observations in surgical patients does not at present appear to be necessary as a routine measure," after setting up a study to evaluate its merits [5]. Some institutions were more enthusiastic and implemented regular recordings of this data during surgeries as early as 1903, as inspired by Cushing's charts. The routine use of measuring physiological signs or charting these measurements was not consistently recommended or described in surgical or anesthesia literature until the 1920s and was not advocated as the standard of care until years later [5].

Though Cushing recognized and promoted the crucial role of intraoperative monitoring, he was no longer able as a young practicing neurosurgeon to record and monitor anesthetic administration as he did while a medical student and intern. His clear recognition of the importance of the role of the anesthetist during neurosurgical operations and his development of a reliable measure of the patient's status while anesthetized served a dual purpose of easing the burden on the anesthetist and decreasing operative risk for the patient [5]:

Were it possible, therefore, under such circumstances for [the anesthetist] to be told with the definiteness which figures alone can give, or for him to read by a glance at a plotted chart that the strength of the cardiac impulse, irrespective of its rapidity, was keeping at a normal level or was affected in one way or another by certain manipulations, not only would this feeling of responsibility be much lightened, but the operative procedure might oftentimes be modified with a consequent lessening of its risks [6].

While studying and operating abroad in England and Switzerland in 1901, Dr. Harvey Cushing not only recognized the importance of Riva-Rocci's sphygmomanometer, but also recognized the importance of integrating laboratory research alongside his surgical practice after studying under Dr. Theodore Kocher [9, 10]. Cushing as a young faculty member of the surgical department at Johns Hopkins was appointed Director of the Hunterian Laboratory by Dr. William Halstead in 1904.

Hunterian Laboratory at Johns Hopkins

The Hunterian Laboratory was established at Johns Hopkins during the early 1900s by Drs. William Welch and William Halstead. In 1904 after being appointed director of the lab, Cushing raised monies and approached the Board of Trustees of Johns Hopkins to build a special building to enlarge and enhance the Hunterian Laboratory. With completion of the new facility, Cushing studied surgical technique on anesthetized dogs and emphasized teaching for medical students. Medical students performing operations on live dogs were taught not only the method of tissue dissection, but also learned the importance of aseptic technique, meticulous recordings of laboratory data, surgical and postoperative notes, and the benefits of postmortem exams [10].

Harvey Cushing modeled the life of a physician, surgeon, and scientist. His work in the Hunterian Laboratory has been described as "one of Cushing's most significant contributions to American surgery" [5]. As Cushing's personal workshop for experimental surgery, the Hunterian Laboratory yielded numerous fundamental discoveries in the field of neuroscience during Cushing's tenure at Johns Hopkins [9]. One such development was a "precordial stethoscope," a tool for monitoring heart sounds without the need for maintaining a hand on the patient's chest in order to palpate the heart rhythm and quality. This was achieved by strapping a transmitter to the anterior chest of dogs and passing a long rubber tube to an aural receiver that the anesthetist could listen through while freeing their hands [5]. The skills practiced in the Hunterian Laboratory were translated into the operating room and paved the way for a safer anesthetic environment for Cushing's and his colleagues' patients. These developments also allowed for more freedom in patient positioning, as vital sign monitoring no longer required continual physical contact with the patient.

Dr. George Washington Crile (Fig. 1.8), a co-founder of the Cleveland Clinic and its first president, carried out extensive blood pressure experiments in a dog lab as well, outlining the effects of adrenaline, saline, and pneumatic pressure in increasing blood pressure (Fig. 1.9). He also recognized and described acidosis as effecting from shock and suggested bicarbonate as an antidote [8]. Crile too, like Cushing, was inspired to improve upon the existing meager knowledge of blood pressure monitoring and shock after he encountered the tragic death of a patient—a young man whose legs had been crushed by a train and who subsequently died of hemorrhagic shock [8]. He is credited with being the first to administer a successful human-to-human blood transfusion in 1906, and his experimentation with volume repletion and blood pressure monitoring in patients with shock are especially noteworthy [8, 11].

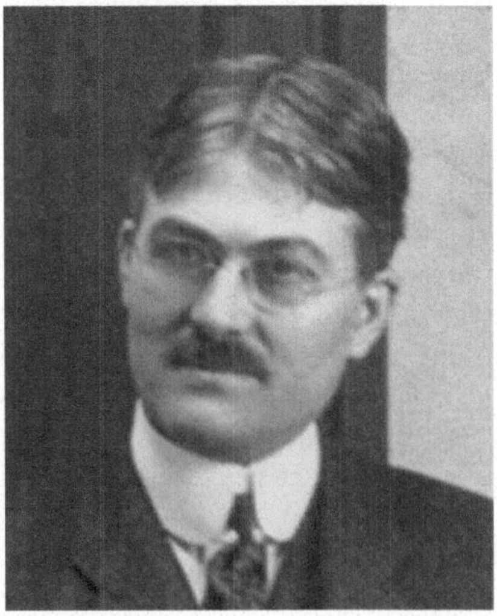

Fig. 1.8 Photography of Dr. George Washington Crile in 1905. Dr. Crile, a general surgeon in Ohio and friend of Cushing's, made great contributions to medicine through his studies of blood pressure and treatments for shock. These advancements allowed for volume repletion during prolonged neurosurgeries or those that caused significant blood loss. He carried out many of these experiments in a dog lab in Cleveland, much like Cushing at the Hunterian Lab [10]

Local Anesthesia

Also stemming from his aversion to improperly administered general anesthetic were Cushing's experimentations with the uses of local anesthetic, in particular cocaine [5]. Though his teacher Halstead had used cocaine for nerve blocking in 1884, Cushing was not largely exposed to its use during his training under Dr. Halsted. Cushing "resurrected" the local nerve block using cocaine and coined the term "regional anesthesia" in 1902 preferentially over "local anesthesia" [5, 8]. Although widely used because of its safety, regional anesthesia had its limitations as noted by Dr. Charles H. Frazier: "No doubt the operation can be performed under local or regional anaesthesia but in our experience the patient welcomes loss of consciousness" [12].

Positioning in Neurological Surgery

Positioning a patient prior to an operation on either the spine, brain, or peripheral nervous system is of utmost importance in neurological surgery. Ideal positioning results in maximum access to the patient for the surgeon and anesthetist and reduces the risk of patient injury. Historical developments in the techniques used to position patients have occurred in congruence with technological and scientific progress in surgery. Many of these advancements occurred through trial and error in the operating room. Hurdles encountered during neurological surgeries have spurred numerous inventions, techniques, surgical approaches, and equipment adjustments. This trend of problem identification and resulting progress has benefits that reach beyond the scope of neurosurgery and has influenced the standards of care in neurosurgical positioning over time.

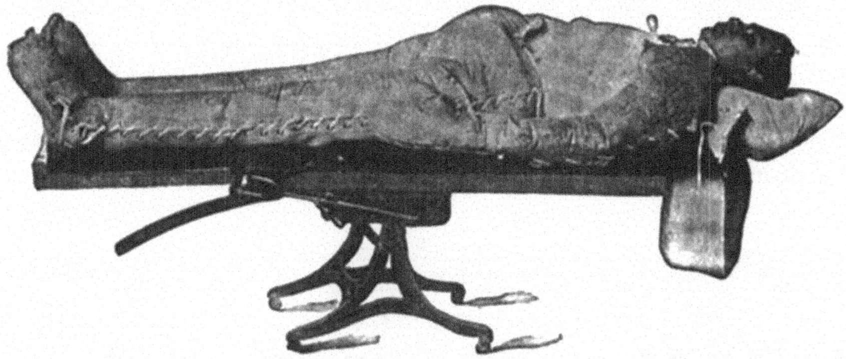

Fig. 1.9 A pneumatic rubber suit invented by Dr. George Washington Crile. This suit was designed to combat shock and was laced on the patient then inflated with a bike tire pump. Although this suit was abandoned by Crile, he worked in conjunction with Goodyear Tire and Rubber Company to adapt this design for antigravity suits used by pilots during World War I [10–12]

Before the patient can be appropriately positioned, they must be transferred to the operating table. Patient transfer assistant devices such as slider boards and roll aids have become implemented since the 1990s and can ease the physical burden of safely transferring patients to the operating table. Prior to this, physical lifting or pushing/pulling the patient horizontally if the patient could not move over to the table themselves was standard. The majority of improvements regarding safety for both the patient and those assisting in the transfer have come in the form of education and courses in proper technique.

Once on the table and anesthetized, special care must be taken to ensure that the patient is sufficiently secured to the table and to prevent development of pressure ulcers or peripheral nerve injury. Points of pressure or traction on the patient's body must be recognized and protected after anesthetizing and prior to sterile draping. From early use of sheets, blankets, and pillows to the use of foam and invention of viscoelastic gel cushioning today, the developments in table padding have significantly reduced the frequency of pressure ulcers caused during surgeries.

Much of the development and changes regarding the supine or prone positions for intracranial surgery have required changes with the operating table, including developments in padding, moveable parts of the table, and increased safety measures (Figs. 1.10 and 1.11). Variations of the supine, lateral, or prone intracranial approaches may involve rotating or flexing the neck to position the head and adjusting the limbs and torso to achieve the desired physiological position for the patient during the surgical procedure. Fixation of the head is critical for positions such as the park-bench, three-quarter (lateral oblique) prone, Concorde, and others. Skeletal fixation of the head may be accomplished with a three- or four-pin fixation. The most commonly used cranial fixation device is the Mayfield frame, which was introduced in the 1970s (Fig. 1.12).

As general anesthetics have become safer and intraoperative monitoring improved over time, patients have tolerated longer and more complex procedures. As the length of surgeries has increased, so have injuries related to positioning. Peripheral nerve injuries such as ulnar or brachial nerve palsies have long been potential adverse outcomes that increase in frequency with the length of each operation. Positioning the arms out laterally during supine operations has allowed the anesthetist easier access to the patient's arms for blood pressure monitoring and administration of drugs and fluids.

Use of the Operating Microscope

Operating microscopes were first utilized in neurosurgery by Dr. Theodore Kurze at UCLA in 1957 for the removal of a CNVII schwannoma from a child [13]. Improvement to the microscope including illumination, stabilization, multiple viewing ports for surgical assistance, increased magnification, mouth piece driving, and imaging integration with MR or CT viewing through the eyepiece has drastically changed the surgeon's ability to more thoroughly and precisely access and visualize intracranial pathology. Through augmentation of surgical access, more complex cases are now being operated on, which can increase the length of operative time. During these cases, it is imperative to pay the utmost

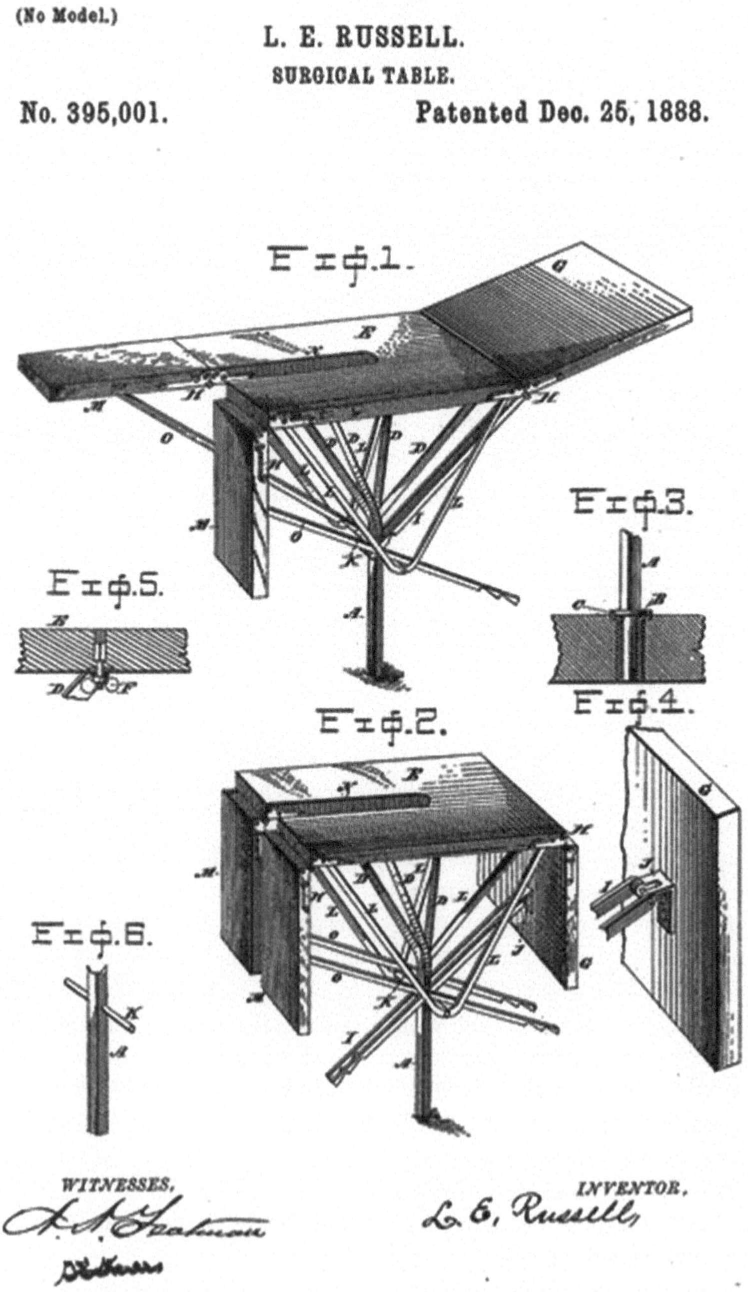

Figs. 1.10 and 1.11 Patents submitted for operating tables in 1888 and 1968. As the complexity and length of neurological surgeries has increased over time, so have the requisite mobility and safety of operating tables [13, 14]

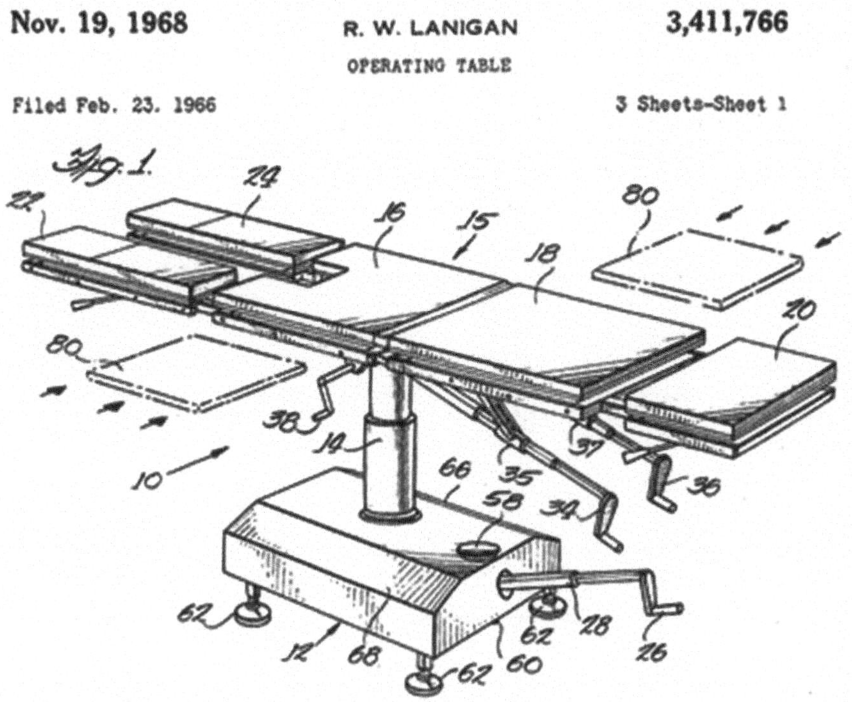

Figs. 1.10 and 1.11 (continued)

attention to preoperative positioning. Once the patient is positioned in anticipation of using the microscope, extensive padding of all the patient's pressure points without inhibiting proper access for anesthesia staff are important for reducing risk of injury.

The operating room layout itself has changed over the last half century to accommodate large operating microscopes and to allow for the surgeon and assistants to sit if desired. Before sterilely prepping and draping the patient, equipment must be gathered and positioned in the best possible formation to prevent unnecessary intraoperative manipulation that could prolong operative and anesthetic time.

Though microscopes were first used for intracranial surgeries within neurosurgery, they are of course widely implemented for spinal procedures as well. In spinal procedures, the operating room layout must adapt not only for the operating microscope, but also the use of imaging with C arm and tables that allow intraoperative maneuvering.

Endovascular Suite

With the advent of newer imaging technologies, neurosurgery has grown to include endovascular interventions that are performed in an endovascular suite which has brought about new positioning considerations. The supine position is preferred for procedures using the angiography machine for easy access to the groin or arms. These tables are fixed and disallow any more than subtle position changes during a procedure, so as to permit free movement of the fluoroscopic C-arms around the patient's head. This limitation is of particular importance when an acute increase in intracranial pressure occurs during a procedure, as the anesthetist cannot simply raise the head of the bed to assist in lowering the pressure, a feature that is easily achievable in modern operating rooms with a standard operating table. Hybrid operating suites with fully mobile operating tables and angiography machines are a modern solution to this problem and are becoming increasingly more common in large care centers.

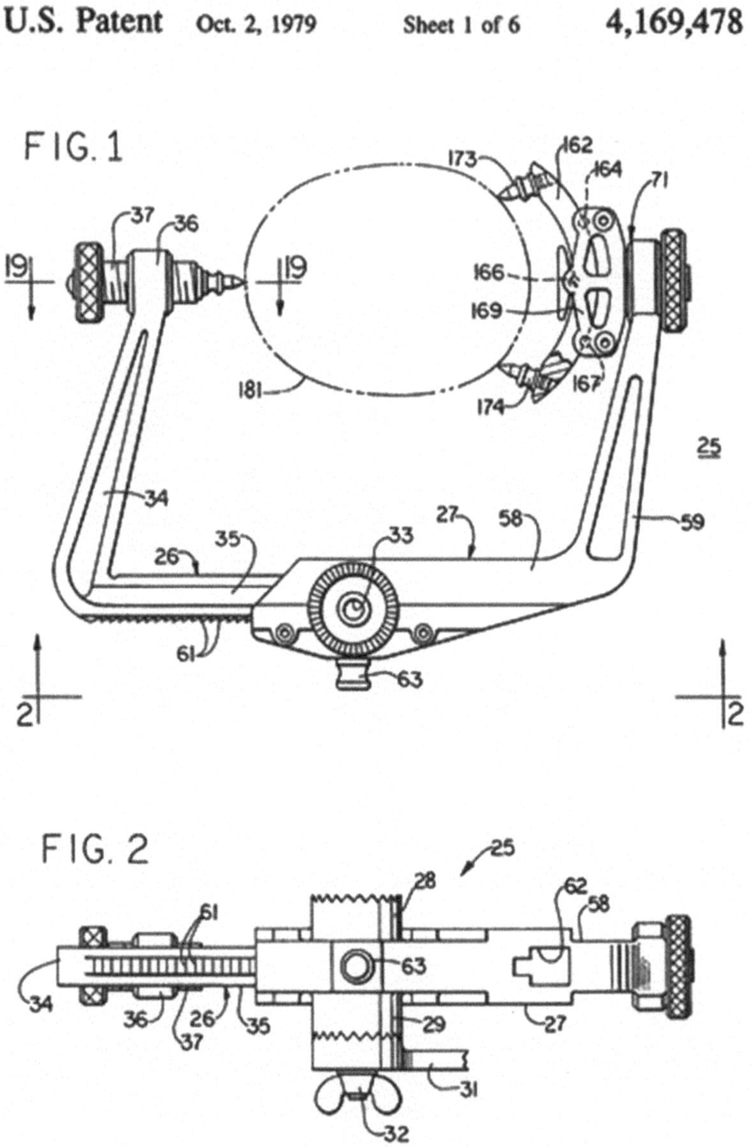

Fig. 1.12 Patent submitted for Surgical Head clamp in 1978. The implementation of the three point headrest has allowed for fixation of the head to the table so as to prevent intraoperative movement [15]

Cranial Procedures

Supine Position

Patient positioning for intracranial surgical procedures is determined by the location of the pathology and surgical approach selected. For all operative positions, care should be taken to decrease the risk of intracranial venous engorgement which could lead to an increase in intracranial pressure. Simply avoiding extreme turning of the head and neck during positioning of the patient and elevating the patient's head after securing the operative position are recommended for all intracranial procedures.

The majority of intracranial procedures are currently and have traditionally been performed with the patient in the supine position. The supine position is chosen for procedures in the frontal, temporal, and anterior parietal areas and for many skull base approaches. The various surgical approaches in the supine position may require turning the patient's head and neck or elevating one shoulder to rotate the upper trunk. Changes in the supine position over time correspond with advancements in operating table, anesthesia, headrest, microscope, and padding technologies.

Lateral Position

A lateral approach with the head maintained in a neutral position may be selected for middle cranial fossa skull base approaches. For surgical approaches to the lateral posterior fossa or craniocervical junction, implementation of the park-bench and three-quarter (lateral oblique) variations of the lateral position provided improved operative exposure. Use of the lateral position lessens blood pooling in the surgical field both through relief of pressure from the abdomen which allows for decreased compression of the vena cava as well as gravitational drainage. Variations of the lateral approach involve rotating or flexing the neck to position the head and adjusting the limbs and torso to achieve the desired physiological position for the patient during the surgical procedure.

Prone Position

The prone position is most commonly chosen for unilateral or bilateral suboccipital craniotomies to address cerebellar or fourth ventricular pathology of the posterior fossa. The three-quarter prone position (lateral oblique or park bench) with the table tilted to elevate the head is used for exposure of the posterior parietal, occipital, lateral suboccipital, and craniocervical junction.

Patients are most often intubated and anesthetized in the supine position on a stretcher and then transferred over to the operating table by rotating them prone. Endotracheal tube positioning is of particular importance in neurosurgery as compared to other areas of anesthesia, as manipulation of the head and neck during positioning puts the tube at greater risk of being kinked or moved [14]. This is particularly important when operating on patients in the prone position, as close monitoring of the endotracheal tube is required when rolling them over after intubation.

One possible alternative to intubating a patient prior to rotating for prone positioning would be to first perform an awake intubation using light sedation and topical anesthetics for the oropharynx before allowing the patient to position themselves comfortably on the operating table [15]. This technique, of course, would require a mobile, cooperative patient who is able to communicate nonverbally and is not widely used for neurosurgical procedures. There is also a risk of slipping and falling in an open table; therefore, only regular operating tables should be considered for this maneuver.

Spine Procedures

Prone Position

The majority of spinal surgeries are routinely approached with the patient in a prone position (Fig. 1.13). Herniated discs were not described as a distinct pathology until 1911 and were thought to represent benign tumors. Operative management of herniated discs by laminotomy with an intradural approach for discectomy was described in 1934. The laminotomy for extradural removal of herniated lumbar and cervical discs has since remained the standard surgical procedure for disc herniations. Once used intracranially, microscopes were quickly adopted for spinal procedures. The first microsurgeries of the spine were described by Yasargil and Caspar in 1977 though lumbar discectomies were being performed under the microscope as early as 1968 [2]. In 1953, the posterior lumbar interbody fusion was first described [2], and over the past three decades there have been

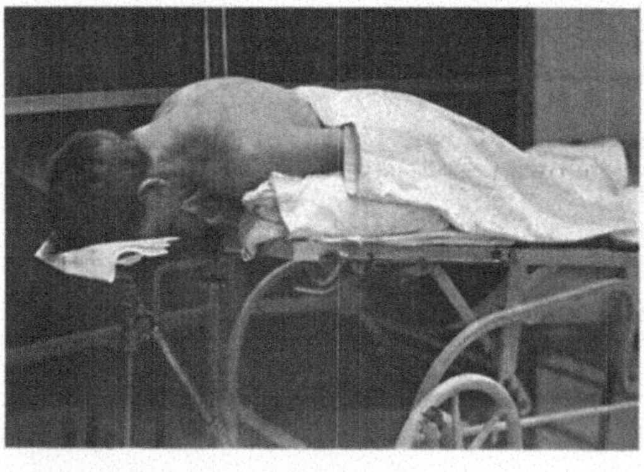

Fig. 1.13 The prone position for a cervical spine operation, described by Dr. Elsber in this 1916 book, *Diagnosis and treatment of surgical diseases of the spinal cord and its membranes* [16]

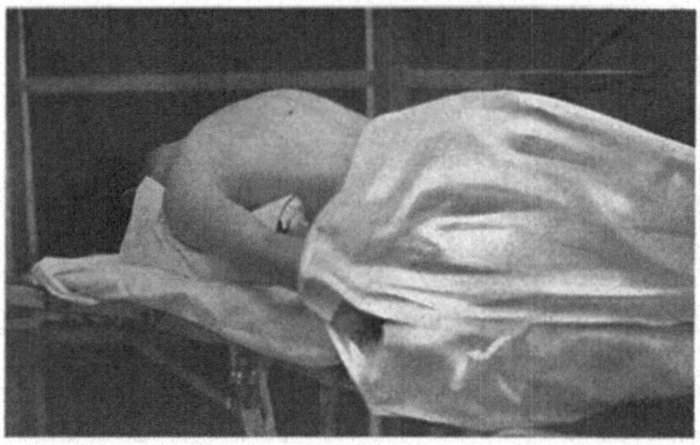

Fig. 1.14 In this photo, the patient is positioned with pillows and blankets underneath the abdomen in order to make the lumbar spine "prominent" for laminectomy, as noted by the author. Though this allowed for better exposure, the increased pressure on the abdomen likely caused increased pressure on the inferior vena cava, and therefore increased bleeding [16].

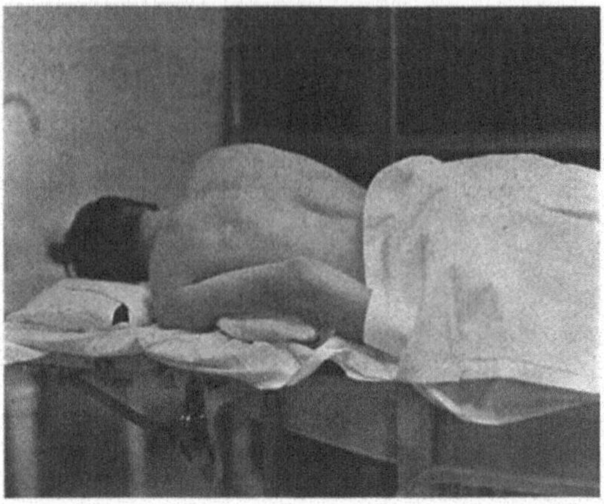

Fig. 1.15 A slight modification of the prone position is the semi-prone, which was used to allow for increased visualization of the surgical field by allowing gravity to draw blood away from the site of operation rather than pooling over the surgical bed [16]

significant advancements in spinal operative approaches, instrumentation, and fusion techniques requiring adjustments in patient positioning and the operating room layout.

A key consideration for surgeries with the patient positioned prone is venous congestion caused by pressure on the abdomen. Despite knowledge of the valveless anatomy of spinal veins, the prone position was not adapted to relieve abdominal pressure until the 1930–1940s (Figs. 1.14 and 1.15) [16]. In 1949, Ecker first described the adaptation of the prone position to account for increased abdominal pressure [17]. Dr. Hunter noted in 1952 that "any improvement in access to the lumbar spine which is attained by mid-line pressure on the anterior abdominal wall is obtained at the expense of quite a serious circulatory upset" [14]. The use of open frames positioned on the operating table has greatly advanced the prone position in the past half century.

Temperature control is attained more readily in the prone patient as compared to a patient in sitting position, as warming blankets can be placed below and on top of the patient [18]. Improvements in the ability to warm the patient include availability of warming machines for blankets, temperature controlled operating rooms, and use of machines that deliver warm air circulated over the patient's body but do not interfere with the sterile field. Concomitant improvement in patient position and padding were important in avoiding pressure injuries, as heat increases the chances of pressure-related injuries.

A variant of the prone position for spine surgery is the kneeling position. This position has been demonstrated to decrease intraoperative blood loss as compared to a traditional prone position but implementation has the trade-off of taking more time to position the patient [19].

Lateral Position

The first mention of lumbar disc surgery in scientific literature comes from the Mayo Clinic in 1937 [17]. Although opening of the spinal canal was a relatively uncommon surgery up until the 1950s, the lateral position was described as being used in 1957 in order to have blood fall away from the surgical field [17]. Improvement in patient positioning devices that relieve pressure from the IVC and thus reduce venous congestion have allowed better visualization of the operative field and a movement away from the lateral position. Positioning patients in a neutral and symmetrical manner is important for spinal operations that involve instrumentation and fixation, which is of course much more prevalent today.

The lateral position is still used for operations such as direct lateral interbody fusions, though positioning decisions are more likely influenced by technical access and exposure, rather than for benefits of decreased blood pooling with midline incisions [20]. The lateral position is not always implemented for this procedure; in the United Kingdom, this operation is at times carried out in a prone position.

Supine Position

Anterior spine surgery comprises a large portion of neurosurgical spine operations. Anterior cervical discectomy and fixation surgeries were first introduced in the mid-1950s. Instrumentation with wiring quickly gave way to plating after its introduction in the 1980s. The anterior lumbar interbody fusion technique was first described in 1956 and allowed for access to the anterior vertebrae while leaving the posterior elements intact [2]. As noted previously, the supine position is the most common and longest-used position in intracranial neurosurgical operations and advances in this position were widely implemented by the time that anterior fixation devices became available and commonly used.

Sitting Position

Positioning patients in a sitting position during neurosurgical procedures was first introduced by Thierry de Martel in 1913 for the removal of a brain tumor and was performed under local anesthesia [21, 22]. The popularity of this position for procedures of the cervical spine and posterior fossa peaked in the 1960s and 1970s. Clear advantages of gravity assist with drainage away from rather than pooling of blood in the surgical site allow for a cleaner procedure and positioning allows for better technical access than the prone position, as well as ease of intraoperative monitoring and drug administration by the anesthetist. Additional benefits include decreased orbital pressure with use of various head holders as compared to a horseshoe in the prone position (Fig. 1.16).

In 1935, Dr. Gardner of the Cleveland Clinic described positioning patients in a dental chair using a cerebellar head rest to the exclusion of using the "horizontal position" for posterior fossa surgeries in all but one case, and in select supratentorial and cervical spine cases [23]. He noted the advantages of decreased intracranial venous pressure and resultant decreased venous bleeding, decreased cerebral edema due to less need for retraction, ease of respiration, better surgical access, as well as better positioning for the anesthetist. Disadvantages included occasional rapid and profound shock and the risk of air embolism [23].

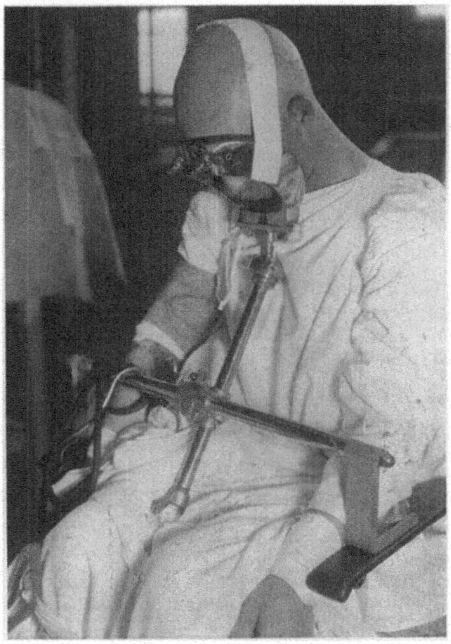

Fig. 1.16 Sitting position for a suboccipital craniotomy. The patient's head is flexed anteriorly for better exposure of the posterior fossa and is secured to the head rest with a strap [18]

Despite the risk of air embolism, some surgeons prefer a semisitting position for operations involving the posterior fossa. The advantages of the semisitting position include improved venous drainage to reduce venous congestion and a decrease in CSF and blood collecting in the depth of the exposure.

Early descriptions of anesthetic concerns when using the sitting position involve carefully avoiding hypotension while the patient's head is elevated, cervical access for jugular massage, access to the precordium for smooth anesthesia delivery as well as monitoring of heart rate and blood pressure, and avoidance of air embolisms during operations [14]. Wrapping of the patient's legs from the ankle to the groin or thigh-high compression hose have been used to increase venous return and avoid postural hypotension in the seated position [24]. Antigravity suits were used in the past to prevent pooling of blood in the extremities and subsequent hypotension [25]. Drs. Gardner and Dohn in the 1950s describe using an antigravity suit to combat hypotension and then improving upon it by creating their own compression device for the legs, pelvis, and abdomen [11, 25]. They noted its effectiveness not only in maintaining blood pressure, but also in increasing venous return and thus decreasing the risk of air embolism [25]. Prior to this in 1903, Dr. Crile first described use of a specially made rubber suit that was double-layered and filled with a bicycle pump to achieve the effect of increasing blood pressure during operations in the semisitting position (Fig. 1.9); Dr. Crile went on to win the Cartwright Prize for his essays in experimentation with blood pressure [25]. Pneumatic compression devices were not widely used in a surgical setting but the antigravity suit's use was resurrected in the late 1960s and early 1970s in Vietnam for emergency resuscitative care in the primitive conditions until transport to a surgical facility was possible [11].

Despite the popularity of the sitting position, many surgeons avoided it altogether due to the increased risk of venous air embolism (VAE) [18, 26, 27]. The first reported case of VAE occurred in 1830 during the removal of a facial mass [22]. Since then, monitoring during operations in the seated position have largely centered around detecting VAEs and intervening to aspirate the air. Blood pressure, heart rate, patient gasp, precordial and esophageal auscultation, end tidal CO_2, central venous pressure monitoring, and EKG have all been used to detect air embolisms, but these measures typically are not positive until physiologic deterioration is already underway. Sensitivity was greatly increased with the common use of Doppler ultrasonography monitoring for VAE by the 1970s [22, 28, 29]. Central venous catheter placement prior to surgery has also allowed for aspiration of air from the heart chambers when it is detected prior to having a detrimental physiologic effect [29]. Operations using alternative positioning techniques are not exempt from VAE risk, which can occur any time that the head is elevated above the heart.

Decreased use of this positioning technique has continued over time [30]. In the 1960s, neurosurgeons in Toronto largely transitioned to prone positioning rather than sitting for operating on posterior fossa pathology [18]. They cite difficulties in positioning as a major contributor to this decision, as problems with patients' slipping down, causing cervical hyperflexion, and dislodging the endotracheal tube were most concerning and alleviated by using the prone position and 15–20° of reverse Trendelenburg.

The use of the sitting position and its variants is largely institution dependent. No concrete criteria exist for preoperative determination of patient positioning, and the choice to use the sitting position is largely dependent on surgeon predilection and training coupled with anesthesia's capabilities. In 1981, 53% of neurosurgical centers in the United Kingdom used the sitting position for patients undergoing posterior fossa surgery and 11% for cervical spine surgeries. Ten years later in 1991, this had decreased to 20% for posterior fossa surgery [22]. This decline was paralleled in the United States; Mayo Clinic reported a greater than 50% decline in its use of the sitting position for posterior fossa surgeries over a 5-year span in the 1980s [22].

Spontaneous respirations were at times preferred for posterior fossa and CPA surgeries in the seated position so as to monitor respiratory effects of brainstem manipulation, though controlled breathing is now widely preferred [18]. The decision to use spontaneous respirations or controlled positive-negative pressure ventilation is especially important when considering the potential for venous air embolism. Air embolisms were found to occur more frequently when patients are in a seated position and breathing spontaneously. This risk is reduced by use of controlled ventilation and even more so when the patient is positioned prone or supine though the risk is still not zero [18]. Over time, with the advent of better monitoring for air embolism beyond vital sign recording, its incidence was found to be higher than was suspected. Ultrasound improves detection a great deal and was implemented by the early 1970s though variation in technology and technique exists amongst hospitals.

Litigation against the neurosurgical team for poor patient outcomes from surgeries performed in the sitting position could be another driving force influencing the frequency with which this position is used. Though cases involving the sitting position have decreased over time, the exact cause for this is uncertain but could involve either a decreased frequency of use for fear of poor outcomes and subsequent litigation, or reflect a better handling of the positioning technique such that poor outcomes are decreased with its increased implementation.

Use of the sitting position, perhaps more than any of the other positions used in neurosurgery, demonstrates the important relationship between the neuroanesthesia team and the surgical team as well as underscores the necessity of preoperative planning and properly informing the patients of the risks associated with any operation.

Partnership Between Neuroanesthetist and Neurosurgeon

Though neurosurgical techniques from various cranial and spinal approaches have greatly improved over time, the concurrent improvements in neuroanesthesia have been of vital importance to decreasing patient mortality and to improving patient outcomes.

> "…in every neurosurgical clinic, operations are begun which cannot be completed for reasons directly traceable to the activities of the anesthetist and that the number of such cases varies inversely with his skill [14]."

The importance of the relationship between a neurosurgeon and his or her partnered anesthetist cannot be overemphasized. Cushing's respect for proper anesthesia delivery and great anesthetists is relevant today. He attributed much of his success as a surgeon to the anesthetist or "etherist" Dr. S. Griffith Davis through implementation of monitoring techniques that Cushing himself created [5]. Dr. Crile worked closely for many years with Agatha Hodgkins who went on to together found one of the first nurse anesthetist schools, again emphasizing the importance and intimacy of the relationship between anesthetist and surgeon [8]. Now there exists amongst neurosurgical teams a better application of patient positioning and perioperative anesthesia management based on patient need.

A Brief History of Semmes-Murphey Neurosurgery in Memphis, Tennessee

Dr. Eustace Semmes (Fig. 1.17) and Dr. Walter Dandy were college classmates and graduated from the University of Missouri (1903–1907). Their college education provided their basic medical training which allowed them to transfer to Johns Hopkins Medical School as second year medical students in 1907. During their medical education, they were strongly influenced by the Hopkins surgical faculty, by the Surgeon in Chief Dr. William Halstead, and by Dr. Harvey Cushing

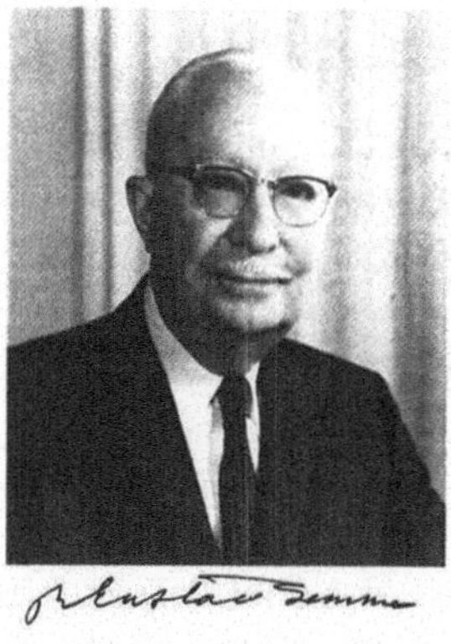

Fig. 1.17 Dr. Eustace Semmes (1885–1982) of Memphis, Tennessee. Dr. Semmes, after training under Dr. Cushing and alongside Dr. Walter Dandy, returned to his hometown to first practice both general and neurological surgery and eventually establish the first dedicated neurosurgical practice in the Mid-South: Semmes-Murphey [20]. (Reproduced from Krier C, Knauff S. Monitoring for neurosurgical procedures in the sitting position. Acta Anaesthesiol Belg. 1980;31(Suppl):101–5. With permission from Acta Medica Belgica)

who at the time was developing the new surgical field of neurosurgery.

In 1908, Cushing removed a tumor from the cerebral cortex of a conscious patient who received neither anesthetic nor experienced pain during the operation. It was reported that Dr. Cushing and the patient conversed during the procedure [31]. Cushing established his neurosurgical preeminence in 1910 in an authoritative address on *The Special Field of Neurological Surgery: Five Years Later* [32].

It was during this seminal period of neurosurgical history that these medical students were introduced to surgical principles and anesthesia methods in the Hunterian Laboratory directed by Dr. Cushing. After graduating from medical school, Dr. Semmes and Dr. Dandy interned at Johns Hopkins. They worked on Dr. Cushing's service caring for his patients and observing his neurosurgical procedures. After completing his internship, and on the recommendation of Dr. Halstead, Dr. Semmes spent one year in New York for a general residency in surgery at the Women's Hospital.

Dr. Eustace Semmes returned in 1912 to his hometown of Memphis, Tennessee after completing his training under Dr. Cushing. His arrival coincided with the opening of a new 150 bed medical facility, Baptist Memorial Hospital just one year after the establishment of the University of Tennessee Medical School in Memphis in 1911. Dr. Semmes received an academic appointment in the University of Tennessee Department of Surgery where he began practicing general surgery but eventually limited his operations to only neurosurgical patients.

Dr. Semmes was the first practicing neurosurgeon in the Mid-South and under his leadership, neurosurgery in Memphis grew to at one point boast the largest number of neurosurgeons per capita than any other city in the United States. In 1932, the University of Tennessee Department of Neurosurgery was established under the Chairmanship of Dr. Semmes. His first neurosurgical trainee was Dr. Francis Murphey who came to Memphis in 1934 following a year of internship in Chicago. Dr. Murphey would become Dr. Semmes future neurosurgical associate, and together they would establish the Semmes-Murphey Clinic.

Safe general anesthesia was not available during the first several decades of Dr. Semmes general surgery and neurosurgical practice. He was influenced by his experience with Dr. Cushing, and preferred local regional anesthesia for many neurosurgical operations, rather than using general anesthetics. A patient treated by Dr. Semmes in her teens for a posterior fossa tumor, returned some 30 years later for treatment of a tumor recurrence. At her preoperative visit, she recalled undergoing her surgery under local anesthesia. She described "watching the blood run from her head and drip down on to Dr. Semmes's shoe" while she lay in a prone position in a horseshoe headrest. Dr. Semmes, in a monolith about lumbar disc operations which he dedicated to his patients, advised, "In working with local anesthesia, the surgeon cannot afford to show any sign of alarm or to lose his temper—which makes it better for the patient, the surgical team, and the surgeon" [33]. As the administration of anesthetics became safer over time with better intraoperative monitoring, the vast majority of both cranial and spine procedures were performed under general anesthesia.

The supine position has been the primary surgical position used by Semmes-Murphey neurosurgeons for cranial surgeries, carotid endarterectomies, and anterior cervical or lumbar spine procedures. Depending upon the cranial approach, head rotation or flexion has been necessary to enhance the surgical exposure. For anterior lumbar spine procedures, general surgery assistance may be needed for transabdominal access. Types of supine positioning employed for neurosurgical cases have included (1) a horizontal supine position used for anterior cervical or lumbar procedures, (2) a lawn chair supine position with 15° of angulation and flexion at the trunk-thigh-knee with proper padding and slight elevation of the head for extended cranial procedures, and (3) a reverse Trendelenburg supine position to elevate the head and trunk when optimal cerebral venous drainage and reduced intracranial pressure is needed.

The preference of the prone position over the sitting position for cranial approaches by Semmes-Murphey neurosurgeons has been limited to lesions of the occipital brain, midline posterior fossa, and pineal region. All surgeries involving the posterior spinal axis have been routinely approached with the patient in a prone position. Unlike the supine position for cranial procedures, two critical maneuvers have been necessary to reduce intracranial venous pressure and excessive blood loss: elevating the patient's head and torso to improve cerebral venous drainage, and the proper use of chest rolls or special table frames (Wilson, Jackson, etc.) to avoid compression of the vena cava. Reduction of spinal epidural venous bleeding during thoracic or lumbar spinal procedures has required the use of chest rolls and special table frames. Head elevation has been necessary for posterior cervical procedures to reduce venous blood loss. The prone Concorde position was used prior to acceptance of the sitting position in Memphis for occipital transtentorial or supracerebellar infratentorial approaches to the pineal region or tentorial notch area.

Early use of the sitting position by Semmes-Murphey neurosurgeons for cervical spine and posterior fossa pathology resulted in several adverse outcomes related to venous air embolism. As a result, the sitting position was largely abandoned in favor of the prone position for many years by Semmes-Murphey physicians and University of Tennessee-trained neurosurgical residents. Close collaboration between the senior author and anesthesia in the early 1980s, with extensive perioperative preparation and intraoperative monitoring, led to a revival in the use of the sitting position for selective neurosurgical cases involving the midline posterior fossa and pineal region. Of all neurosurgical positions employed, the success of the sitting position for neurosurgical cases was found to be dependent upon close communication at all stages of the surgical procedure between the operating neurosurgeon and the anesthetist.

The lateral position was traditionally used in Memphis for cranial approaches involving the temporal lobe, lateral supratentorial skull base, posterior fossa at the cerebellopontine angle, and craniocervical junction. The major limitation of the lateral position was with ventilation though it did provide the added benefit of removing pressure from the abdomen and allowing blood to flow away from the surgical field. When employing any of the lateral positions, one should apply the appropriate padding of the torso and extremities, and secure the patient on the operating table. This will prevent movement of the patient if the table should be rotated by the surgeon to gain additional surgical exposure.

Conclusion

As was mentioned in anesthesia guidelines set out in 1952, proper control of intracranial pressure and venous pressure are of critical importance during neurosurgical cases and are first manipulated during positioning. As such, "the responsibility of the neurosurgical anesthetist is thus far heavier than that of his colleagues in other fields [14]." Charles Robert Allen, Professor Emeritus with the Department of Anesthesiology at the University of Texas noted in 1942 in his Forward to the Second Edition of *Positioning in Anesthesia and Surgery*:

> *On physiologic analysis it became evident that some patients were going into shock, not because of the anesthetic and surgical procedures per se, but because of the physiologic distress that occurred when anesthetic depression and surgical trauma were superimposed upon respiratory and cardiovascular impairment produced by improperly positioning patients on operating tables.*

We now understand the physiology behind these events better and, more importantly, consider the possible consequences before we position patients. Do we have standard of care methods extant for positioning of neurosurgical patients to prevent the problems that our patients continue to manifest? No, and perhaps rightly so as neurosurgery is constantly evolving with new approaches demanding different positioning. We can, however, learn from prior complications and make note of new problems that arise with changes in the field of neurosurgery in order to prevent future mistakes.

References

1. Chivukula S, Grandhi R, Friedlander RM. A brief history of early neuroanesthesia. Neurosurg Focus. 2014;36(4):E2.
2. Samartzis D, Shen FH, Perez-Cruet MJ, Anderson DG. Minimally invasive spine surgery: a historical perspective. Orthop Clin North Am. 2007;38(3):305–26; abstract v.
3. Frost EAM. A history of neuroanesthesia. Wondrous story of anesthesia. New York: Springer Science & Business Media; 2014. p. 871–85.
4. Bacon DR, Ament R. Ralph Waters and the beginnings of academic anesthesiology in the United States: the Wisconsin Template. J Clin Anesth. 1995;7(6):534–43.
5. Shephard DA. Harvey Cushing and anaesthesia. Can Anaesth Soc J. 1965;12(5):431–42.
6. Cushing H. On routine determinations of arterial tension in operating room and clinic. Boston Med Surg J. 1903;148:250–6.
7. Moore FD. Harvey Cushing. General surgeon, biologist, professor. J Neurosurg. 1969;31(3):262–70.
8. Nathoo N, Lautzenheiser FK, Barnett GH. George W. Crile, Ohio's first neurosurgeon, and his relationship with Harvey Cushing. J Neurosurg. 2005; 103(2):378–86.
9. Sampath P, Long DM, Brem H. The Hunterian Neurosurgical Laboratory: the first 100 years of neurosurgical research. Neurosurgery. 2000;46(1):184–94. discussion 94-5.
10. Dutta A. Harvey Cushing (1869-1939) and the Hunterian laboratory: a revolution in surgical training. J Med Biogr. 2010;18(4):183–5.
11. Cutler BS, Daggett WM. Application of the "G-suit" to the control of hemorrhage in massive trauma. Ann Surg. 1971;173(4):511–4.
12. Frazier CH. Operation for the radical cure of trigeminal neuralgia: analysis of five hundred cases. Ann Surg. 1928;88(3):534–47.
13. Uluc K, Kujoth GC, Baskaya MK. Operating microscopes: past, present, and future. Neurosurg Focus. 2009;27(3):E4.
14. Hunter AR. The present position of anaesthesia for neurosurgery. Proc R Soc Med. 1952;45(7):427–34.
15. SD W, Yilmaz M, Tamul PC, Meeks JJ, Nadler RB. Awake endotracheal intubation and prone patient self-positioning: anesthetic and positioning considerations during percutaneous nephrolithotomy in obese patients. J Endourol. 2009;23(10):1599–602.
16. Edgcombe H, Carter K, Yarrow S. Anaesthesia in the prone position. Br J Anaesth. 2008;100(2):165–83.
17. Anderton JM. The prone position for the surgical patient: a historical review of the principles and hazards. Br J Anaesth. 1991;67(4):452–63.
18. Humphreys RP, Creighton RE, Hendrick EB, Hoffman HJ. Advantages of the prone position for neurosurgical procedures on the upper cervical spine and posterior cranial fossa in children. Childs Brain. 1975;1(6):325–36.
19. Bostman O, Hyrkas J, Hirvensalo E, Kallio E. Blood loss, operating time, and positioning of the patient in lumbar disc surgery. Spine (Phila Pa 1976). 1990;15(5):360–3.
20. Gragnaniello C, Seex K. Anterior to psoas (ATP) fusion of the lumbar spine: evolution of a technique facilitated by changes in equipment. J Spine Surg. 2016;2(4):256–65.
21. Bucy PC. Scotland: the birthplace of surgical neurology. J Neurol Neurosurg Psychiatry. 1985;48(10): 965–76.
22. Porter JM, Pidgeon C, Cunningham AJ. The sitting position in neurosurgery: a critical appraisal. Br J Anaesth. 1999;82(1):117–28.
23. Gardner WJ. Intracranial operations in the sitting position. Ann Surg. 1935;101(1):138–45.
24. Ecker A. Use of standard cerebellar frame for neurosurgical operations in sitting position. J Neurosurg. 1948;5(1):104.
25. Dohn DF, Gardner WJ. The antigravity suit (G-suit) in surgery; control of blood pressure in the sitting position and in hypotensive anesthesia. J Am Med Assoc. 1956;162(4):274–6.
26. Gale T, Leslie K. Anaesthesia for neurosurgery in the sitting position. J Clin Neurosci. 2004;11(7):693–6.
27. Hunter AR. Air embolism in the sitting position. Anaesthesia. 1962;17:467–72.
28. Gildenberg PL, O'Brien RP, Britt WJ, Frost EA. The efficacy of Doppler monitoring for the detection of venous air embolism. J Neurosurg. 1981;54(1): 75–8.
29. Krier C, Knauff S. Monitoring for neurosurgical procedures in the sitting position. Acta Anaesthesiol Belg. 1980;31(Suppl):101–5.
30. Dallier F, Di Roio C. Sitting position for pineal surgery: some anaesthetic considerations. Neurochirurgie. 2015;61(2–3):164–7.
31. Thomas H, Cushing H. Removal of a subcortical cystic tumor at a second-stage operation without anesthesia. JAMA. 1908;50(12):847–56.
32. Cushing H. The special field of neurological surgery: five years later. Bull Johns Hopkins Hosp. 1910;1910(21):325–38.
33. Semmes ER. Ruptures of the lumbar intervertebral disc: their mechanism, diagnosis, and treatment. Springfield: Charles C Thomas; 1964. 80p.

2 Biomechanics and the Mathematics of Positioning

George F. Young

The proper flow of blood and other bodily fluids is crucial to achieving successful surgical outcomes and maintaining patient health. In general, neutral positions of the body, head, and neck are recommended in order to achieve optimum blood flow [1]. Despite this, other positions may be necessary or preferred for particular surgeries, and in these cases it is important to understand how these positions affect flows in the head and brain.

The major flows in the head and brain can be modeled by considering the major sources and sinks of fluid, namely arterial flow into the head, venous flow out of the head, and cerebrospinal fluid (CSF) production. Let P_a denote the mean (carotid) arterial pressure, P_d denote the mean pressure in the dural venous sinuses (equivalent to the pressure at the top of the internal jugular), and P_{CSF} denote the component of intracranial pressure (ICP) due to the formation of CSF. Then the ICP is given by [2]

$$P_{ICP} = P_{CSF} + P_d, \tag{2.1}$$

the cerebral perfusion pressure (CePP) is given by

$$P_{CePP} = P_a - P_{ICP} = P_a - P_d - P_{CSF}, \tag{2.2}$$

and the capillary perfusion pressure (CaPP) in the head is given by

$$P_{CaPP} = P_a - P_d. \tag{2.3}$$

Following [2], $P_{CSF} = R_{out} I_{formation}$, where R_{out} is the resistance to outflow of CSF and $I_{formation}$ is the formation rate of CSF. $I_{formation}$ can be expected to be around 0.45 mL/min [3] while values of R_{out} below 13 mmHg/(mL/min) are considered normal [4]. Thus, P_{CSF} can be expected to be around 5.8 mmHg or below. In [2], average P_{CSF} was 5.7 mmHg. Under normal circumstances, P_{CSF} can be taken to be constant [5], and hence we only need to determine the effects of position on the arterial and venous pressures. Furthermore, P_{CePP} and P_{CaPP} differ by a constant amount and so any trend in one is also displayed in the other.

It is now necessary to define some geometrical parameters to describe the position of the patient as well as their head and neck. We can first describe the patient's basic position as supine, prone, or lateral. In general, the arterial pressure is not affected by this basic position [6–8], while the venous pressure can be expected to be the same in either the supine or lateral position, but raised by about 2 mmHg in the prone position [6, 7]. By ignoring the arrangement of the patient's arms and legs, their remaining body position can be described by a single parameter, namely the *tilt angle* τ. τ is the angle between the horizontal and the line from the heart through the center of the neck and head (see Fig. 2.1), with positive values corresponding to head-up tilt and negative values corresponding to head-down tilt.

G. F. Young (✉)
Germantown, TN, USA

A. Arthur et al. (eds.), *Perioperative Considerations and Positioning for Neurosurgical Procedures*,
https://doi.org/10.1007/978-3-319-72679-3_2

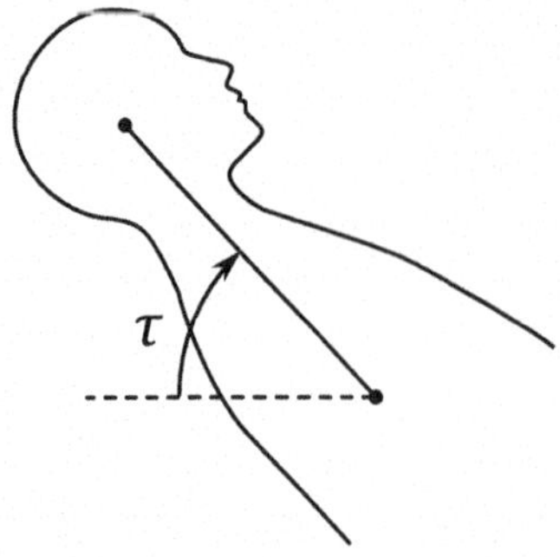

Fig. 2.1 The *tilt angle* τ that describes the angle of the patient's body relative to the horizontal (supine position shown)

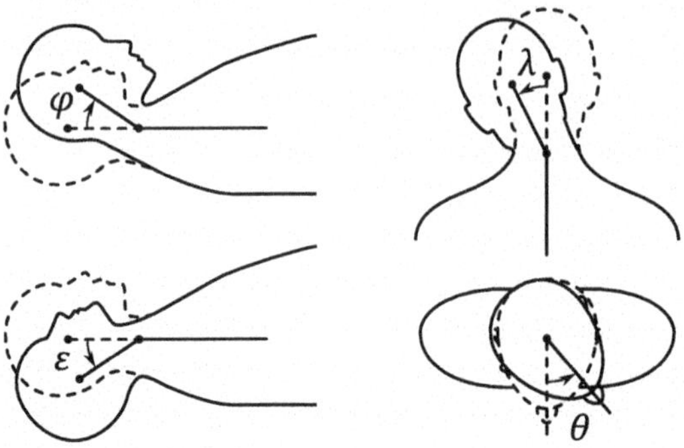

Fig. 2.2 The four angles that describe the position of the patient's head relative to their body. These are the *flexion angle* φ, the *extension angle* ε, the *lateral flexion angle* λ, and the *rotation angle* θ

Four angles can be used to describe the position of the head and neck. These are the *flexion angle* φ, the *extension angle* ε, the *lateral flexion angle* λ, and the *rotation angle* θ (see Fig. 2.2). Although the flexion and extension of the neck could be described by a single angle, the following model of blood pressure becomes simpler when two separate angles are used. Furthermore, for simplicity we will assume that the neck is never rotated and laterally flexed at the same time. Then λ is the angle between the line from the heart to the top of the neck (extended) and the line from the top of the neck to the top of the head, projected into the coronal plane. Positive values of λ correspond to lateral flexion toward the patient's right and negative values correspond to lateral flexion to the patient's left. θ is the angle between the line from the center of the head through the center of the face, projected into the transverse plane, and the line through the center of the head perpendicular to the coronal plane. Positive values of θ correspond to head rotation toward the patient's left, and negative values correspond to rotation to the right.

Finally, φ is the angle between the line from the top of the neck to the center of the head and the intersection of the coronal plane with the transverse plane of the head, whenever the head is bent toward the chest (and thus φ is always either positive or zero). ε is the angle between the line from the top of the neck to the center of the head and the intersection of the coronal plane with the transverse plane of the head, whenever the head is bent toward the back (and thus ε is always positive or zero).

It is a well-established principle that within a communicating fluid system[1], gravity will create a hydrostatic pressure gradient [9]. The hydrostatic pressure difference between two points in the system is given by

$$\Delta P = \rho g \Delta h, \tag{2.4}$$

where ρ is the fluid density, g is the acceleration due to gravity, and Δh is the difference in height between the two points. Thus, we can expect that both the arterial and venous pressures will decrease toward the head for positive tilt angles, and increase toward the head for negative tilt angles. By itself, this understanding is only sufficient to determine pressure differences rather than actual pressure at any point in the body (particularly since the circulatory system is able to respond to changes in body position). To proceed, we must utilize the concept of a *hydrostatic indifference point* (HIP), that is, a point at which the hydrostatic pressure remains the same no matter the orientation of the system [9]. Then, if the blood pressure at a zero tilt angle is known (i.e., when there is no hydrostatic gradient present), the pressure change to any given body orientation is governed by the change in height relative to the HIP.

[1]A fluid system is called communicating if fluid is freely able to pass between any two points in the system.

The HIP for arterial flow to the head is located just above heart level [9], and so the heart location can reasonably be taken to represent the arterial HIP. The venous HIP, in contrast, is located around the level of the diaphragm [2]. Thus, we can model the effect of tilt angle on arterial pressure as

$$P_a = P_a(0^\circ) - \rho g L_{heart} \sin(\tau), \tag{2.5}$$

where $P_a(0^\circ)$ is the arterial pressure at zero tilt angle—i.e., in a "standard" supine, prone, or lateral position, ρ is the density of blood, g is the acceleration due to gravity, and L_{heart} is the distance between the center of the head and the heart. Based on standard values, $\rho g \approx 78$ mmHg/m.

The model for venous pressure is complicated by the fact that as venous pressure in the jugular falls to zero, the vein can collapse and divide the venous flow in the head from the rest of the body [10]. In this case, the reference point for venous pressure in the head is no longer the venous HIP, but the point of collapse of the jugular. Although there are other venous pathways flowing out from the head (thus maintaining *some* communication with the rest of the venous system), observations indicate that blood flow is divided between those and the jugular so as to maintain zero pressure at the point of jugular collapse [2]. Thus, the effect of tilt on venous pressure becomes

$$P_d = \begin{cases} P_d(0^\circ) - \rho g \left(L_{heart} + L_{heart-HIPvein} \right) \sin(\tau), \tau < \tau_{collapse} \\ -\rho g L_{collapse} \sin(\tau + \eta), \tau \geq \tau_{collapse} \end{cases} \tag{2.6}$$

where $P_d(0^\circ)$ is the venous pressure at zero tilt angle, $L_{heart-HIPvein}$ is the distance between the heart and the venous HIP (around the level of the diaphragm [2]), $L_{collapse}$ is the distance between the center of the head and the point of collapse of the jugular,

$$\eta = \begin{cases} \varphi - \varepsilon, \text{supine position} \\ \varepsilon - \varphi, \text{prone position} \\ \lambda, \text{left lateral position} \\ -\lambda, \text{right lateral position} \end{cases} \tag{2.7}$$

is the neck tilt angle and $\tau_{collapse}$ is the tilt angle at which the jugular first collapses. Note that $P_d(0^\circ)$ can be expected to be around 2 mmHg higher in the prone position compared to the supine or lateral positions [6, 7]. From the definition of the various parameters, we can solve for $\tau_{collapse}$ as

$$\tau_{collapse} = \sin^{-1}\left(\frac{P_d(0^\circ)}{\rho g \left[L_{heart} + L_{heart-HIPvein} - L_{collapse} \right]} \right). \tag{2.8}$$

Based on fitting done in [2], we can assume that in general, $L_{heart-HIPvein} \approx 0.09$ m and $L_{collapse} \approx 0.11$ m. The neck tilt angle is only required for calculations following collapse of the jugular since the reference point in this case is located within the neck. Note that according to Eq. (2.6), P_d will be negative for a range of tilt angles (even for some angles below $\tau_{collapse}$). There is no theoretical problem with this since all pressures are measured relative to ambient (i.e., atmospheric) pressure and so negative values simply indicate pressures below ambient.

We can reproduce some trends seen in the literature when we apply this model of gravitational effects to the expressions for ICP and CePP. As reported in numerous studies (e.g., see [2, 11–14]), ICP decreases with increasing tilt angle. This effect is seen in the model by the hydrostatic decrease in venous pressure with increasing tilt angles. However, CePP has been reported both to decrease with tilt angle in some studies (e.g., [13]) and to be unaffected by tilt angle in others (e.g., [11, 12]). An examination of the current model shows that CePP can actually be expected to *increase* with tilt angle for $\tau < \tau_{collapse}$ (due to the greater distance between the head and the venous HIP compared to the arterial HIP) but then decrease with tilt angle for $\tau > \tau_{collapse}$. Furthermore, the value of $\tau_{collapse}$ can vary significantly between individuals [2], presumably due to the wide variation in venous pressure at zero tilt. Thus, the differences between studies can be attributed in part to individual patient differences and in part to other factors that influence blood flow (e.g., the study in [13] was conducted on

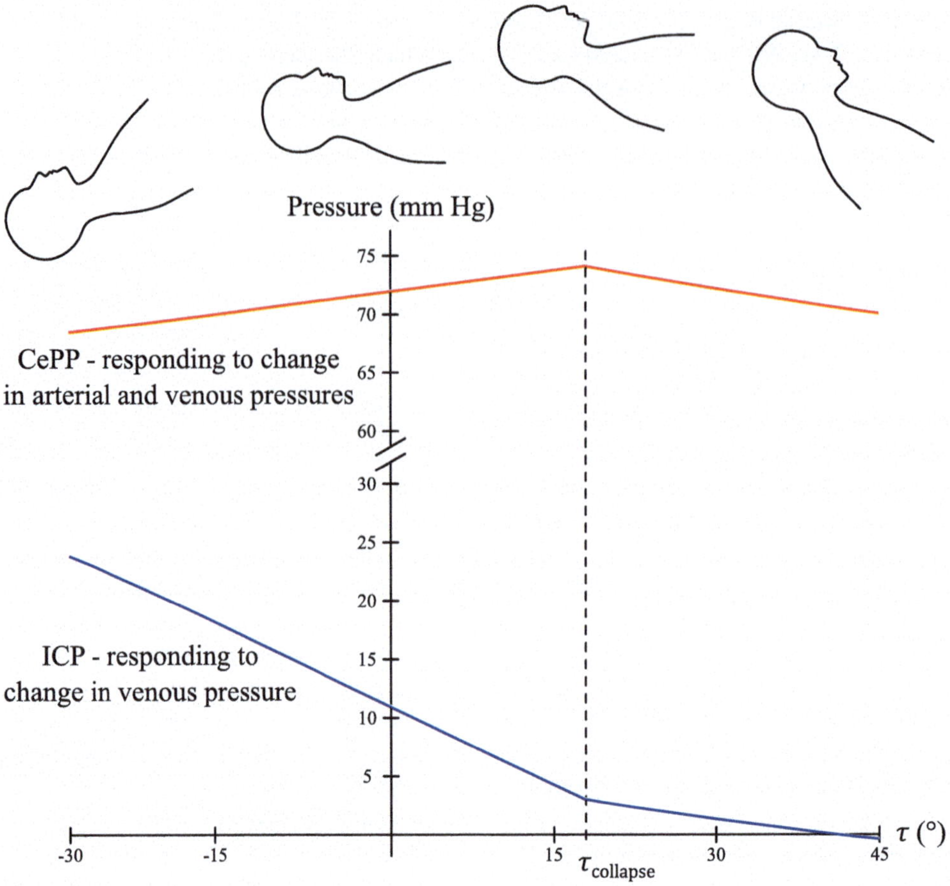

Fig. 2.3 A numerical example of the effects of tilt angle τ on intracranial pressure (ICP) and cerebral perfusion pressure (CePP). In this example, the patient is supine with their neck in a neutral position, $P_a(0^\circ) = 83$ mmHg, $P_d(0^\circ) = 5.3$ mmHg, $P_{CSF} = 5.7$ mmHg, $L_{heart} = 0.24$ m, $L_{heart-HIPvein} = 0.09$ m, and $L_{collapse} = 0.09$ m. ICP always decreases as τ increases, but the rate of decrease diminishes for $\tau > \tau_{collapse}$. CePP, and thus flow through the brain, has a maximum at $\tau = \tau_{collapse}$

patients who had suffered middle cerebral artery stroke). See Fig. 2.3 for an example of ICP and CePP changing with τ.

In contrast to the effects seen in this model for positive tilt angles, negative tilt angles can be expected to increase the ICP (due to the hydrostatic increase in venous pressure) and decrease the CePP (due to the venous pressure increasing more rapidly than the arterial pressure). Thus, this model predicts that in general, any position with head-down tilt can be expected to impair blood flow in the head.

While the hydrostatic effects of body position on blood pressure are relatively well understood, the effects of head and neck position are more difficult to model. The dominant effect of neck flexion, extension, rotation, and lateral flexion on blood flow appears to be the bending and compression of the blood vessels in the neck [14–19]. In principle, this should manifest as increased resistance to flow and thus greater pressure drops in these vessels. This increased resistance arises from the fact that the ratio of the perimeter to cross-sectional area of a blood vessel increases as the vessel is compressed, as well as the fact that increased blood velocity through the narrower section will lead to increased frictional losses. Therefore, it is reasonable to expect that any head motion away from a neutral position could decrease P_a and increase P_d (since the pressure drops occur in the direction of flow), leading to increases in ICP and decreases in CePP and CaPP. Furthermore, since veins are much more compliant than arteries, we can expect that the effects on venous pressure to be more significant than those on arterial pressure. In fact, for general patients, normal neck motions appear not to have a significant effect on vertebral arterial flow [17] or central venous and arterial pressure [14]. Moreover, while neck motion can change the geometry of the arteries in the neck and the distribution of flow between them, these effects vary between individuals and there does not appear to be a general trend or a significant effect on flow into the head [20]. This suggests that there is no need to model the effects of neck motion on arterial flow into the head.

Perhaps due to the lower pressures involved and increased vascular compliance, neck motion can have a significant effect on venous pressure and hence ICP [14, 21]. In one study that examined neck flexion, extension, lateral flexion, and rotation [21], every motion away from the neutral position resulted in an increase in ICP, although not all of these individually achieved statistical significance. Nevertheless, the trends were consistent enough to warrant a model that captures effects of each considered motion. Rotation-induced pressure increases were observed to usually be linear with increasing rotation angle [14]. Therefore, in the absence of contrary evidence, we will assume that venous pressure increases linearly with each motion of the neck. Next, it was found that the combination of flexion/extension with lateral flexion or rotation decreased the influence of the second motion [21]. One possible explanation for this is that flexion of the neck slackens the blood vessels somewhat, reducing the bending or compression required for the second motion (lateral flexion or rotation). In contrast, extension of the neck can stretch the blood vessels somewhat, decreasing their compliance and thus decreasing the effects of the second motion. Since the effect of neck motion is to change the resistance to flow of the venous system, the induced change in pressure should be proportional to the pressure difference that is driving flow through the head. Together, all of these effects suggest the following model for venous pressure in response to neck position.

$$P_{\mathrm{d}} = P_{\mathrm{d}}(\text{neutral}) + \frac{P_{\mathrm{a}} - P_{\mathrm{d}}(\text{neutral})}{\Delta P_{\mathrm{ref}}} \begin{bmatrix} P_{\varphi_{\mathrm{lim}}} \dfrac{\varphi}{\varphi_{\mathrm{lim}}} + P_{\varepsilon_{\mathrm{lim}}} \dfrac{\varepsilon}{\varepsilon_{\mathrm{lim}}} + \\ \dfrac{\lambda}{\lambda_{\mathrm{lim}}} \left(P_{\lambda_{\mathrm{lim}}} - P_{\lambda_{\mathrm{dec}}} \left(\dfrac{\varphi}{\varphi_{\mathrm{lim}}} + \dfrac{\varepsilon}{\varepsilon_{\mathrm{lim}}} \right) \right) + \\ \dfrac{\theta}{\theta_{\mathrm{lim}}} \left(P_{\theta_{\mathrm{lim}}} - P_{\theta_{\mathrm{dec}}} \left(\dfrac{\varphi}{\varphi_{\mathrm{lim}}} + \dfrac{\varepsilon}{\varepsilon_{\mathrm{lim}}} \right) \right) \end{bmatrix}, \quad (2.9)$$

where ΔP_{ref} is a reference arterial to venous pressure difference and for each variable x, x_{lim} is a limiting value of the angle and $P_{x_{\mathrm{lim}}}$ is the pressure increment observed at that limiting value (when $P_{\mathrm{a}} - P_{\mathrm{d}}(\text{neutral}) = \Delta P_{\mathrm{ref}}$). Furthermore, $P_{\lambda_{\mathrm{dec}}}$ and $P_{\theta_{\mathrm{dec}}}$ are the decreases in pressure increments for lateral flexion and rotation, respectively, when the neck is flexed or extended to its limiting angle. There is no *a priori* reason why $P_{\lambda_{\mathrm{dec}}}$ and $P_{\theta_{\mathrm{dec}}}$ should apply to both flexion and extension of the neck, instead of requiring separate parameters for each motion (particularly as the two motions individually have different effects on pressure). However, the data collected in [21] suggested that both flexion and extension cause equivalent decreases in the effect of rotation and the effect of lateral flexion. The values for P_{a} and $P_{\mathrm{d}}(\text{neutral})$ in Eq. (2.9) should be those given by Eqs. (2.5) and (2.6), respectively. Since jugular collapse significantly changes the flow through the venous system (and renders any other distal geometrical changes to the jugular irrelevant), the parameter values in Eq. (2.9) can be expected to change for $\tau \geq \tau_{\mathrm{collapse}}$.

Equation (2.9) does not include any direct dependence on blood viscosity because even with geometrical changes to the blood vessels, vascular resistance should be proportional to viscosity. Therefore, even though the resistance of the altered neck vasculature will increase with increased viscosity, the resistance of the rest of the cerebral system will also increase in proportion, leading to the same distribution of pressure. However, since increased blood viscosity leads to decreased flow, patients with higher blood viscosities can be expected to have higher arterial pressures as the body attempts to maintain cardiac output. This will, in turn, increase the effects on neck motion on venous pressure and thus lead to higher values of ICP.

Based on the results in [21], we can estimate that for general patients and $\tau < \tau_{\text{collapse}}$, $\Delta P_{\text{ref}} \approx 80$ mmHg, $P_{\varphi_{\text{lim}}} \approx 4.8\text{mmHg}$, $\varphi_{\text{lim}} \approx 45^\circ$, $P_{\varepsilon_{\text{lim}}} \approx 1.5\text{mmHg}$, $\varepsilon_{\text{lim}} \approx 60^\circ$, $P_{\lambda_{\text{lim}}} \approx 2.6\text{mmHg}$, $\lambda_{\text{lim}} = 45^\circ$, $P_{\lambda_{\text{dec}}} \approx 1.4\text{mmHg}$, $P_{\theta_{\text{lim}}} \approx 4.2\text{mmHg}$, $\theta_{\text{lim}} \approx 60^\circ$, and $P_{\theta_{\text{dec}}} \approx 1.9\text{mmHg}$, where some angles are taken from the original study and others are estimated according to the patients' age range using [22]. This suggests that the largest increases in P_{d} and ICP occur with flexion and rotation of the neck, while extension of the neck can actually reduce the pressure rise from rotation. See Fig. 2.4 for an example of how various neck positions affect ICP and CePP. There does not appear to be any existing studies that would allow for the estimation of parameter values for $\tau \geq \tau_{\text{collapse}}$.

Although only rotation was considered in [14], their results suggested a potentially much larger value of $P_{\theta_{\text{lim}}}$, up to 12.5 mmHg. This discrepancy can potentially be attributed to the different patient populations in the two studies, with [21] excluding patients with high ICP, increased CSF volume or any impairment on the Glasgow Coma Scale, while [14] only included patients with intracranial tumors. Since the numerical value of arterial pressure was not reported in [14], it is possible (but unknown) that patient hypertension contributed to the observed effects. Furthermore, the patients with the highest initial ICP in [14] exhibited the largest (and nonlinear) pressure increases. This, coupled with the amount of individual variation seen in arterial studies (e.g., [18, 20]) suggests that this model of the effects of neck motion will not apply to any

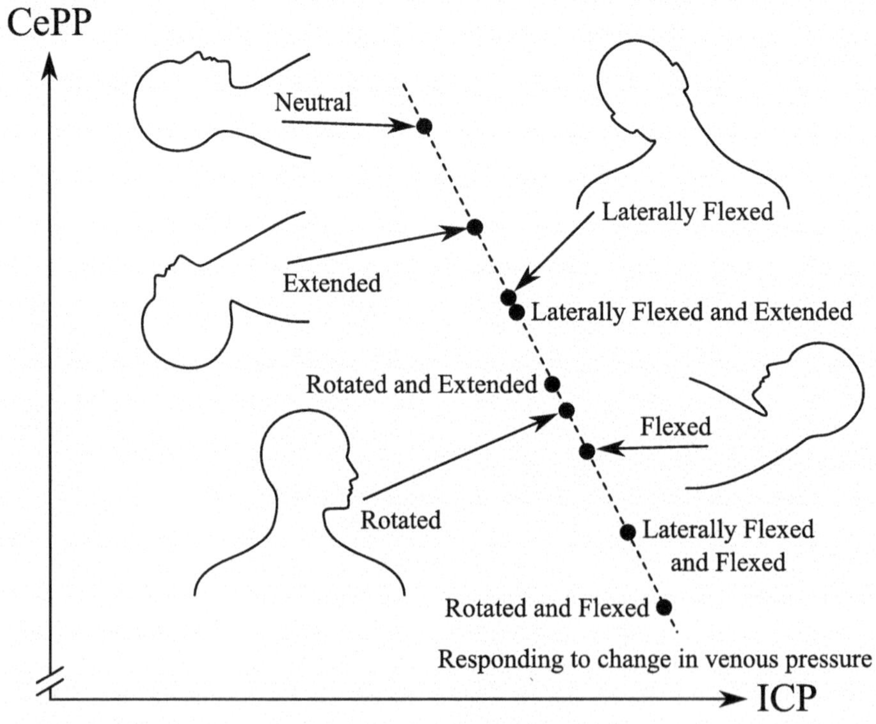

Fig. 2.4 An example of the effects of different neck positions on intracranial pressure (ICP) and cerebral perfusion pressure (CePP). In this example, the patient is supine with zero tilt angle. Compared to the neutral position, any other neck position increases ICP and decreases CePP. All cases shown correspond to the limiting values of the angles used in Eq. (2.9)

patient with existing impairments in blood flow to the head and neck. In principle, any disease state distal to the neck should not influence the model, but only if they do not induce any changes to the geometry or distribution of flow in the neck. Finally, the amount of variation seen in studies of neck motion suggest that there is an increased possibility that positioning the patient's neck without due care could adversely affect blood flow to the head. In particular, moving the head and neck past their normal range of motion (e.g., by hyperextending the neck [23]) can be expected to increase the risk of complications.

References

1. Recommended practices for positioning the patient in the perioperative practice setting. In: Perioperative standards and recommended practices. Denver, CO: AORN; 2014. p. 481–99.
2. Qvarlander S, Sundström N, Malm J, Eklund A. Postural effects on intracranial pressure: modeling and clinical evaluation. J Appl Physiol. 2013;115: 1474–80.
3. Nilsson C, Stahlberg F, Thomsen C, Henriksen O, Herning M, Owman C. Circadian variation in human cerebrospinal fluid production measured by magnetic resonance imaging. Am J Physiol Regul Integr Comp Physiol. 1992;262(1):R20–4.
4. Czosnyka M, Pickard J. Monitoring and interpretation of intracranial pressure. J Neurol Neurosurg Psychiatry. 2004;75(6):813–21.
5. Andersson N, Malm J, Eklund A. Dependency of cerebrospinal fluid outflow resistance on intracranial pressure. J Neurosurg. 2008;109(5):918–22.
6. Kose G, Hatipoglu S. Effect of head and body positioning on cerebral blood flow velocity in patients who underwent cranial surgery. J Clin Nurs. 2012;21(13-14):1859–67.
7. Jang E, Lee S, Choi J, Cho S. Changes in the hemodynamic parameters between the prone and supine positions measured by an arterial pulse contour cardiac output monitoring system. Anesth Pain Med. 2015;10:291–4.
8. Edgcombe H, Carter K, Yarrow S. Anaesthesia in the prone position. Br J Anaesth. 2008;100(2):165–83.
9. Hinghofer-Szalkay H. Gravity, the hydrostatic indifference concept and the cardiovascular system. Eur J Appl Physiol. 2011;111:163–74.
10. Gisolf A, van Lieshout J, van Heusden K, Pott F, Stok W, Karemaker J. Human cerebral venous outflow pathway depends on posture and central venous pressure. J Physiol. 2004;560(1):317–27.
11. Feldman Z, Kanter M, Robertson C, Contant C, Hayes C, Sheinberg M, et al. Effect of head elevation on intracranial pressure, cerebral perfusion pressure, and cerebral blood flow in head-injured patients. J Neurosurg. 1992;76:207–11.
12. Schneider G, van Helden A, Franke R, Lanksch W, Unterberg A. Influence of body position on jugular venous oxygen saturation, intracranial pressure and cerebral perfusion pressure. In: Unterberg A, Schneider G, Lanksch W, editors. Monitoring of cerebral blood flow and metabolism in intensive care. Vienna: Springer; 1993. p. 107–12.
13. Schwarz S, Georgiadis D, Aschoff A, Schwab S. Effects of body position on intracranial pressure and cerebral perfusion in patients with large hemispheric stroke. Stroke. 2002;33:497–501.
14. Hung O, Hare G, Brien S. Head elevation reduces head-rotation associated increased ICP in patients with intracranial tumours. Can J Anaesth. 2000;47(5):415–20.
15. Hulme A, Cooper R. The effects of head position and jugular vein compression (JVC) on intracranial pressure (ICP). A clinical study. In: Beks J, Bosch D, Brock M, editors. Intracranial pressure III. Berlin: Springer; 1976. p. 259–63.
16. Højlund J, Sandmand M, Sonne M, Mantoni T, Jørgensen H, Belhage B, et al. Effect of head rotation on cerebral blood velocity in the prone position. Anesthesiol Res Pract. 2012;2012:647258.
17. Thiel H, Wallace K, Donat J, Yong-Hing K. Effect of various head and neck positions on vertebral artery blood flow. Clin Biomech. 1994;9:105–10.
18. Toole J, Tucker S. Influence of head position upon cerebral circulation: studies on blood flow in cadavers. AMA Arch Neurol. 1960;2(6):616–23.
19. Wang L, Zhao F, Wang D, Hu S, Liu J, Zhou Z, et al. Pressure drop in tortuosity/kinking of the internal carotid artery: simulation and clinical investigation. Biomed Res Int. 2016;2016:2428970.
20. Aristokleous N, Seimenis I, Georgiou G, Nicolaides A, Anayiotos A. The effect of head rotation on the geometry and hemodynamics of healthy vertebral arteries. Ann Biomed Eng. 2015;43(6):1287–97.
21. Mavrocordatos P, Bissonnette B, Ravussin P. Effects of neck position and head elevation on intracranial pressure in anaesthetized neurosurgical patients: preliminary results. J Neurosurg Anesthesiol. 2000;12(1):10–4.
22. Youdas J, Garrett T, Suman V, Bogard C, Hallman H, Carey J. Normal range of motion of the cervical spine: an initial goniometric study. Phys Ther. 1992;72(11):770–80.
23. Tsai Y, Doufas A, Huang C, Liou F, Lin C. Postoperative coma in a patient with complete basilar syndrome after cervical discectomy. Can J Anaesth. 2006;53(2):202–7.

Anesthesia and Patient Positioning

3

C. Wayne Hamm

Introduction

Of all the surgical specialties, neurosurgery most frequently employs positioning that not only impacts the administration and choice of the anesthetic, but can also remove the anesthesia provider from access to the intravenous tubing, and the airway itself. This chapter will examine the specific issues associated with positioning the patient for neurosurgical procedures, both spinal and cranial, in the supine, sitting, lateral and prone positions.

The goal of this chapter is to sensitize the anesthesia provider to the considerations that must be applied to the planing for general anesthesia specific to positioning in neurosurgical procedures. Thus, an extensive discussion of the specific anesthesia medications and techniques identified with neurosurgical procedures will not take place. Additionally, preanesthesia evaluation of the patient to entertain the specific positions in neurosurgical procedures will be discussed at length in Chap. 4.

Basic monitoring for neurosurgical cases includes, but is not limited to: precordial/esophageal stethoscope, blood pressure measurement, end-tidal carbon dioxide monitoring, pulse oximetry, and temperature measurement. Additions to the monitoring will appear as indicated for specific procedures/positions.

> "Knowledge, planning, teamwork, and housekeeping, all equally important, are the key ingredients of safe positioning of a surgical patient upon an operating table. As trite and pompous as identifying these components may seem, ignoring or being casual about any of them can easily render the care team inept, bring harm to the patient, and endanger the institution." [1].

Supine Position

Spinal Procedures

In the neurosurgical operating room, patient positioning must be a collaborative effort that includes the anesthesiologist, neurosurgeon, and nursing staff [2]. When patients are positioned supine for spinal procedures, the most common procedure involves an anterior approach to the cervical spine.

Patients with cervical spine pathology should have the following items in agreement between the anesthesia provider, the patient, and the neurosurgeon: (1) The correct side—the patient and their physical findings are specific for that side, (2) The stability of the neck and the integrity of the spinal cord are consistent with laryngoscopic endotracheal intubation, and (3) The

C. Wayne Hamm (✉)
Medical Anesthesia Group, Germantown, TN, USA
e-mail: whamm3@gmail.com

A. Arthur et al. (eds.), *Perioperative Considerations and Positioning for Neurosurgical Procedures*,
https://doi.org/10.1007/978-3-319-72679-3_3

patient must demonstrate neck movement consistent with intubation without symptomatology. Any disagreement must be resolved prior to proceeding with the anesthetic. Once agreed and noted, one peripheral intravenous line for most anterior cervical spine cases is sufficient. Obese patients with arms at the side will likely have trouble with conventional blood pressure cuffs. Often, an arterial line will be indicated.

Anesthesia induction and maintenance should be based primarily on the patient's underlying medical condition, the anticipated intraoperative conditions, and the preference of the anesthesia provider [3]. If electrophysiologic monitoring is planned, an awareness of the effects of anesthetics on such monitoring is essential. Appropriate explanation of changes encountered are dependent on a stable intraoperative anesthetic depth [3].

There is much variety in the management of the head for these approaches. The head can be placed in a halter traction, Gardner-Wells tongs, a horseshoe (cerebellar headrest), a gel doughnut, etc. Extension of the head can be achieved by cervical traction, taping the chin back or placing a roll behind the neck. Because anesthesia is placed remote to the head and airway, Securing and maintaining the airway are critical issues. For anterior cervical procedures below the level of the third cervical vertebra, oral intubation is sufficient.

Much has been written regarding maintaining endotracheal tube cuff pressures less than 20 mmHg for anterior cervical procedures. Following placement of self-retaining retractors, the cuff is fully deflated and reinflated until seal is reestablished at our institution. With removal of the retractor system, additional air will usually be required to reestablish the seal.

Limit the bite block to approximately the size of the endotracheal tube as larger blocks will limit the cephalad surgical exposure. Depending on the body habitus of the patient, for anterior cervical procedures at and above the third cervical vertebra, placement of a nasotracheal tube may be indicated. Insertion of bite blocks in these patients may compromise cephalad surgical exposure. Secure the endotracheal tube to the contralateral side. A nasopharyngeal temperature probe is inserted into the esophagus for temperature monitoring and also aids with surgical identification of the esophagus. If halter traction is used with a bite block of insufficient thickness or with no bite block in procedures using orotracheal tubes, compression of the endotracheal tube can occur. Additionally, when head holding devices such as halo or cerebellar head rest are used, the endotracheal tube is likely to be kinked by the weight of the drapes weighing down on the tube and kinking the tube at the corner of the mouth. The weight of the drapes in combination with surgical retraction make iatrogenic extubation possible, which must be prevented. If the head is supported otherwise, consider use of viscoelastic gel pads and/or round head holders. This is important in patients with traction as the pressure on the occipital area is greater. By virtue of the eyes' close proximity to the surgical site in combination with being hidden by the drapes, cephalad retraction should be evaluated often by anesthesia for possible globe compression.

For suggested airway management of patients with unstable cervical spines, please refer to the ASA Difficult Algorithm [4]. Much has been written on this topic with less than complete consensus. Gary Stier summarizes the literature, "… there is no evidence that any particular airway management technique is either safe or dangerous in a patient with an unstable cervical spine." [3] Further he notes, "The method for definitive airway control should be based primarily on the operator's skill and experience rather than on the fear of inflicting cervical cord damage." [3] The presence of an unstable cervical spine is sufficient indication for a urinary catheter and invasive arterial monitoring.

The supine position has three major variations: traditional, contoured, and the frogleg. We will not consider the frogleg position as it is not usually encountered in neurosurgical procedures [5]. The contoured position we will discuss in regard to cranial procedures in the supine position. In the traditional version, the patient lies on their back with their head on a head holder. The arms are comfortably restrained alongside the trunk. This position usually places the hips and knees in extension which may be poorly tolerated for long periods of time [5]. As the shoulders are often taped in a caudad manner with the head placed in extension, we have found it useful to bend the arms slightly and place the hands at the pubic level fixed in place with the draw sheet (papoose fashion) (see Fig. 3.1).

For transoral approaches to the spine, in the absence of a tracheostomy, we have used armored endotracheal tubes. We have secured these by stitching them to the surgeon-requested side (see Fig. 3.2). We have traditionally done these procedures with the patient in a halo vest. The front vest is removed with the back remaining intact. The arms are placed papoose fashion. The endotracheal tube is also attached to the halo to avoid the possibility of extubation.

These are usually long procedures often requiring a posterior approach for fusion. Thus, we typically place at least two peripheral IVs, a urinary catheter and invasive arterial monitoring.

The maintenance of the anesthetic is dictated by the electrophysiologic monitoring employed. Transoral procedures usually anticipate an overnight intubation and full airway evaluation before extubation if the patient does not have a pre-existing tracheostomy.

Complications Associated with the Supine Position

Patients who must lie immobile for prolonged periods in a supine position often complain of backache [5, 6]. During prolonged procedures, the heels and plantar flexor tendons are especially at risk for developing blisters and ischemic pressure areas [5]. Prolonged compression of the hair follicles may produce hair loss [7]. The alopecia may not occur until several days to weeks after the operation is done [8–10]. Probably, the single most reported neuropraxic complication is ulnar neuropathy [11].

Cranial Procedures

The most common cranial procedures performed on patients in the supine position are subdural hematoma drainage and pituitary tumor removal [3]. The contoured supine position or lawn chair position as coined by John Martin is frequently used [5]. The lawn chair position is an alternative supine position in which the hips and knees are slightly flexed into positions that are more neutral. This contoured position is similar to that assumed when resting in an adjustable reclining

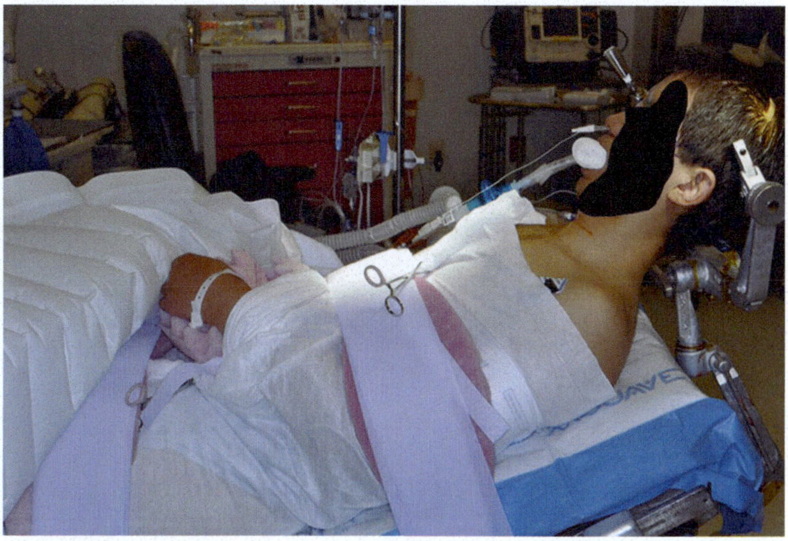

Fig. 3.1 Note how the hands are placed in the suprapubic area with the arms flexed with all snuggly secured by the draw sheet (Papoosing of the arms)

chair. The supine position is the easiest for the anesthesiologist because the need to move the patient, catheters, and monitors is minimized [3].

Subdural hematoma evacuations are not generally lengthy procedures and are not given the same positioning considerations as long combined craniofacial surgery. Pituitary removal can put anesthesia very remote to the airway owing to localizing equipment such as X-ray.

Significant blood loss or cranial nerve reflex elicitation requires continuous arterial monitoring, a urinary catheter (mandatory for pituitary tumors) and an additional IV. If the use of hypertonic solutions is anticipated, a central venous line is placed after intubation.

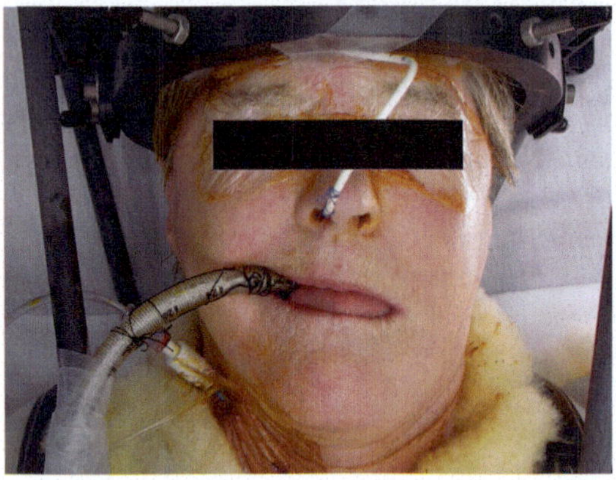

Fig. 3.2 Transoral odontoidectomy patient with tube stitched into the corner of the mouth

Placement of a skull pin skeletal fixation apparatus is as painful as the surgical incision and requires additional anesthesia for its application. The advantage of the skull pins is that it immobilizes the patient's head and neck while providing superior access to the surgical field. Anesthesia-related problems which can cause unexpected movement after the device is applied can result in injury to the cervical spine or severe lacerations if the head is forcibly pulled out of the clamp [3]. Nonelective extubation while in the frame may make reestablishment of the airway difficult if not impossible until the frame is removed.

Although poor positioning may be tolerated with little issue in patients having brief surgical procedures, a small overlooked detail may result in long-term or permanent injury and disability after a long neurosurgical procedure [3]. Prolonged supine neurosurgical procedures include combined head and neck surgery with neurosurgery for extensive craniofacial surgery. These surgeries will often require that anesthesia be placed at the foot of the table. For these procedures, we often stitch the endotracheal tube to the jaw (see Fig. 3.3). For other procedures where surgical exposure of the maxilla is not involved, we will secure the endotracheal tube with a bridal technique. This is accomplished by passing an aspiration catheter via the nare and pulling it from the posterior pharynx and attaching to the

Fig. 3.3 Maxillotomy approach to a clival chordoma with the endotracheal tube stitched to the corner of the mouth. Anesthesia was positioned at the patient's feet

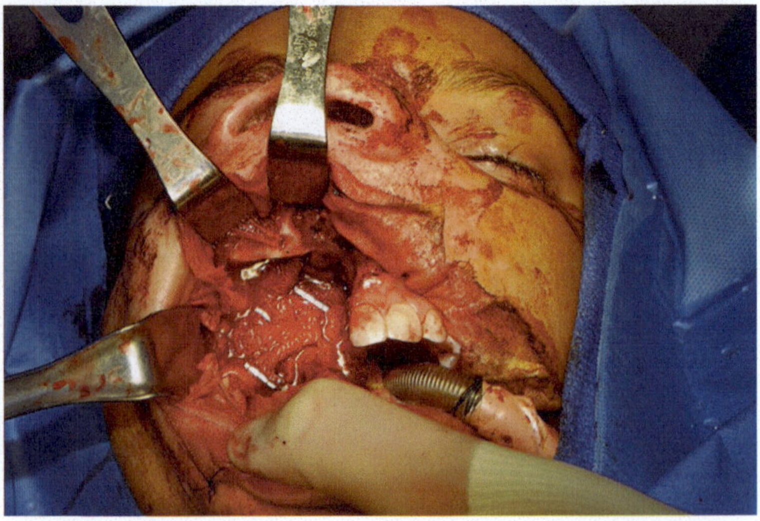

a b

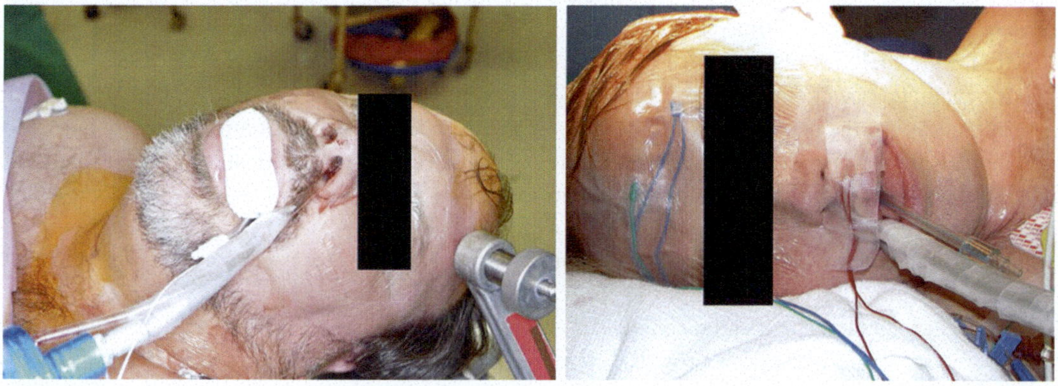

Fig. 3.4 (**a**) A plastic catheter inserted through the nose and removed from the back of the throat. (**b**) It is then taped securely to the endotracheal tube

endotracheal tube (see Fig. 3.4a, b). Venous air embolism (VAE) during cranial procedures in the contoured supine position has not been an issue at our institution. We do take all VAE prophylaxis steps when cranial exposure is over a major venous sinus. This includes precordial Doppler and placement of an air aspiration catheter in the right atrium.

Each 2.5 cm change of vertical height from the reference point at the level of the heart leads to a decrease of 2 mmHg in the blood pressure at the level of the heart [8]. Thus, we always measure blood pressure at the level of the tragus.

Sitting Position

Use of the sitting position in neurosurgery has long been a matter of some debate [12]. The use of the sitting position for patients having posterior fossa and cervical spine surgery facilitates surgical access but presents unique physiological challenges for the anesthesia provider with the potential for serious complications [13]. This patient position provides optimum access to midline lesions, improves cerebral venous decompression, lowers intracranial pressure, and promotes gravity drainage of blood and cerebral spinal fluid [14]. The presence of a patent foramen ovale is an absolute contraindication to the sitting position. Preoperative contrast echocardiography should be used as a screening technique to detect the population at risk of paradoxical air embolism [12]. Modern techniques to prevent, monitor, diagnose, and rapidly treat these complications can potentially improve outcome [15]. This is supported by a number of recent series that have demonstrated reduced rates of complications, particularly VAE, relative to older studies [16–18]. These results suggest that rather than abandoning this procedure as has occurred in many centers, modern techniques aimed as recognizing VAE may mitigate complications associated with the sitting position, improving its safety [19]. In the most recent series, Himes reports a modern series of 1792 procedures performed in the sitting position. He concludes that when appropriately used with modern anesthesia techniques, the sitting position provides a safe means of surgical access [19].

Spinal Procedures

The sitting cervical position affords advantages over prone positioning for elective posterior cervical decompression and fusion. In a modern series of 560 cervical procedures performed in the sitting position Sandwell et al. demonstrated no VAE. They concluded that many surgeons at their institution prefer the sitting position. The position provided a dry surgical field, easily verified spinal alignment prior to fusion, and superior visualization on intraoperative X-rays due to reduced shoulder artifact [20].

Monitoring includes placement of an arterial line for accurate measurement of the blood pressure at the level of the head.

The patient should be informed of the specific risks of venous air embolism, quadriparesis, and peripheral nerve injuries. Appropriate charting of patient information provided and special consent issues are essential at some institutions [12].

Choice of induction agent and techniques is at the discretion of the anesthesia provider. After induction and intubation, intraoperative monitoring for VAE is established. Precordial Doppler ultrasonography is standard at our institution for cervical procedures. Doppler ultrasonography is the most sensitive of the generally available monitors capable of detecting intracardiac air [14, 21]. Unless venous lakes are reasonably anticipated in the cervical exposure or dural opening is expected, right atrial lines are not placed.

After accounting for the pain of the placement of the Mayfield, the patient is slowly raised into the sitting position. The arterial line is placed at the level of the tragus at all times. The hydrostatic effect of gravity may produce a decrease in systemic arterial pressure because of venous pooling. The volume of blood accumulating in the venous system may be influenced by patient factors (i.e., body mass index, intravascular volume status, pre-existing hypertension) and factors related to anesthesia. As much as 1500 mL may be sequestered in the venous system of the lower limbs [22].

After the patient has been placed in the sitting position, special attention should be placed on protecting and padding the boney prominences; particularly before a prolonged procedure. The arms should be supported in order to prevent brachial plexus injury. The ulnar nerve should be padded to prevent compression. The knees should also be flexed to prevent stretching of the sciatic nerve [23].

Should VAE be encountered, the surgeon is notified, the surgical field flooded, and the position changed if ineffective. Jugular venous compression has been demonstrated to be effective in reducing air entry [24, 25]. Use of positive end expiratory pressure, advocated by some may impair surgical conditions, decrease venous return, and increase the chance that right atrial pressure will exceed left atrial pressure and predispose an at-risk patient to paradoxical air embolus [26].

Cranial Procedures

This position is most commonly utilized for posterior fossa surgery, in particular lesions in the pineal region via a supracerebellar infratentorial approach. Relative contraindications to the sitting position include: open ventriculoatrial shunt, signs of cerebral ischemia when upright and awake, right-to-left shunt (patent foramen ovale), and cardiac instability [27].

The patient should be informed of the specific risks of venous air embolism, quadriparesis, and peripheral nerve injuries. Appropriate charting of patient information provided and special consent issues are essential in some centers [12].

Intraoperative monitoring for patients undergoing complex intracranial neurosurgical procedures in the sitting position should include a urinary catheter invasive arterial monitoring with the transducer placed at the level of the tragus [12]. The use of nitrous oxide is debated in the literature. We have found it easy to avoid nitrous oxide in these cases.

After induction and intubation, we place a thick gauze bite block. Avoidance of oral airways and oropharyngeal tubes in patients where the head is placed in flexion may help prevent macroglossia. We place a multi-orifice air aspiration catheter via the internal jugular circulation which is removed at the conclusion of surgery. We double-stick the internal jugular for placement of a triple lumen catheter (see Fig. 3.5). The tip is localized using intravascular electrocardiography with the P wave large and negative and no positive component [28]. Observation of the ECG configuration to confirm proper catheter placement in the right atrium in some studies is more precise than chest radiography [29]. If there is any question, a chest X-ray is made to confirm

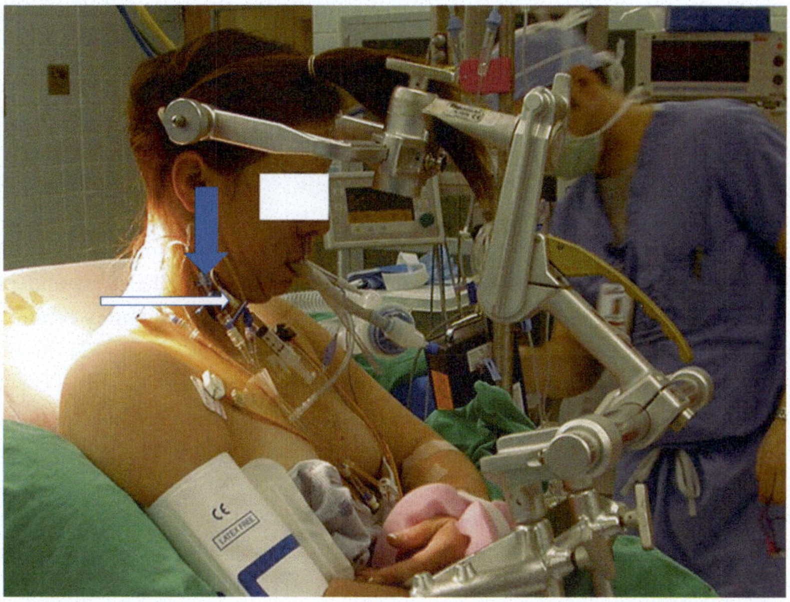

Fig. 3.5 Small arrow pointing to the 16 gauge air aspiration catheter. Large arrow pointing to the triple lumen catheter

position at the caval-atrial junction as data suggest this is the most efficacious site for air removal [30]. Multi-orifice catheters have been designed to enhance bubble recovery [31].

Supplementary monitoring is directed toward prompt detection and early treatment of VAE. This monitoring includes precordial Doppler, right heart catheters, transesophageal echocardiography (TEE), fractional excretion of nitrogen (FEN2), capnography, esophageal stethoscope, and transcutaneous oxygen measurement [12]. TEE is the most sensitive monitor to detect air in the right atrium and paradoxical embolization of the air to the left atrium through a patent foramen ovale [32]. A minimum of three monitoring techniques are recommended [14]. TEE and Doppler were found to be equally sensitive with respect to air detection [33]. The classic method of monitoring for air with an esophageal stethoscope for a change in heart sounds or a "mill-wheel" murmur is dependent on large amounts of intracardiac air and provides little advance warning of cardiovascular collapse [12]. It is recommended that the esophageal stethoscope be retained because of its noninvasive nature and mechanical simplicity [12]. Thus, the esophageal stethoscope, precordial Doppler, capnography, right atrial catheter, and transcutaneous oxygen measurement represent our usual monitoring. TEE is available. If used, it is not maintained for prolonged periods of time. Unless, indicated by preexisting comorbidities, we usually do not place a pulmonary artery catheter.

Maintenance of anesthesia is accomplished with controlled positive-pressure ventilation with paralysis. This allows for lighter levels of anesthesia, hyperventilation, which diminishes $PaCO_2$, thereby decreasing both sympathetic stimulation and blood pressure at any given depth of anesthesia, cerebral vasoconstriction, less bleeding, lower ICP, less cardiovascular depression, and less likely patient movement [26]. Excessive decreases in inhaled agent concentration as a strategy to combat hypotension may allow awareness [26]. There is no information that demonstrates that the sitting position alters the minimal alveolar concentration necessary for anesthesia [26, 34]. If electrophysiologic monitoring involving motor-evoked responses are anticipated, muscle relaxation is avoided and anesthesia levels adjusted accordingly.

If Doppler ultrasonography changes occur or $ETCO_2$ shows a sudden drop, the surgeon should be informed. Aspiration of the RAC should be initiated as it has been demonstrated effective in reducing morbidity from VAE [35–38]. Have the surgeon flood the field with fluid. Patient position should be changed to lower the head to heart level when possible. Provide cardiovascular support [26]. External cardiac massage has been shown to be effective in disrupting a large air lock in the event of cardiovascular collapse [39].

The incidence and severity of VAE may be decreased by the use of controlled positive-pressure ventilation, adequate hydration, proper wrapping of the lower extremities, positioning so the head is the lowest possible while still providing good exposure, liberal use of bone wax, avoidance of nitrous in patients with known intracardiac defects and avoidance of drugs that may increase venous capacitance (nitroglycerine) [26]. The anesthetic goals during emergence are to prevent abrupt rises in blood pressure, effect rapid awakening, return motor strength and minimize coughing and straining on the endotracheal tube [26]. Extubation is dependent on the manipulation of medullary structures and the patient's pre-existing comorbidities. The airway should be maintained until the patient is awake, following commands and demonstrating return of protective airway reflexes.

Complications Associated with the Sitting Position

Hypotension is the most frequent complication of the sitting position [40].

The greater the pressure gradient between cerebral veins and the right atrium and the lower the central venous pressures, the greater is the tendency for air to enter venous openings at the craniotomy site [26]. The vertical distance between the head and heart may range from 20 to 65 cm, depending on the procedure [41]. The incidence of venous air embolism ranges from 25% [42] to 50% [43] in studies using precordial Doppler monitoring. Transesophageal echo monitoring has indicated an incidence as high as 76% [44]. A paradoxical air embolism is most likely the result of right-to-left shunting through an intracardiac defect. A patent foramen ovale has an incidence of 20–30% in the population [45]. The calculated risk of paradoxical air embolism is 5–10%.

Tension pneumocephalus has been reported in association with posterior fossa exploration in the sitting position [46, 47] with an incidence of 3% in one study [18]. Pneumocephalus can lead to delayed emergence, postoperative lethargy, headaches, confusion, cranial nerve deficits, and hemiparesis.

Extreme flexion of the head with the chin resting on the chest and prolonged presence of an oral airway may promote macroglossia in the sitting position [12]. Five unreported cases of mid-cervical quadriplegia after acoustic neuroma resection in the sitting position were referred to in an editorial comment by Hitselberger and House [12, 48]. Wilder claimed knowledge of more than 20 such unreported cases [12, 49]. Quadriparesis has been associated with sitting position in a patient with severe cervical stenosis [50]. Peripheral nerve injuries associated with the sitting position for neurosurgery include damage to the common peroneal nerve, resulting in foot drop and rarely, recurrent laryngeal nerve palsy [12]. The incidence of common peroneal nerve neuropathy in a series of 488 patients was less than 1% [18]. Recurrent laryngeal nerve palsy has been described in association with the use of transesophageal echo who underwent craniotomy in the sitting position [33].

Lateral Position

The decubitus position is defined as "the position of an individual lying on a horizontal surface, designated according to the portion of the body resting on the surface…" [51]. The lateral decubitus position is referred to as right or left depending on which side is down. Monitoring blood pressure in the lateral decubitus position presents unique problems related to the type and placement of the sensors. The discrepancy in blood pressure between the up-side and down-side arm could be as much as 32 mmHg [52]. The lateral decubitus position shifts the mediastinum toward the down side and rotates the heart on its axis which can interfere with venous return and cardiac output [52]. Marked reductions in arterial pressures occur with almost all lateral positions during anesthesia. The lowest mean arterial blood pressure has been noted in those patients placed in the right lateral decubitus [53].

Flexion and extension of the adult neck after initial placement of the endotracheal tube will move its tip more than an inch within the trachea [54]. Movement of the head during the turning process demands reassessment of the airway placement. The anesthetized patient in the lateral decubitus position with a closed chest exhibits an increased mismatch of ventilation and perfusion. The up-side lung is well ventilated, but poorly perfused. If the chest wall and pleura are opened, further ventilation/perfusion mismatch occurs. This is because positive-pressure ventilation is now required, the upper lung becoming more compliant and receiving additional ventilation and positive atmospheric pressure on the up-side lung causes a downward displacement [52].

Lawson cites three general principles for attaining the lateral decubitus position with little risk of problems. He identifies the anesthesiologist as the most appropriate person to coordinate the move primarily because he controls the airway and holds the relaxed head and neck. The next principle is that the shoulders and pelvis of the paralyzed anesthetized patient must be maintained in the same plane during the turn to avoid torsional stress on the spine. The last principle requires that a minimum of two team members plus the anesthesiologist are needed for a safe turn [52].

Spinal Procedures

The lateral position is used for surgical approach for patients requiring the retroperitoneal approach to the thoracolumbar spine. Retropleural thoracotomy is an appropriate approach for localized ventral thoracic and thoracolumbar vertebral lesions between T3 and L2 [34, 55]. Fourney found that for simultaneous anterior-posterior approach to the thoracic and lumbar spine for the radical resection tumors advantages of the approach include direct visualization of adjacent neurovascular structures, the ability to achieve complete resection of lesions involving all three columns simultaneously, and the ability to perform excellent dorsal and ventral stabilization in one operative session [56].

The anesthesia choices will be dictated by the type of monitoring and the necessity of isolated lung anesthesia. With electrophysiologic monitoring requiring motor-evoked capability, we use a total intravenous anesthetic (TIVA). If the electrophysiologic monitoring will not require motor-evoked responses or will not be used, we conduct these cases with muscle relaxation, inhalation agent, and narcotics.

All patients undergoing thoracic opening in the lateral position should be preoperatively evaluated for the ability to maintain the lateral position and if necessary, one-lung anesthesia. We institute one-lung anesthesia for spinal procedures in the lateral position at and above T10.

Additional intraoperative monitoring for patients undergoing complex spinal neurosurgical procedures in the lateral position includes urinary catheter and invasive arterial monitoring. Vascular access requirements are specific to the procedure, but any metastatic disease requires at least two 14-gauge peripheral intravenous lines and a 7–9-Fr introducer with blood available [57]. Induction of the anesthetic is consistent with the requirements of the monitoring and a left-sided endobronchial tube is placed if surgery at T10 or above.

Patients to be placed in lateral position should have the following items in agreement between the anesthesia provider, the patient, and the neurosurgeon: (1) The correct side, (2) the patient and their physical findings are specific for that side, (3) the stability of the neck and the integrity of the spinal cord are consistent with laryngoscopic endotracheal intubation and lastly, the patient demonstrates neck movement consistent with intubation without symptomatology. Any disagreement must be resolved prior to proceeding with the anesthetic.

After induction and intubation, the patient is positioned in the lateral decubitus position with a viscoelastic axillary roll placed to prevent dependent brachial plexus stretching. The head is positioned in a neutral position taking care to avoid lateral bending of the cervical spine which may result in stretching of the nondependent brachial plexus, especially if the shoulders are taped to facilitate positioning [57]. Placement of the pulse oximeter on the down-side arm is recommended [58]. Double lumen tube position must always be confirmed after intubation and reconfirmed before surgery since tubes are easily displaced while moving the patient to the lateral decubitus position [59]. The tension in the pilot balloon of the bronchial cuff should be noted after first inflating that cuff [60]. Confirmation of correct tube placement by use of the fiberoptic bronchoscope is recommended. The tube is considered to be in an ideal position when the proximal edge of its bronchial cuff is immediately below the carina in the appropriate bronchus [61]. Confirmation is also accomplished by physical examination of the chest, including auscultation and observation of chest wall movement and measurement of peak inspiratory pressures during independent ventilation of each lung.

During intrathoracic procedures in which the operated lung is selectively collapsed, hemodynamic stability and oxygenation must be maintained while ventilating only one lung. A completely atelectatic lung eliminates the need for vigorous retraction during surgery, so there is less intraoperative lung trauma. Regional hypoxia in the lungs causes arteriolar constriction with diversion of blood flow away from a hypoxic segment to areas that are better oxygenated. This hypoxic pulmonary vasoconstriction (HPV) can be depressed by inhalational anesthetics. In clinical practice, the overall effects by inhalational and intravenous anesthetic agents on HPV during one-lung anesthesia are small [62, 63]. There is no difference in oxygenation between a TIVA (propofol-alfentanil) anesthetic which spares the HPV, and an inhalational anesthetic (isoflurane) which depresses HPV during one-lung ventilation [64]. If electrophysiologic monitoring in effect, it is most important to not vary the level of anesthesia.

During one-lung ventilation, monitoring oxygenation by oxygen saturation in otherwise healthy patients should be adequate [65]. But, we prefer to monitor arterial blood gases on an hourly basis while in one-lung ventilation as these can often be lengthy procedures and incur major blood loss.

Prior to reinflating the collapsed lung, both lumens of the double lumen tube should be suctioned to remove any mucus, blood, or debris from each lung. Both lungs must be fully re-expanded and the mediastinum must be midline at the completion of one-lung ventilation. Following total collapse, the down-side lung will re-expand unevenly during inflation. Alterations in pulmonary surfactant occur during one-lung ventilation and this necessitates the application of high-sustained pressures in order to reopen the atelectatic lung, but once the lung has been fully reinflated, subsequent inflation will require lower pressures consistent with normal surfactant activity.

Emergence and extubation are as per any major surgery with extubation expected unless there are pre-existing comorbidities or intraoperative misadventures which would contraindicate doing so.

Cranial Procedures

The lateral position is used for neurosurgical approaches in patients requiring temporal bone craniotomy, skull base, and posterior fossa procedures [27]. The lateral position lends itself well to approaches to the cerebellopontine angle and other lateral lesions as well as lesions of the clivus and lateral foramen magnum and other lesions requiring an infracerebellar approach. Gravity-assisted retraction of the cerebellum is especially useful for exposure of the cerebellopontine angle for acoustic tumors and microvascular decompression procedures [66].

Additional intraoperative monitoring for patients undergoing complex cranial neurosurgical procedures in the lateral position includes a urinary catheter and invasive arterial monitoring. In lateral cranial procedures, we also place external pacing pads in anticipation of cranial nerve/brainstem stimulation-induced bradycardia. Vascular access requirements are specific to the case with two peripheral intravenous lines a minimum. As with the spinal procedures in the lateral position, choice of induction and maintenance anesthetic agents and techniques are dependent on electrophysiologic monitoring and if it will involve motor-evoked responses.

Prior to any cranial surgery in the lateral position, the following items should be in agreement between the anesthesia provider, the patient, and the neurosurgeon: (1) The correct side—the patient and their physical findings are specific for that side, (2) The stability of the neck and the integrity of the spinal cord are consistent with laryngoscopic endotracheal intubation, and (3) The patient demonstrates neck movement consistent with intubation without symptomatology. Any disagreement must be resolved prior to proceeding with the anesthetic.

We secure the endotracheal tube with a bridle maneuver and place a large gauze bite block between the teeth after induction and intubation. We place a triple lumen line in the internal jugular vein in anticipation of possible hypertonic solution administration. In the lateral position, the head is most often supported by an appropriate headrest that does not compress the downside ear necessitating an increase in anesthesia to accommodate the stimulation. A roll is placed immediately caudal to the axilla to support the chest and to avoid axillary neurovascular compression. The dependent arm is placed along the patient's side or across the chest. The patient's legs are positioned with the dependent leg strait and the upper leg flexed on pillows [66]. For the three-quarter prone position, skull pins are used for head position. The dependent arm is positioned along the patient's side, and a longitudinal roll is placed under the thorax on the contralateral side. The park-bench position has the patient's head in skull pins with their back at 45°. The dependent arm is now placed flexed in a sling and suspended over the head of the table (see Fig. 3.6). For the three-quarter prone position, skull pins are used for head position. The dependent arm is positioned along the patient's side, and a longitudinal roll is placed under the thorax on the contralateral side. The park-bench position has the patient's head in skull pins with their back at 45°. The dependent arm is now placed flexed in a sling and suspended over the head of the table [67]. The patient is secured to the table with a minimum of three Velcro straps. The table is then articulated to the extent deemed necessary by the surgeon prior to prepping and draping to assure the patient's security.

Unless contraindicated by the electrophysiologic monitoring, anesthesia is maintained with controlled positive-pressure ventilation with muscle relaxation. We use a combination of inhalation agent plus a continuous infusion of narcotic. TIVO is used if required by monitoring.

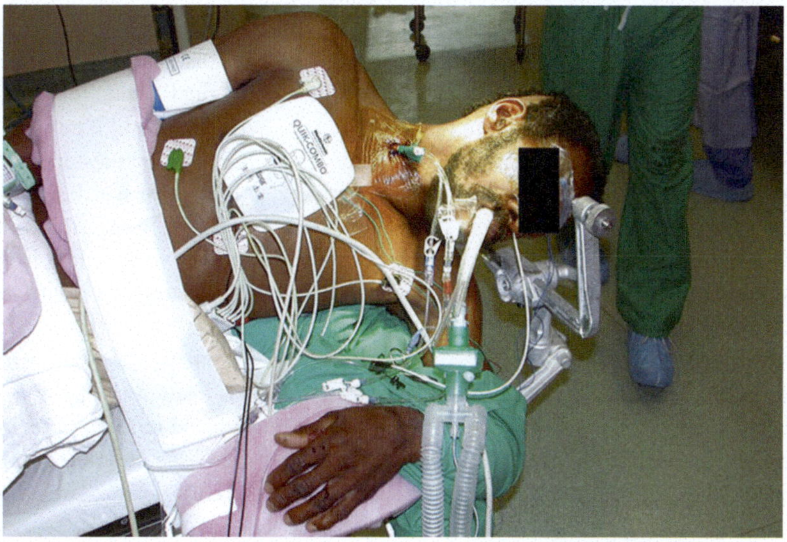

Fig. 3.6 Patient placed in park-bench position with endotracheal tube "bridled" into position. A gauze bite block will be placed between the teeth

We use a combination of an infusion of Propofol and a narcotic (remifentanil) with intermittent doses of midazolam.

Depending on the location of the pathology, manipulation of cranial nerves V and/or X or manipulation of the brainstem can result in bradyarrhythmias that can be usually treated by informing the surgeon who can then avoid manipulation of the nerve. If not, pharmacological intervention may be necessary or use of the external pacemaker is available.

Emergence is accomplished by discontinuing the anesthetic agents. Not infrequently, these patients emerge with hypertension that we treat with a nicardipine infusion titrated to effect. Unless contraindicated by surgical manipulation, misadventure, or pre-existing comorbidity, the patients muscle relaxant is reversed and extubated after the removal of the Mayfield.

Complications Associated with the Lateral Position

The source of many complications in the lateral decubitus position is usually attributed to abnormal pressure or stretch or both [68–70]. Pressure injuries to the skin, soft tissues, and ligaments are probably the most common positional injuries that the lateral position shares with other positions [71]. Baldness after long operations with associated hypotension. Backache is a common complaint for patients who have had surgery in the lateral decubitus position. The incidence is lower than that observed for the prone, lithotomy, or supine position, but still may be related to stretched lumbosacral ligaments [52, 72]. Whiplash injury to the cervical spine is a reported complication of undue tension on the cervical ligaments in the lateral position [73]. Horner's syndrome [74] and postoperative parotitis [75, 76] have also been reported in association with lateral positioning.

In the lateral decubitus position, compression is the major cause of damage to the brachial plexus. This occurs when the lower arm and shoulder are allowed to remain directly under the rib cage. The presence of a cervical rib will increase the vulnerability of the brachial plexus. The properly placed axillary roll prevents this [52]. Stretch becomes a factor if there is excessive dorsal extension of the neck, suspension of the up-side arm on a Mayo tray or anesthesia screen that stretches the brachial plexus around the clavicle, and postural instability allowing too much patient movement [52]. Although clinical practice permits maximum abduction to the arm to 90°, injuries have occurred with as little as 60° when accompanied by forearm rotation [77, 78].

If the laterally positioned patient shifts ventral during surgery, the down-side arm is forced ventromedially and may stretch the suprascapular nerve [79]. The median and ulnar nerves can be damaged if the arm is allowed to hang over the edge of the operating table [52].

The long thoracic nerve may be stretched by lateral angulation the neck and head away from the up-side shoulder producing a "winged-scapula" [52].

Prone Position

In the 1930s and 1940s spinal surgery, pioneers were hampered because no effort was made to avoid abdominal compression when positioning the patient prone. This is somewhat surprising given that the valve less nature of the venous system was well understood at the time. Increased intra-abdominal pressure forced blood from the inferior vena cava into the extradural venous plexus, resulting in increased bleeding and a poor surgical field [80]. Ecker provided the first description of a new position which attempted to account for the increased abdominal pressure in 1949, with his description of the kneeling position [81]. Since that time no less than 16 variations have appeared in the literature [80].

Turning a patient into the prone position also affects the cardiovascular system, the most consistent is a reduction in the cardiac index. This has been attributed to reduced venous return and reduced left ventricular compliance secondary to increased thoracic pressure. Obstruction of the inferior vena cava is a complication of the prone position and is worsened by any degree of increased abdominal pressure. The net result is decreased cardiac output, increased bleeding, venous stasis, and consequent thrombotic complications [80].

In the prone position, there is an increase in the functional residual capacity with alterations in the distribution of both ventilation and perfusion throughout the lungs.

For patients with pre-existing tracheostomies, the table or frame may put either pressure or retraction on the tracheal appliance when placed prone. An endotracheal tube may be placed orally if the patient has a fresh tracheostomy or use a flexible armored endotracheal tube placed via the tracheal stoma if there is a mature tracheostomy. This tube is then stitched into place.

Turning a patient prone requires a level of anesthesia that preserves autonomic compensation, allows sufficient analgesia to avoid sympathetic activity and includes sustained relaxation to allow gentle positioning. No specific drugs or regimens are clearly superior for these purposes. Choices are specific to the patient and the team [82].

In order to turn the patient prone, two receivers stand against the free side of the operating table/frame. Two turners face them at the free side of the patient bed. The arms are kept at the patient's side. At the signal from the anesthesiologist and after disconnection of the airway, the receivers extend their arms across the table to receive the patient. The turners begin to rotate the patient slowly from supine to prone onto the arms of the receivers. The head is maintained firmly in the sagittal plane of the body. The airway is reconnected and the patient's head placed on its holder. The arms are positioned as desired with appropriate restraining tapes and straps [82]. The patient bed is not removed from the room until the vital signs are stable and the security of the airway assured. We keep the head midline and neither flexed or extended on a cushion or device designed to hold the head.

When turning a patient prone whose cervical spine is unstable spontaneous breathing may be used as an evaluation of cord function. Somatosensory-evoked potentials or motor-evoked potentials may be employed with general anesthesia with testing done before, during, and after the turn [83, 84]. The use of a collar provides significant benefit in limiting spine motion that is observed in the axial rotation [85]. It is important to keep the head and spine in a neutral position during the positioning. Once the prone position has been attained, access to the head and endotracheal tube is restricted. Use of a flexible armored endotracheal tube is advocated to avoid the risk of tube kinking [3].

"When the continuity of the cervical spine is at risk, whether the patient is awake or asleep, it is prudent and customary to have the responsible surgeon (1) maintain the stable alignment of the head with the body during the turn, (2) position the pronated head to his or her satisfaction, and (3) personally assure that intact neurologic function has been retained once the patient is situated or that the position is optimized if neurologic function cannot be assessed" [82].

Spinal Procedures

There is a long list of spinal procedures performed in the prone position from simple lumbar discectomy to complex spinal fusions. Patients presenting for surgery of the spine may manifest peripheral neuropathy, paraplegia, or spine instability, each with its attendant complications and anesthetic considerations.

Patients with rheumatoid arthritis, cervical myelopathy, or spinal cord injury are at an increased risk for further neurologic injury if a controlled airway management approach by an experienced anesthesiologist is not performed. If an awake intubation is preferred, it should be discussed with the patient. It should always be brought to the patient's attention that the potential for further neurologic injury exists.

Difficult laryngoscopy has been reported as high as 20% in patients with cervical spinal disease [12]. Patients with occipito-atlanto-axial complex disease have a higher incidence of difficulty than those with subaxial (C3–C7) disease [86]. Patients with symptomatic spinal stenosis (cervical myelopathy) may benefit from an awake fiberoptic intubation or induction with the head stabilized and intubation performed under fiberoptic guidance with use of spinal cord monitoring [3]. For most other patients scheduled for cervical spine surgery, who have a reasonable range of motion, difficulty with intubation is no higher than with other types of surgery.

Unless pre-existing comorbidities argue otherwise, additional anesthesia monitoring for most posterior spinal discectomies is not indicated. Complex spinal procedures involving blood loss and prolonged time require additional monitoring to include an arterial line, urinary catheter, and additional line access as indicated.

An acute spinal cord injury that disrupts sympathetic outflow and may result in unopposed vagal stimulation and myocardial depression will require the standard monitors plus a urinary catheter, arterial catheter, and placement of external pacemaker pads. Some advocate for placement of a pulmonary artery catheter [3]. When using transesophageal echo in acute spinal cord injury patients, we must consider the potential difficulty in placing the probe with the cervical spine immobilized, the theoretical possibility of cervical movement when the probe is placed and moved to obtain views and the potential for an associated esophageal injury in trauma patients with a high spinal cord injury [3].

Patients being positioned prone for neurosurgical spinal procedures should have the following items in agreement between the anesthesia provider, the patient, and the neurosurgeon: (1) The correct side—the patient and their physical findings are specific for that side, (2) The stability of the neck and the integrity of the spinal cord are consistent with laryngoscopic endotracheal intubation, and (3) The patient demonstrates neck movement consistent with intubation without symptomatology.

Induction of anesthesia for spinal procedures in the prone position shares the same issues as any other general anesthetic. Induction must consider the choice of airway management and any electrophysiologic monitoring consideration. Muscle relaxation must be used with consideration of possible hyperkalemic response in the case of succinylcholine.

After the airway is obtained, securing the endotracheal tube will depend on how the head is held. If using skull pins, we use a bridle to secure the tube. A plastic tube is passed via one nare and pulled from the throat. The tube is then taped to the ends of the plastic thus securing the tube to the maxilla. If simple head holding pillows are used, taping is sufficient. A bite block must be inserted that is large enough to protect the tongue and substantial enough to withstand repeated biting from motor-evoked potentials. Tongue bite injuries can occur even with a bite block in place [87]. There is no consensus on the type and number of bite blocks to prevent this problem. The basic principles of head positioning include avoidance of hyperextension, hyperflexion, and extreme rotation of the cervical spine. For posterior procedures in the cervical spine, the position of the head is managed by the surgeon. For posterior approaches to the middle to lower thoracic, lumbar, or sacral spine, the head is typically placed on a soft foam or gel pad with preconfigured cutouts or a horseshoe headrest that allows midline orientation of the face and head. The eyes should be protected with no source of external compression. The nose should be free from surfaces.

Maintenance of anesthesia for spinal procedures in the prone position should be based on the patient's underlying medical condition, the anticipated intraoperative conditions, and the preference of the individual anesthesia provider. An awareness of the various anesthetic effects on neurophysiologic monitoring is essential and the anesthesia consistent with the requirements of the monitoring employed. A stable operative anesthetic depth is essential for accurate monitoring [3].

If an intraoperative wake-up test is required, either a total intravenous anesthetic or a balanced technique consisting of low doses of a volatile agent together with opioids is effective [88]. It should be noted and included in patient interview that there is an associated 25% incidence of intraoperative awareness and recall of the awakening event. The recall is not regarded as unpleasant in most instances [89].

Emergence and extubation are in accordance with the level of severity and length of the surgery, pre-existing comorbidities, and experience of the anesthesiologist. All posterior cervical procedures deserve special consideration as fusion procedures may make the patient, who has no problem to intubate preoperatively, difficult after the fusion. Prone position procedures done in association with anterior cervical or transoral procedures will result in edema in the neck or posterior pharynx that will preclude immediate extubation.

Cranial Procedures

The prone position is commonly used for approaches to the posterior fossa, pineal and suboccipital regions, and posterior parietal and occipital regions.

Monitoring for these procedures includes invasive arterial pressure monitoring, a urinary catheter, and additional line access as indicated. Electrophysiologic monitoring may be indicated according to the procedure planned.

Induction of anesthesia must be cognizant of the monitoring requirements, the pre-existing comorbidities of the patient, and the specific needs of the patient. A total intravenous anesthetic technique or a balanced anesthesia technique incorporating both an inhalation agent with an opioid are discussed in the literature. Patients being positioned prone for neurosurgical cranial procedures should have the following items in agreement between the anesthesia provider, the patient, and the neurosurgeon: (1) The correct side—the patient and their physical findings are specific for that side, (2) the stability of the neck and the integrity of the spinal cord are consistent with laryngoscopic endotracheal intubation, and (3) the patient demonstrates neck movement consistent with intubation without symptomatology.

Intubation is accomplished using a flexible armored endotracheal tube using the bridle technique previously noted. A bite block of rolled gauze substantial enough to withstand spasmodic biting induced by evoked monitoring (if employed) and broad enough to maintain the tongue in the mouth is secured.

After induction and intubation, an esophageal stethoscope and nasopharyngeal temperature probe are placed. A central venous catheter is then placed. The prone position is associated with a lower incidence of venous air embolism, [90, 91] but the risk is not eliminated. Thus, if the surgical opening is planned to be over the torcula or a major venous sinus, we additionally double-stick the internal jugular vein and place a multi-orifice air aspiration catheter using the intravascular electrocardiography with the P wave large and negative and no positive component. If unclear, a chest X-ray is made. External pacemaker pads are applied to the chest. Additional anesthesia is given when skull pins are applied.

The patient is turned prone and positioned (see Fig. 3.7). If placed in flexed position, be cognizant of the possibility of macroglossia postoperatively. The head should be placed in such a manner that the shoulders are at or above the edge of the operating table. This will prevent the face from becoming compressed against the cephalad edge of the operating table when elevated [26]. After turning and positioning, the right atrial line should be checked again for placement and a precordial Doppler placed. Unless dictated otherwise by electrophysiologic monitoring requirements, anesthesia is maintained with controlled positive-pressure ventilation with muscle relaxation. TIVA may be employed if preferred or required by monitoring.

Emergence is aimed at preventing abrupt rises in blood pressure. To this end, we start all our posterior fossa cases on nicardipine and titrate accordingly. Rapid awakening with reversal of muscle relaxation and minimal coughing on the endotracheal tube are all goals. Extubation is dependent on the extent and nature of the brainstem manipulation and/or cranial nerve involvement [92, 93]. Agreement between surgeon and anesthesiologist is recommended.

a b

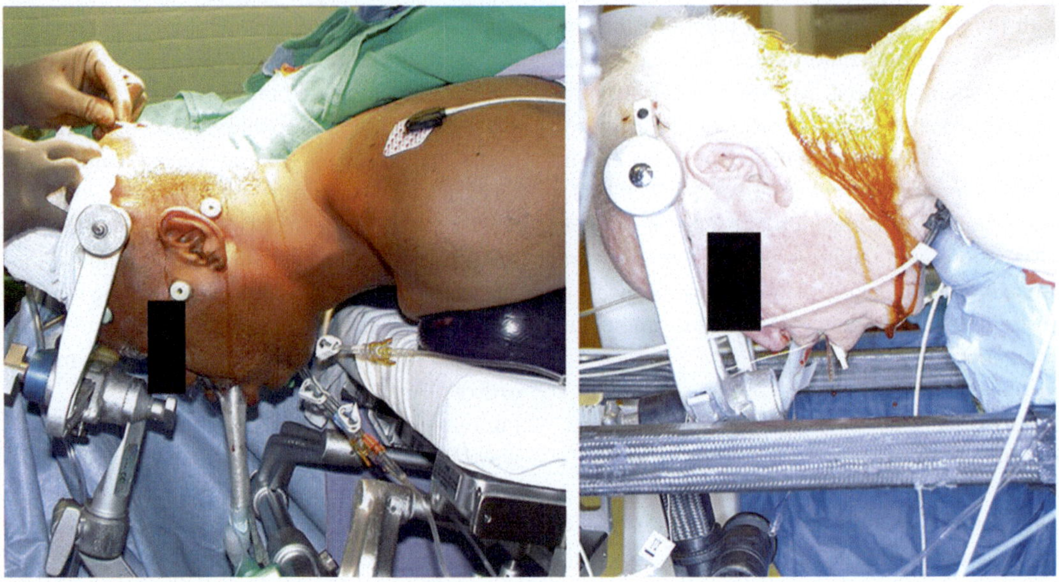

Fig. 3.7 Note the distance between the chin and the edge of the table

Complications of the Prone Position

Dropping the patient during the turn can happen as a result of an uncoordinated or unskilled team of turners, too few team members to accommodate the weight of the patient, or unexpected separation of the operating table and transport cart just as the patient is in the lateral phase of the turn and not well supported by the table or the bed [82].

Loss of airway, vascular access lines, catheters, and monitors can and does happen.

The prone position can result in injuries to the central nervous system. These can be classified according to the underlying mechanism—arterial occlusion, venous occlusion, air entrainment, cervical spine injury, or the effect of undiagnosed neoplasms. Failure to avoid excessive neck movement and allowing normal blood flow in the carotid and vertebral arteries can lead to carotid dissection and infarction [94]. A stroke has been reported in a patient after prone spine surgery with the head turned and unrecognized carotid stenosis [95].

Occlusion of the vertebral arteries has been reported in at least four cases. In one the patient developed a lateral medullary syndrome immediately after surgery [96]. A sudden quadriplegia developed a few hours after surgery in the knee-chest position with the head rotated. The MRI screening showed infarcts in the upper cervical cord and at watershed areas between anterior and posterior cerebral circulations. The authors propose that temporary occlusion of the vertebral artery led to stasis, thrombosis, and embolism [97]. A single report with a similar mechanism occurred during scoliosis repair [98]. Another prone surgery patient with the head rotated developed vertebral artery dissection and cerebellar infarct [99].

Four patients after cervical laminectomy in the prone position supported by chest rolls developed neurological deficits immediately after the operation. Two developed hemiparesis, one developed quadraparesis, and one paraparesis [100]. The authors proposed that the use of chest rolls caused a degree of increased venous pressure combined with mild arterial hypotension leading to decreased perfusion pressure in the spinal cord and ischemia [80]. A similar mechanism may explain a quadriplegia which occurred after thoracolumbar decompression, [101] and two reports of thoracic level paraplegia after lumbar spine surgery [102]. Two reports of injury involving venous occlusion occurred in the context of abnormal venous anatomy [80].

Bilateral jugular venous infarcts developed in the cerebellum of an achondroplastic dwarf thought the result of stenosis of the jugular foramen (a recognized feature of achondroplasia). The patient had 9 h of surgery head down on a Wilson Frame [103]. A patient with an occipital meningioma which had obliterated the superior sagittal sinus, such that the venous drainage from the cerebral hemispheres occurred through the anterior emissary veins into the scalp. When turned, prone onto the horseshoe headrest, these veins were compressed leading to venous stasis and rupture into the frontal extradural space [104].

Introduction of air into the cranial cavity is common after neurosurgical procedures and occurs in all positions [80]. In spite of the frequency, only two reported cases of tension pneumocephalus have been observed in prone position cases [105, 106]. A single case of pneumorrhachis (air in the spinal canal) after posterior fossa exploration [107].

There have been a large number of case reports of venous air embolism [80]. There are four reported cases of fat embolism in patients undergoing spine procedures in the prone position [80].

Excessive neck flexion in a patient for an 8.5-h operation in prone position with the neck flexed and chin approximately one finger-breadth from the sternum resulted in complete and permanent C5/6 sensory and motor deficit level [108]. A patient having lumbar spinal surgery awoke with a T6 sensory level as a result of a prolapsed disc at C6/7 [109].

Space-occupying lesions within the spinal canal or cranium can become symptomatic as a result of the prone position [80]. Although the mechanism involved was uncertain, spinal arachnoid cysts, [110] spinal metastases, [111] and frontal lobe tumors [112] have become symptomatic following surgery in prone position. Bradycardia and fatal neurogenic edema occurred when an undiagnosed neurofibroma in the posterior fossa fell anteriorly in a patient turned prone, thus compressing the medulla and pons [113].

Four cases of brachial nerve damage have been reported which occurred after prone positioning [114–117]. An isolated axillary nerve injury occurred following lumbar spine surgery [118]. Musculocutaneous [119] and radial nerve injury [120, 121] have also been reported. Damage to the lateral cutaneous nerve of the thigh is a commonly recognized complication of the prone position [80, 120]. A patient thought to have incurred inadvertent jaw retraction in the prone position reported damage to the lingual and buccal nerves [122].

Supra orbital nerve injuries have been reported in three patients [123, 124]. Phrenic nerve [125] and recurrent laryngeal nerve injury [126] has been reported with overextension or rotation of the neck while prone. One case series describes injury to the dorsal nerves of the penis in two patients prone on a fracture table [84, 127].

Direct pressure in the prone position is a common cause of anesthesia-related injury. The affected skin areas include the malar regions, iliac crests, chin, eyelids, nose, and tongue [128–135].

Placement of the head in a PronePositioner™ has been reported to cause contact dermatitis [136].

There have been four reported cases of tracheal compression during prone position cases [137–140]. All were associated with thoracic scoliosis and the proposed mechanism involved a reduced anterior-posterior diameter of the chest [80]. In three of the patients, an underlying connective tissue defect was found, either Marfan syndrome [138, 139] or tracheomalacia [140].

Salivary gland swelling has been reported after surgery in the prone position with the head rotated [141].

Anterior dislocation of the shoulder has been reported [142]. In this case it was only noticed because it led to compression of the axillary artery and loss of the pressure trace in the radial arterial line [80]. Shoulder pain has been reported in a larger series of patients [143].

There have been reports of macroglossia in prone position patients [144–146]. One developed massive swelling of the tongue, soft palate, lateral pharynx, and arytenoids after a craniotomy

[144]. One case for a posterior cervical decompression had swelling of the tongue and oropharynx after surgery requiring emergency tracheostomy [145].

Two case reports describe severe hypotension resulting from compression of the right ventricle against an abnormal sternum [147, 148].

A case has been reported of aorto-coronary vein graft compression and occlusion from prone position [149]. Another case reports transient obstruction of a Rastelli conduit during scoliosis surgery [150].

Hepatic ischemia, with progressive metabolic acidosis and elevated enzymes, has been described after prolonged prone surgery [151, 152]. Pancreatitis is a recognized complication of scoliosis surgery [80].

Three patients undergoing decompressive spinal surgery in the prone position using a hypotensive anesthetic technique demonstrated avascular necrosis of the femoral head [153].

Compartment syndrome has been reported in multiple patients after spinal surgery in some variation of the prone position involving flexion of the hips and the knees [154–159]. Rhabdomyolysis has been reported in the absence of compartment syndrome in prone-positioned patients. These have involved prolonged spinal surgery with flexion of hips and knees [159–161].

With regard to postoperative visual loss (POVL) after non-ocular surgery, spinal surgery performed prone may be associated with ophthalmic injury. Ophthalmic complications have been reported to occur in less than 0.2% of spine surgeries [162–166].

The two injuries most frequently described are ischemic optic neuropathy [167, 168] and central retinal artery occlusion [169, 170]. Other complications appearing in the prone patient include multiple reports of transient and permanent ophthalmoplegia [123, 124, 170–172]. Cavernous sinus thrombosis, [173] central retinal vein occlusion, [166] unexpected presentation of an orbital hemangioma, [174] painful orbital compartment syndrome, [175] bilateral angle closure glaucoma, [176] non-traumatic subperiosteal orbital hemorrhage, [177] amaurosis, [178] dislocated intraocular lens, [179] and fixed mydriasis [180] have all been associated with prone position spinal cases.

Prone position studies demonstrate a relationship between operation time and position complications. Only three prone position studies reported complications following procedures of less than 120 min, seven studies reported complications following mean operative times of 121–240 min, and nine additional studies reported complications following mean operative times greater than 240 min [181].

Dr. G. Edge in evaluating the Third Edition of Martin and Warner's *Positioning in Anesthesia and Surgery* made the following comments:

> "Patient positioning is a subject of prime concern to the anaesthetist and surgeon; it is also occasionally a cause of conflict between the anaesthetist attempting to maintain parameters within physiological limits while the surgeon attempts to push anatomical considerations to their limits in an attempt to achieve optimum access to the surgical target. Indeed, the preface to this the third, edition of this book notes that in the earlier editions the presentation of major topics by surgical and anaesthetic authors deliberately resulted in varied opinions—a factor overcome in this current edition by excluding the surgeons. However, this simple recipe for operating room harmony cannot be applied to the operating theatre where, frequently, the anaesthetist's role is to accept the patient position decreed by the surgeon then institute a damage limitation exercise" [182].

A deliberate effort has been made throughout this chapter to emphasize the word "agreement." Often, because of the infrequency of some procedures and some positions, anesthesia providers will be unfamiliar with conducting an anesthetic in a given position. It is incumbent on the part of the anesthesia providers to make their concerns known to the neurosurgeon. The neurosurgeon then has the option to modify the intended approach, request another anesthesia provider, or cancel the case. The neurosurgeon must believe that the pathology and the pre-existing morbidities of the patient make the position selected is the best choice for that patient. The anesthesia provider must believe that they can conduct a safe anesthetic that delivers optimum operating and monitoring conditions while being fully aware of and prepared for complications associated with the position, the procedure, and the interaction between the two. The neurosurgeon and the anesthesiologist must be in agreement.

References

1. Martin JT. General principles of safe positioning. In: Martin JT, Warner MA, editors. Positioning in anesthesia and surgery. 3rd ed. Philadelphia: W. B. Saunders; 1997. p. 5.
2. Cheney FW, Domino KB, Caplan RA, Posner KL. Nerve injury associated with anesthesia: a closed claims analysis. Anesthesiology. 1990;90(4):1062–9.
3. Stier G, Gabriel CL, Cole DJ. Neurosurgical diseases and trauma of the spine and spinal cord: anesthetic considerations. In: Cottrell J, William Y, editors. Cottrell and Yung's neuroanesthesia. 5th ed. Philadelphia: Mosby Elsevier; 2010. p. 343–89.
4. Apfelbaum J, Hagberg C, Caplan R, Blitt CD, Connis RT, Nickinovich DG, et al. Practice guidelines for management of the difficult airway: an updated report by the American Society of Anesthesiologists Task Force on Management of the Difficult Airway. Anesthesiology. 2013;118:251–70.
5. Supine WM. Positions. In: Martin J, Warner M, editors. Positioning in anesthesia and surgery. 3rd ed. Philadelphia: W. B. Saunders; 1997. p. 39.
6. Brown EM, Elman DS. Postoperative backache. Anesth Analg. 1961;40:683–5.
7. Wiles JC. Postoperative (pressure) alopecia. J Am Acad Dermatol. 1985;12:195–8.
8. Courington F, Little DM Jr. The role of posture in anesthesia. Clin Anesth. 1968;3:24–54.
9. Abel R, Lewis G. Postoperative alopecia. Arch Dermatol. 1960;81:34–42.
10. Patel K, Henschel E. Postoperative alopecia. Anesth Analg. 1980;59:311–3.
11. American Society of Anesthesiologists. Task force on the prevention of perioperative. Peripheral neuropathies: practice advisory for the prevention of perioperative peripheral neuropathies. Anesthesiology. 2000;92:1168–82.
12. Porter J, Pidgeon C, Cunningham A. The sitting position in neurosurgery: a critical appraisal. Br J Anesth. 1999;82:117–28.
13. Slbin MS, Babinske M, Maroon JC, Jannetta P. Anaesthetic management of posterior fossa surgery in the sitting position. Acta Anaesthesiol Scand. 1976;20:117–28.
14. Black S, Cucchiara R. Tumor surgery. In: Cucchiara R, Michenfelder J, editors. Clinical neuroanaesthesia. Edinburg: Churchill Livingstone; 1990. p. 285–308.
15. Gale T, Leslie K. Anaesthesia for neurosurgery in the sitting position. J Clin Neurosci. 2004;11:693–6.
16. Ganslandt O, Merkel A, Schmitt H, Tzabazis A. The sitting position in neurosurgery: indications, complications and results. A single institution experience of 600 cases. Acta Neurochir (Wein). 2013;155(10):1887–93.
17. Hooper A, Okum M, Foote K, Haq IU, Fernandez HH, Hegland D, et al. Venous air embolism in deep brain stimulation. Stereotact Funct Neurosurg. 2009;87(10):1887–93.
18. Standefer M, Bay J, Trusso R. The sitting position in neurosurgery: a retrospective analysis of 488 cases. Neurosurgery. 1984;14(6):649–58.
19. Himes B, Grant W, Arnoley S, Pasternak J. Contemporary analysis of the intraoperative and perioperative complications of neurosurgical procedures performed in the sitting position. J Neurosurg. 2017;127(1):182–8.
20. Sandwell S, Kimmell K, Silberstein H, Rodenhouse T, Maurer PK, Pilcher WH, et al. Safety of the sitting cervical position for elective spine surgery. Neurosurgery. 2016;63(CN_suppl_1):203.
21. Gildenberg P, O'Brien P, Brett W, Frost E. The efficach of Doppler monitoring for the detection of venous air embolism. J Neurosurg. 1981;54(1):75–8.
22. Michenfelder J. Complications during neurosurgery. Anesthesia and the neuromuscular system II. Anesthesiology. 1974;16:17.
23. Silverman R. Positioning for neurosurgery. In: Ruskin K, Rosenbaum S, Rampil I, editors. Fundamentals of neuroanesthesia: a physiologic approach to clinical practice. New York: Oxford University Press; 2014. p. 279.
24. Grady M, Bedford R, Park T. Changes in superior sagittal sinus pressure in children with head elevation, jugular venous compression and PEEP. J Neurosurg. 1986;65(2):199–202.
25. Toung TJ, Miyabe M, McShane AJ, Rogers MC, Traystman RJ. Effect of PEEP and jugular venous compression on canine cerebral blood flow and oxygen consumption in the head elevated position. Anesthesiology. 1988;68(1):53–8.
26. Smith D. Anesthetic management for posterior fossa surgery. In: Cottrell J, Young W, editors. Cottrell and Young's neuroanesthesia. 5th ed. Philadelphia: Mosby Elsevier; 2010. p. 204–17.
27. Rozet I, Vavilala M. Risks and benefits of patient positioning during neurosurgical care. Anesthesiol Clin. 2007;25(3):631.
28. Martin T. Neuroanesthetic adjuncts for surgery in the sitting posiiton: III. Intravascular electrocardiography. Anesth Analg. 1970;49:588.
29. Mongan P, Peterson R. Pressure monitoring can accurately position catheters for air embolism aspiration. J Clin Monit. 1992;8(2):121–5.
30. Cucchiara R, Bowers B. Air embolism in children undergoingsuboccipitalcraniotomy. Anesthesiology. 1982;57(4):338–9.
31. Bunegin L, Albin M, Hesel P, Hoffman A, Hung TK. Positioning the right atrial catheter. A model for re-appraisal. Anesthesiology. 1981;55(4):343–8.

32. Cucchiara R, Seward J, Nishimura R, Nugent M, Faust R. Identification of patent foramen ovale during sitting position craniotomy by transesophageal echocardiography with positive airway pressure. Anesthesiology. 1985;63(1):107–9.
33. Cucchiara R, Nugent M, Steward J, Messick JM. Air embolism in upright neurosurgical ptients: detection and localisation by two-dimensional transesophageal echocardiography. Anesthesiology. 1984;60(4):353–5.
34. Marshall B. Air embolism in neurosurgical anesthesia; its diagnosis and treatment. Can Anaesth Soc J. 1965;12:255–61.
35. Adornato D, Gildenberg P, Ferrario C, Ferrario CM, Smart J, Frost EA. Pathophysiology of intravenous air embolism in dogs. Anesthesiology. 1978;49(2):120–7.
36. Michenfelder J, Martin J, Altenburg B, Rehder K. Air embolism during neurosurgery: an evaluation of right atrial catheters for diagnosis and treatment. JAMA. 1969;208(8):1353–8.
37. Alvaran S, Toung J, Graff T, Benson DW. Venous air embolism: comparative merits of external cardiac massage, intracardiac aspiration, and left lateral decubitus position. Anesth Analg. 1978;57(2):166–70.
38. Colley P, Artu A. Bunegin-Albin catheter improves air retrival and resuscitation from lethal venous air embolism in upright dogs. Anesth Analg. 1969;68(3):298–301.
39. Ericsson J, Gottlieb J, Sweet R. Closed-chest cardiac massage in the treatment of venous air embolism. N Engl J Med. 1964;270:1353–4.
40. Milde L. The head-elevated positions. In: Martin J, Warner M, editors. Positioning in anesthesia and surgery. W. B. Saunders: Philadelphia; 1997. p. 82.
41. Albin M. Air embolism. Anesth Clin N Am. 1993;11:1–24.
42. Albin M, Babinski M, Maroon J, Jannetta P. Anaesthetic management of posterior fossa surgery in the sitting position. Acta Anaesthesiol Scand. 1976;20((2)):117–28.
43. Voorhies R, Fraser A, Van P. Prevention of air embolism with positive expiratory pressure. Neurosurgery. 1983;12(5):503–6.
44. Papadopoulos G, Kuhly P, Brock M, Rudolph KH, Link J, Eyrich K. Venous and paradoxical air embolism in the sitting position. A prospective study. Acta Neurochir. 1994;126(2-4):140–3.
45. Hagan P, Scholz D, Edwards W. Incidence and size of patent foramen ovale during the first 10 decades of life: an autopsy study of 965 normal hearts. Mayo Clin Proc. 1984;59(1):17–20.
46. Kitahata L, Katz J. Tension pneumocephalus after posterior-fossa craniotomy, a complication of the sitting position. Anesthesiology. 1976;44(5):448–50.
47. Toung T, Donham R, Lehner A, Alano J, Campbell J. Tension pneumocephalus after posterior fossa craniotomy: a report of four additional cases and a review of postoperative pneumocephalus. Neurosurgery. 1983;12(2):164–8.
48. Hitlelberger W, House W. A warning regarding the sitting position for acoustic tumour surgery. Arch Otolaryngol. 1980;106(2):69.
49. Wilder B. Hypothesis: the etiology of mid-cervical quadriplegia after operration with the patient in the sitting position. Neurosurgery. 1982;11(4):530–1.
50. Matjasko J, Petrozza P, Cohen M, Steinberg P. Anaesthesia and surgery in the seated position: analysis of 554 cases. Neurosurgery. 1985;17(5):695–702.
51. Dorland W. Illustrated medical dictionary. Philadelphia: W. B. Saunders; 1981.
52. Lawson N, Meyer D. Lateral positions. In: Martin J, Warner M, editors. Positioning in anesthesia and surgery. 3rd ed. Philadelphia: W. B. Saunders; 1997. p. 140.
53. WNE G Jr, DeGroot W, Tanner C, Leonard J. Hemodynamic changes associated with various surgical positions. JAMA. 1963;185:1–5.
54. Conrady P, Goodman L, Lainge F, Singer M. Alteration of endotracheal tube position: flexion and extension of the neck. Crit Care Med. 1976;4(1):8–12.
55. McCormick PC. The retropleural approach to the ventral thoracic and thoracolumbar spine. In: Benzel EC, editor. Spine surgery, techniques, complication avoidance and management. Philadelphia: Churchill Livingstone; 1999. p. 293.
56. Fourney D, Agi-Said D, Rains L, Walsh G, Lang FF, McCutcheon IE, et al. Simultaneous anterior-posterior approach to the thoracic and lumbar spine for the radical resection of tumors followed by reconstructiona and stabilization. J Neurosurg. 2001;94(2 Suppl):232–44.
57. Mahla M, Horlocker T. Vertebral column and spinal cord surgery. In: Cucchiara R, Black S, Michenfelder J, editors. Clinical neuroanesthesia. 2nd ed. New York: Churchill Livingstone; 1998. p. 434.
58. Hagberg C, Welch W, Bowman-Howard M. Anesthesia and surgery for spine and spinal cord procedures. In: Albin M, editor. Textbook of neuroanesthesia with neurosurgical and neuroscience perspectives. New York: McGraw-Hill; 1997. p. 1067.
59. Saito S, Dohi S, Naito H. Alteration of double-lumen endobronchial tube position by flexion and extension of the neck. Anesthesiology. 1985;62(5):696–7.
60. Araki K, Nomura R, Urushibara R, Hatano Y. Displacement of the double-lumen endobronchial tube can be detected by bronchial cuff pressure change. Anesth Analg. 1997;84(6):1349–53.
61. Smith G, Hirsch N, Ehrenwerth J. Placement of double-lumen endobronchial tubes. Correlation between clinical impressions and bronchoscopic findings. Br J Anaesth. 1986;58(11):1317–20.
62. Satho D, Sato M, Kaise A, Hagiwara Y, Saishu T, Hashimoto Y. Effects of isoflurane on oxygenation during one-lung ventilation in pulmonary emphysema patients. Acta Anaesthesiol Scand. 1998;42(10):1145–8.

63. Slinger P, Scott W. Arterial oxygenation during one-lung ventilation: a comparison of enflurand and isoflurane. Anesthesiology. 1995;82:940–6.
64. Reid C, Slinger P, Lenis S. A comparison of the effects of propofol-alfentanil versus isoflurane anesthesia on arterial oxygenation during one-lung ventilation. J Cardiothrac Vasc Anesth. 1996;10(7):860–3.
65. Brodsky J, Shulman M, Swan M, Mark J. Pulse oximetry during one-lung ventilation. Anesthesiology. 1985;63(2):212–4.
66. Wen D, Haines S. Posterior fossa: surgical considerations. In: Cottrell J, Smith D, editors. Anesthesia and neurosurgery. 3rd ed. St. Louis: Mosby; 1994. p. 333.
67. Calliauw L, Rolly G, Rolly G, Verbeke L. The position of the patient during neurosurgical procedures on the posterior fossa. Acta Neurochir. 1987;85(3-4):154–8.
68. Britt B, Gordon R. Peripheral nerve injuries associated with anesthesia. Can Anaesth Soc J. 1964;11:514–36.
69. Smith J, Pellicci P, Sharrock N, Mineo R, Wilson PD Jr. Complications after total hip replacement: the contralateral limb. J Bone Joint Surg Am. 1989;71(4):528–35.
70. Targa L, Droghetti G, Caggese R. Rhabdomyolysis and operating position. Anaesthesia. 1991;46(2): 141–3.
71. Rommel F, Kabler R, Moward J. The crush syndrome: a complication of urological surgery. J Urol. 1986;135(4):809–11.
72. Clarke A, Stillwell S, Paterson M, Getty C. Role of the surgical position in the development of postoperative low back pain. J Spinal Disord. 1993;6(3):238–41.
73. Britt B, Joy J, Mackay M. Positioning trauma. In: Orkin F, Cooperman L, editors. Complications in anesthesiology. Philadelphia: J.B. Lippincott; 1983.
74. Jaffe T, McLesky C. Position induced Horner's syndrome. Anesthesiology. 1982;56(1):49–50.
75. Katayama T, Katou F, Motegi K. Unilateral parotid swelling after general anesthesia. J Craniomaxillofac Surg. 1990;18(5):229–32.
76. Kimura H, Watanabe Y, Mizukoshi K, Yamamoto Y, Araki S. Six cases of anesthesia mumps. Nippon Jibinkoka Gakkai Kaiho. 1993;96(11):1915–21.
77. Cuschieri A. Thorascopic subtotal oesophagectomy. Endo Surg Allied Tech. 1994;2(1):21–5.
78. Gothard J, Branthwaite M. Principles of anesthesia for thoracic surgery. In: Gothard J, Branthwaite M, editors. Anesthesia for thoracic surgery. Oxford: Blackwell Scientific; 1982.
79. Kopoll H, Thompson W. Suprascapular nerve. In: Thompson W, editor. Peripheral entrapment neuropathies. New York: Krieger; 1976.
80. Edgcombe H, Carter K, Yarrow S. Anesthesia in the prone position. Br J Anesth. 2008;100(2):165–83.
81. Eker A. Kneeling position for operations on the lumbar spine. Surgery. 1949;25(1):112.
82. The MJ. Ventral decubitus (prone) positions. In: Martin J, Warner M, editors. Positioning in aesthesia and surgery. 3rd ed. Philadelphia: W. B. Saunders; 1997. p. 172.
83. Lesser R, Raudzens P, Luders H, Nuwer MR, Goldie WD, Morris HH, et al. Postoperative neurologic deficits may occur despite unchanged intraoperative somatosensory evoked potentials. Ann Neurol. 1986;19(1):22–5.
84. Edmonds H, Paloheimo M, Backman M, Johnson JR, Holt RT, Shields CB. Transcranial magnetic motor evoked potentials for functional monitoring of motor pathways during scoliosis surgery. Spine. 1989;14(7):683–6.
85. Diaola M, DiPaola C, Conrad B, Horodyski M, Horodyski M, Del Rossi G, et al. Cervical spine motion in manual versus Jackson table turning methods in a cadaveric global instability model. J Spinal Disord Tech. 2008;21(4):273–80.
86. Calder I, Calder J, Crockard H. Difficult direct laryngoscopy with cervical spine disease. Anaesthesia. 1995;50(9):756–63.
87. Williams A, Singh G. Tongue bite injury after use of transcranial electric stimulation motor-evoked potential monitoring. J Anaesthesiol Clin Pharmacol. 2014;30(3):439–40.
88. Raw D, Beattie J, Hunter J. Anaesthesia for spinal surgery in adults. Br J Anaesth. 2003;91:886–904.
89. Abbott T, Bentley G. Intraoperative awakening during scoliosis surgery. Anaesthesia. 1980;35(3):298–302.
90. Black S, Ockert D, Oliver W, Cucchiara RF. Outcome following posterior fossa craniotomy in patients in the sitting or horizontal positions. Anesthesiology. 1988;69(1):49–56.
91. Albin M, Carroll R, Maroon J. Clinical considerations concerning detection of venous air embolism. Neurosurgery. 1978;3(3):380–4.
92. Artru A, Cucchiara R, Messick J. Cardiorespiratory and cranial nerve sequelae of surgical porcedures involving the posterior fossa. Anesthesiology. 1980;52(1):83–6.
93. Howard R, Mahoney A, Thurlow A. Respiratory obstruction after posterior fossa surgery. Anaesthesia. 1990;45(3):222–4.
94. Gould DB, Cunningham K. Internal carotid artery dissection after remote surgery. Iatrogenic complications of anesthesia. Stroke. 1995;25:1276–8.
95. Wang L, Liou J, Liu FC, Hsu JC, Liu PW. Fatal ischemia stroke in a patient with an asymptomatic carotid artery occlusion after lumbar spine surgery—a case report. Acta Anaesthesiol Taiwanica. 2004;42(3):179–82.
96. Chu Y, Tsai S, Chan K, Kao S, Liang C, Lin S. Lateral medullary syndrome after prone position for general surgery. Anesth Analg. 2002;95:1451–3.
97. Langmayr J, Ortler M, Obwegeser A, Felber S. Quadriplegia after lumbar disc surgery. A case report. Spine. 1996;21:1932–5.

98. Tettenborn B, Caplan L, Sloan M, Estol CJ, Pessin MS, DeWitt LD, et al. Postoperative brainstem and cerebellar infarcts. Neurology. 1993;43:471–7.
99. Shermak M, Shoo B, Deune E. Prone positioning precautions in plastic surgery. Plast Reconstr Surg. 2006;117(5):1584–8.
100. Bhard A, Long D, Ducker T, Toung T. Neurologic deficits after cervical laminectomy in the prone position. J Neurosurg Anesthesiol. 2001;13(4):314–9.
101. Deem S, Shapiro H, Marshall L. Quadriplegia in a patient with cervical spondylosis after thorocolumbar surgery in the prone position. Anesthesiology. 1991;75(3):527–8.
102. Turker R, Slack D, Regan Q. Thoracic paraplegia after lumbar spinal surgery. J Spinal Disord. 1995;8:195–200.
103. Elmaci I, Ain M, Wright M, Lee RR, Sheppard JM, Rigamonti D, et al. Perioperative intracranial hemorrhage in achondroplasia: a case report. J Neurosurg Anesthesiol. 2000;12(3):217–20.
104. Chandra P, Jaiswal A, Mahapatra AK. Bifrontal epidural haematomas following surgery for occipital falcine meningioma: an unusual complication of surgery in the prone position. J Clin Neurosci. 2002;9:582–4.
105. Olympio M, Wo B. Venous air embolism after craniotomy closure: tension pneumocephalus implicated. J Neurosurg Anesthesiol. 1994;6:35–9.
106. Wronski M, Ferber J, Wronski J. Acute tension pneumocephalus as a complication of surgical procedures of the posterior cranial fossa in prone position. Neurol Neurochir Pol. 1987;21:167–70.
107. Prabhakar H, Bithal P, Ghosh IDH. Pneumocchachis presenting as quadriplegia following surgery in the prone position. Br J Anaesth. 2006;97:901–3.
108. Rau C, Liang C, Lui C, Lee T, Lu K. Quadriplegia in a patient who underwent posterior fossa surgery in the prone position. A case report. J Neurosurg. 2002;96:101–3.
109. Chen S, Hui Y, Yu C, Niu C, Niu CC, Lui PW. Paraplegia by acute cervical disc protrusion after lumbar spine surgery. Chang Gung Med J. 2005;28:254–7.
110. Valls P, Naul L, Kanter S. Paraplegia after a routine lumbar laminectomy: report of a rare complication and successful. Neurosurgery. 1990;27:638–40.
111. Kim C, Blank J, McClain B. Transient paraparesis after general anesthesia in a patient in the prone position. Anesthesiology. 1994;81:775–7.
112. Gercek A, Konya D, Babayev R, Ozgen S. Delayed recovery from general anesthesia from intracranial tumor. Anesth Analg. 2007;104:235–6.
113. Van Aken H, Scherer R, Lawin P. A rare intraoperative complication in a child with von Recklinghausen's neurofibromatosis. Anaesthesia. 1982;37:827–9.
114. Winfree C, Kline D. Intraoperative positioning nerve injuries. Surg Neurol. 2005;63:5–18.
115. Schwartz D, Drummond D, Hahn M, Ecker M, Dormans J. Prevention of positional brachial plexopathy during surgical correction of scoliosis. J Spinal Disord. 2000;13(2):178–82.
116. Jackson L, Keats A. Mechanism of brachial plexus palsy following anesthesia. Anesthesiology. 1965;26:190–4.
117. Anderton J, Schady W, Markham D. An unusual cause of postoperatie brachial plexus palsy. Br J Anaesth. 1994;72:605–7.
118. Gwinnutt C. Injury to the axillary nerve. Anaesthesia. 1988;43:529.
119. Abbott K, Nesathurai S. Musculocutaneous nerve palsy following traumatic spinal cord injury. Spinal Cord. 1998;36(8):588–90.
120. Parks B. Postoperative peripheral neuropathies. Surgery. 1973;74(3):348–57.
121. Schmidt C, Lincoln J. Peripheral nerve injuries with anesthesia: a review and report of three cases. Anesth Analg. 1966;45:748–53.
122. Winter R, Munro M. Lingual and buccal nerve neuropathy in a patient in the prone position: a case report. Anesthesiology. 1989;71(3):452–4.
123. Wolfe S, Lospinuso M, Burke S. Unilateral blindness as a complication of patient positioning for spinal surgery. A case report. Spine. 1992;17(5):600–5.
124. Hollenhorst R, Svien H, Benoit C. Unilateral blindness occurring during anesthesia for neurosurgical operations. AMA Arch Opthalmol. 1954;52(6):819–30.
125. Wakeno M, Sakamoto S, Asai T, Hirose T, Shingu K. A case of diaphragmatic paralysis in a patient with diabetes mellitus after surgery in prolonged prone position. Masui. 2001;50(9):1019–21.
126. Ono S, Nishiyama T, Hanaoka K. Harseness after endotracheal intubation caused by submucosal hemorrage of the vocal cord and recurrent nerve palsy. Masui. 2000;49(8):881–3.
127. Hofmann A, Jones R. Pudendal-nerve neuropraxia as a result of traction on the fracture table. A report of four cases. J Bone Joint Surg Am. 1982;64(1):136–8.
128. Anderton J. The prone position for the surgical patient: a historical review of the principles and hazards. Br J Anaesth. 1991;67(4):452–63.
129. Drummond J. Macroglossia, deja vu. Anesth Analg. 1999;89(2):534–5.
130. Jain V, Bithal P, Rath G. Pressure sore on malar prominences by horseshoe headrest in prone position. Anaesth Intensive Care. 2007;35(2):304–5.
131. Moore D, Edmunds L. Prone position frame. Surgery. 1950;27:276–9.
132. Ray C. New kneeling attachment and cushoned face rest for spinal surgery. Neurosurgery. 1987;20(2):266–9.
133. Roth S, Tung A, Ksiazek S. Visual loss in a prone-positioned spine surgery patient with the head on a foam headrest and goggles covering the eyes: an old complication witha new mechanism. Anesth Analg. 2007;104(5):1185–7.
134. Smith R. One solution to the problem of the prone position for surgical procedures. Anesth Analg. 1976;53(2):221–4.
135. Weis K. Threatening necrosis of the tip of the tongue during long-term anaesthesia in the prone position. Der Anaesthetist. 1964;13:241.

136. Jericho B, Skaria G. Contact dermatitis after the use of the PronePositione. Anesth Analg. 2003;97:1381–95.
137. Bagshaw O, Jardine A. Cardiopulmonary complications during anesthesia and surgery for severe lordoscoliosis. Anaesthesia. 1995;50(10):890–2.
138. Kai Y, Yamaoka A, Zaitsu A, Takahashi S. Transient tracheal obstruction during surgical correction of scoliosis in a patient with Marfan's. Masui. 1995;44:868–73.
139. Mesrobian R, Epps J. Midtracheal obstruction after Harrington rod placement in a patient with Marfan's syndrome. Anesth Analg. 1986;65(4):411–3.
140. Rittoo D, Morris P. Tracheal occlusion in the prone position in an intubated patient with Duchenne muscular dystrophy. Anaesthesia. 1995;50(8):719–21.
141. Hans P, Demoitie J, Collignon L, Bex V, Bonhomme V. Acute bilateral submandibular swelling following surgery in prone position. Eur J Anaesthesiol. 2006;23:83–4.
142. Ali A, Breslin D, Hardman H, Martin G. Unusual presentation and complication of the prone position for spinal surgery. J Clin Anesth. 2003;15(6):471–3.
143. Sutterlin C, Rechtine G. Using the Heffington frame in elective lumbar spinal surgery. Orthop Rev. 1988;17:597.
144. Pivalizza E, Katz J, Singh S, Liu W, Liu W, McGraw-Wall B. Massive macroglossia after posterior fossa surgery in the prone position. J Neurosurg Anesthesiol. 1998;10(1):34–6.
145. Sinha A, Agarwal A, Gaur A, Pandey C. Oropharyngeal swelling and macroglossia after cervical spine surgery in the prone position. J Neurosurg Anesthesiol. 2001;13(3):237–9.
146. Tsung Y, Wu C, Hsu C, Yeh C, Lin S, Wong CS. Macroglossia after posterior fossa surgery in the prone position—a case report. Acta Anaesthesiol Taiwanica. 2006;44:43–6.
147. Teoh D, Williams D. Adult Klippel-Feil syndrome: haemodynamic instability in the prone position and postoperative respiratory failure. Anaesth Intensive Care. 2007;35(1):124–7.
148. Alexianu D, Skolnick E, Pinto A, Ohkawa S, Roye DP Jr, Solowiejczyk DE, et al. Severe hypotension in the prone position in a child with neurofibromatosis, scoliosis and pectus excavatum presenting for posterior spinal fusion. Anesth Analg. 2004;98(2):334–5.
149. Weinlander C, Coombs D, Plume S. Myocardial ischemia due to obstruction of an aortocoronary bypass graft by intraoperative positioning. Anesth Analg. 1985;64:933–6.
150. Hiraga Y, Maruoka H, Yamamoto M. Compression of the graft during corrective surgery for scoliosis in a patient who has undergone a Rastelli's operation: a case study. Masui. 1992;41(9):1490–3.
151. Yuen M, Chow B, Irwin M. Severe hypotension and hepatic dysfunction in a patient undergoing scoliosis surgery in the prone position. Anaesth Intensive Care. 2005;33(3):393–9.
152. Ziser A, Friedhoff R, Rose S. Prone position: visceral hypoperfusion and rhabdomyolysis. Anesth Analg. 1996;82(2):412–5.
153. Orpen N, Walker G, Fairlie N, Coghill S, Birch N. Avascular necrosis of the femoral head after surgery for lumbar spinal stenosis. Spine. 2003;28(18):E364–7.
154. Aschoff A, Steiner-Milz H, Steiner H. Lower limb compartment syndrome following lumbar discectomy in the knee-chest position. Neurosurg Rev. 1990;13(2):155–9.
155. Geisler FH, Laich DT, Goldflies M, Shepard A. Anterior tibila compartment syndrome as a positionig complication of the prone-sitting position for lumbar surgery. Neurosurgery. 1993;33:1117.
156. Gordon B, Newman W. Lower nephron syndrome following prolonged knee-chest position. J Bone Joint Surg Am. 1953;35:764–8.
157. Keim HA, Weinstein JD. Acute renal failure—a complication of spine fusion in the tuck positional a case report. J Bone Joint Surg Am. 1970;52:1248–50.
158. Kuperwasser B, Zaid B, Ortega R. Compartment syndrome after spinal surgery and use of the Codman frame. Anesthesiology. 1995;82(3):793.
159. Cruette D, Navarre M, Pinaquy C, Siméon F. Rhabdomyolysis after prolonged knee-chest position. Ann Fr Anesth Reanim. 1986;5:67–9.
160. Foster M. Rhabdomyolysis in lumbar spine surgery: a case report. Spine. 2003;28(1):67–9.
161. Prabhu M, Samra S. An unusual cause of rhabdomyolysis following surgery in the prone position. J Neurosurg Anesthesiol. 2000;12:359–63.
162. Chang S, Miller N. The incidence of vision loss due to perioperative ischemic optic neuropathy associated with spine surgery: the Johns Hopkins Hospital experience. Spine. 2005;30(11):1299–302.
163. Patil C, Lad E, Lad S, Ho C, Boakye M. Visual loss after spine surgery: a population-based study. Spine. 2008;33(13):1491–6.
164. Roth S, Barach P. Postoperative visual loss: still no answers—yet. Anesthesiology. 2001;95:575–7.
165. Shen Y, Drum M, Roth S. The prevalence of perioperative visual loss in the United States: a 10-year study from 1996 to 2005 of spinal, orthopedic, cardiac, and general surgery. Anesth Analg. 2009;109(5):1534–45.
166. Stevens W, Glazer P, Kelley S, Lietman T, Lietman TM, Bradford DS. Opthalmic complications after spinal surgery. Spine. 1997;22(12):1319–24.
167. Ho V, Newman N, Song S, Ksiazek S, Roth S. Ischemic optic neuropathy following spine surgery. J Neurosurg Anesthesiol. 2005;17(1):38–44.
168. Kamming D, Clarke S. Postoperative visual loss following prone spinal surgery. Br J Anaesth. 2005;95:257–60.
169. Grossman W, Ward W. Central retinal artery occlusion after scoliosis surgry with a horshoe headrest. Case report and literature review. Spine. 1983;18(9):1226–8.
170. Halfon M, Bonardo P, Valiensi S, Zaffaroni MC, Pardal MMF, Ayerza DR, et al. Central retinal artery occlusion and opthalmoplegia following spinal surgery. Br J Opthalmol. 2004;88(10):1350–2.

171. Kumar N, Jivan S, Topping N. Blindness and rectus muscle damage following spinal surgery. Am J Opthalmol. 2004;138(5):889–91.
172. West J, Askin G, Clarke VS. Loss of vision in one eye following scoliosis surgery. Br J Opthalmol. 1990;74(4):243–4.
173. Anand S, Mushin A. Cavernous sinus thrombosis following prone position anaesthesia. Eye. 2005;19(7): 803–4.
174. Greenberg R, Tymms A. Alert for perioperative visual loss: an unusual presentation of an orbital haemangioma during spinal surgery. Anaesth Intensive Care. 2003;31(6):679–82.
175. Leibovich I, Casson R, Laforest C, Selva D. Ischemic orbital compartment syndrome as a complication of spinal surgery in the prone position. Opthalmology. 2006;113(1):105–8.
176. Gordon-Bennett P, Ung T, Stephenson C, McClelland HK, Claoué C. Misdiagnosis of angle closure glaucoma. Br Med J. 2006;333:1157.
177. Yang Y, Lee Y, Lai H. Nontraumatic subperiosteal orbital haemorrhage in an anaesthetised patient with surgery in the prone position. Anaesth Intensive Care. 2007;35:1–158.
178. Katzman S, Moschonas C, Dzioba R. Amaurosis secondary to massive blood loss after lumbar spine surgery. Spine. 1994;14(4):468–9.
179. Kiran S, Gombar SCB, Gombar K. Another hazard of the prone position. Anesth Analg. 1997;85:949.
180. Caricato A, Pennisi M, Pappalardo F, Iodice F, Lepore D. Bilateral fixed mydriasis reversible during orthopedic surgery in the prone position. Anesthesiology. 1999;90(6):1777–8.
181. Shriver M, Zeer V, Alentado V, Mroz TE, Benzel EC, Steinmetz MP. Lumbar spine surgery positioning complications: a systematic review. Neurosurg Focus. 2015;39(4):E16.
182. Edge G. Positioning in anesthesia & surgery. Anaesthesia. 1998;53(1):102–3.

Check for updates

Preoperative Assessment of the Patient for the Planned Position

4

C. Wayne Hamm and Jaafar Basma

Introduction

In this chapter, we will adopt the preanesthesia evaluation model described in "A Practice Advisory for Preanesthesia Evaluation," published by the American Society of Anesthesiologists (ASA) in 2012, to address the specific evaluation of neurosurgical patients' ability to assume and sustain the desired position for the planned procedure. ASA Practice Advisories are not intended as standards, guidelines, or absolute requirements, and their use cannot guarantee any specific outcome. They may be adopted, modified, or rejected according to clinical needs and constraints and are not intended to replace local institutional policies [1].

According to this model, a thorough preanesthesia evaluation aimed at evaluation of assumption and sustainability of anticipated neurosurgical position will include all of the following:

1. Describing the process of surgery and anesthesia and developing a rapport with the patient.
2. Review of readily accessible medical records.
3. A patient interview.
4. Preoperative tests when indicated.
5. Other consultations when appropriate.
6. At a minimum, a directed preanesthetic physical examination should include an assessment of the airway, lungs, and heart.

C.W. Hamm (✉)
Medical Anesthesia Group, Germantown, TN, USA

J. Basma
University of Tennessee Health Sciences Center, Memphis, TN, USA

Describing the Process of Surgery and Anesthesia and Developing Rapport with the Patient

Although many of the same general principles for preoperative evaluation apply to neurosurgical patients as to patients undergoing other types of procedures, neurosurgical patients suffer from unique pathologic conditions and are undergoing procedures that require tailored evaluation and monitoring in the perioperative period.

Discuss the anticipated position the patient will assume and maintain with the patient/family. Review the anticipated postoperative issues that may be associated with the position such as possible painful extended extremities, back pain, dependent edema, and pressure points unique to the position assumed. For example, neurosurgical patients to be positioned in the supine position may experience antecubital pain associated with tucked arms. Neck pain associated with sustained head turning may also be encountered. Patients who must lie immobile for prolonged

A. Arthur et al. (eds.), *Perioperative Considerations and Positioning for Neurosurgical Procedures*,
https://doi.org/10.1007/978-3-319-72679-3_4

periods in a supine position often complain of backache [2, 3]. During prolonged procedures, the heels and plantar flexor tendons are especially at risk for developing blisters and ischemic pressure areas [3]. Prolonged compression of the hair follicles may produce hair loss [4]. The alopecia may not occur until several days to weeks after the operation have passed [5–8]. Probably the single most reported neuropraxic complication is ulnar neuropathy [9]. Time spent discussing these issues will go far in establishing rapport and confidence in the patient.

The timing of an initial preanesthesia evaluation is guided by such factors as patient demographics, clinical conditions, type and invasiveness of procedure, and the nature of the healthcare system. For supine patients undergoing an awake craniotomy, early preoperative evaluation is critical. Awake craniotomies require preanesthesia evaluation in order to determine if the patient is a suitable candidate for the procedure. It is essential that the preoperative education for a patient undergoing an awake craniotomy be thorough, frank, and conducted in such a manner that both the patient and the anesthesia provider believe that the anticipated procedure should and can be accomplished in an awake state.

The anesthesia provider directly responsible for the conduct of the awake craniotomy should meet with the patient at a date prior to the surgery. Meeting within a week of surgery allows issues to be fresh in the minds of all parties. The anesthesia provider should assess the suitability of the patient for an awake craniotomy. Only those patients with the ability to clearly understand risks and benefits of the surgery and who, in the opinion of the neurosurgeon and the anesthesia provider, will cooperate during surgery should be considered as candidates for an awake craniotomy.

The preoperative education of the patient should address what the patient should expect from a sensory standpoint. This includes a visual description of the operating room as well as what the patient will see when he emerges under the drapes, whom he will see, and how people in the operating room will be dressed. Pictures, PowerPoint, or video are all helpful in this explanation. The patient should be advised to expect possible offensive odors, particularly where electrocautery will be used. Tastes or flavors encountered with the use of airway devices and medications should also be explained. Touch should focus on how the patient will be positioned and the use of the Mayfield/pinion head holder, the awkward body positioning with the need for minimal movement and the potential for significant discomfort. Special emphasis should be placed on the sounds a patient should expect to hear. Usually, patients are emerging during the removal of the bone flap. The drilling sound is conducted directly to the ear and can be quite loud and disturbing to the patient.

The preoperative education should also address the activities in which the patient will participate during the surgery. What is involved in the mapping of aphasia and anomia should be clearly explained to the patient with attention placed on how the Ojemann stimulation can result in temporary aphasia.

The preoperative education should next focus on how intraoperative issues will be addressed. The patient's seizure history should be thoroughly addressed to assess the presence of "aura," time of day when most seizures occur and medications. The anesthesia provider must have a clear understanding of the type of seizure the patient has historically and its presentation.

The patient should be fully informed of all plans for dealing with seizures encountered during the procedure. The potential for nausea should also be discussed with anticipated plans for dealing with it. The potential for emergent intubation and general anesthesia should the patient become uncooperative and have persistent seizure activity, airway compromise, or hemodynamic instability should also be discussed. The anesthesia provider should ascertain patient wishes with regard to the possible abandonment of the awake technique for a general anesthetic. If the patient and the neurosurgeon maintain that the awake technique is the only way to accomplish the surgical goals, the patient must understand that conditions which dictate airway control and a general anesthetic during the time of the awake phase of the procedure will result in the cancellation of surgery if the surgical situation will permit. All additional questions should be addressed and a written outline of all of the above should be provided to the patient for their further review.

The importance of this preoperative education for both the patient and the anesthesia provider cannot be overemphasized. Arguably, the single most important element in the successful awake craniotomy is the well-motivated, well-informed patient. In our experience, early communication with the patient, describing the process of the surgery and the anesthesia actions provides an opportunity for the patient to consider what he has been told, ask appropriate questions.

For outpatient supine spinal procedures, describing the process of surgery and anesthesia and developing rapport with the patient can easily be accomplished at the time of admission on the day of surgery.

For neurosurgical patients to be positioned prone, possible numbness and tingling in ulnar distribution associated with their arms placed at the head. Facial/tongue edema may be anticipated if prolonged procedure with anticipated major fluid shifts. Red areas may appear around the forehead or chin associated with the use of the head pillow. Red areas appearing at the pressure points of the supporting device in the shoulder, leg, and hip areas should be discussed. Obstruction of the inferior vena cava is a complication of the prone position and is worsened by any degree of increased abdominal pressure. The net result is decreased cardiac output, increased bleeding, venous stasis, and consequent thrombotic complications [10].

Preoperative education for neurosurgical patients to be positioned in the lateral position should include a discussion that numbness and tingling down the arm may occur. The patient may also experience redness or pain associated with the ischial tuberosity on the down side. Facial edema may occur. Anesthesia mumps is a unique clinical entity characterized by acute transient postoperative swelling of the parotid gland may be associated with the lateral position. Neck and shoulder pain may be associated with the maintained position of the head.

Neurosurgical patients to be positioned in the sitting position should be advised that possible cranial nerve dysfunction remote to the surgical site may occur. Facial/tongue edema requiring postoperative ventilation is possible. The need for additional monitoring and placement of catheters for evacuation of venous air aspiration should also be explained.

Content of the Preanesthetic Evaluation Includes but is not Limited to Readily Accessible Medical Records

A review of the patient's past medical records, including any current diagnoses, current medications and therapies, and medical conditions, will often reveal if the anticipated position for the neurosurgical procedure is feasible or not. For example, the presence of a septal defect in the heart would preclude the sitting position.

In patients to be positioned supine, the prior medical history should be evaluated for possible mediastinal mass, severe congestive heart failure/cor pulmonale, or severe chronic obstructive pulmonary disease. Where these conditions are present, assumption and maintenance of the position may not be possible, may not be maintainable for long periods of time, or may demand increased levels of postoperative care.

In patients to be positioned prone, a prior medical history of intrathoracic tumor, pulmonary problems, prior abdominal procedures with stomas, prior placement of vascular access devices, implanted cardiac pacemaker/defibrillator devices and implantable pumps, the presence of ventriculo-peritoneal shunts, arm/shoulder injuries or symptomatology should be vetted. Intrathoracic tumors may move when turned prone and result in occlusion or partial occlusion of bronchi or great vessels.

Patients who have had prior coronary bypass surgery, depending on the revascularization procedure, may have problems with the prone position. A case has been reported of aorto-coronary vein graft compression and occlusion from prone position [11]. Another case reports transient obstruction of a Rastelli conduit during scoliosis surgery [12]. Two case reports describe severe hypotension resulting from compression of the right ventricle against an abnormal sternum [13, 14]. Evaluation of patients with sternal abnormality such as pectus excavatum or carinatum as well as rib fractures or any lack of rib sternum stability should be done before prone position is established in all these at risk patients.

There have been four reported cases of tracheal compression during prone position cases [15–18]. All were associated with thoracic scoliosis and the proposed mechanism involved a reduced anterior-posterior diameter of the chest [10]. In three of the patients, an underlying connective tissue defect was found, either Marfan's syndrome [16, 17] or tracheomalacia [18].

The prone position can result in injuries to the central nervous system. These may be classified according to the underlying mechanism—arterial occlusion, venous occlusion, air entrainment, cervical spine injury, or the effect of undiagnosed neoplasms. Failure to avoid excessive neck movement and allowing normal blood flow in the carotid and vertebral arteries can lead to carotid dissection and infarction [19]. A stroke has been reported in a patient after prone spine surgery with the head turned and unrecognized carotid stenosis [20].

Occlusion of the vertebral arteries associated with the prone position has been reported in at least four cases [21–24].

There have been four reports of patients developing neurological deficits immediately after cervical laminectomy in the prone position supported by chest rolls [25]. In another case where the patient was an achondroplastic dwarf, bilateral venous infarcts developed in the cerebellum following thoraco-lumbar surgery in the prone position, possibly as a result of stenosis of the jugular foramen (a recognized feature of achondroplasia) [26].

Introduction of air into the cranial cavity is common after neurosurgical procedures and occurs in all positions and there have been a large number of reports of venous air embolism associated with the prone position [10]. Only two reported cases of tension pneumocephalus have been observed in prone position cases [27, 28]. A single case of pneumorrhachis (air in the spinal canal) after posterior fossa exploration has been reported in the prone position [10].

Severe restrictive pulmonary disease can require even higher ventilatory pressures in the prone position. Prior creation of abdominal stomas requires thought on how to position so that there is neither obstruction nor pressure on the stoma itself. If placed in a position such that the accessed vascular devices such as Port-a-Cath can rub the patients skin. Erosion of the skin at that site is possible. Placing patients with implanted cardiac devices may require magnet placement. The location and padding of such equipment should be discussed prior to turning patient. The location of implanted pumps should be assessed to assure that the position does not put so much pressure on the skin above the pump that it causes ischemia, or the position occludes the delivery catheter. Place those patients with ventriculo-peritoneal shunts prone in such a manner that the distal catheter is under no compression. Patients with prior arm/shoulder pathology should be assessed for their ability to assume the prone position. If pain is encountered, alternative positioning should be considered. Any preoperative symptomatic extremity issues should be noted. It is important to consider the size of the patient. If they are obese, it may not be possible to obtain descent of the abdomen. Additionally, the size of the patient may exceed the capabilities of the equipment. An increase of intra-abdominal pressure in the prone position of more than 12 mmHg creates a high risk for abdominal compartment syndrome, as visceral compression and intra-abdominal hypertension cause dropped perfusion pressure resulting in multi-organ failure. Patients with previous abdominal surgeries are at particularly high risk as tight abdominal closures can reduce abdominal compliance, increasing abdominal pressure. Previous abdominal surgeries are at risk for incisional hernia, particularly if the patient is obese [2].

Preoperative ophthalmologic evaluation should be considered if the patient has personal or family history of acute angle-closure glaucoma [6]. The prone position test is also recommended to properly identify a patient's risk of developing acute angle-closure glaucoma because of the test's superior sensitivity and specificity. The prone position can shift the lens-iris diaphragm forward, impinging on the drainage angle recess and obstructing the aqueous humor outflow and increased intraocular pressure and optic nerve injury [6]. An 8-mmHg rise in intraocular pressure over 60 min is considered significant [6]. Anatomical factors, including ethnicity (Asians, Canadians, Eskimos), female sex, shorter axial length of eyes, and a thicker, anteriorly located lens, seem to substantially increase the risk of increased intraocular pressure and may contraindicate use of the prone position in some patients [6, 7]. One hour of prone positioning in these high-risk individuals may result in acute angle glaucoma, substantially threatening the patient's vision [6, 7]. Several studies have discussed postoperative vision loss due to prone position. The rate of this complication is estimated to be between 0.05 and 1% [3–5]. The onset of acute angle-closure glaucoma in a patient complaining of persistent unilateral eye pain, nausea, and vomiting is typically 2 days following lumbar fusion surgery [6].

Patients with preexisting tracheostomies need to be evaluated for possible obstruction of the airway. There are currently no guidelines in the medical literature regarding perioperative management of patients with a tracheostomy requiring the prone position for surgery. We usually remove the tracheostomy tube and place an armored endotracheal tube during surgical procedures in the prone position.

In patients who are to assume a lateral position for their neurosurgical procedure a prior medical history of ipsilateral metastatic disease in the chest may result in movement of the thoracic tumor in such a manner to either obstruct or occlude a bronchus or vessel. Pulmonary disease may compromise further ventilation perfusion mismatch associated with the lateral position.

Consider patients who have cochlear implant devices on the down side as needing special padding to avoid compression of the cochlear device with possible ischemia of the skin flap. Necrosis of the down side ear has been reported [8].

The skin over the lower iliac crest is particularly at risk from pressure necrosis in long operations. In emaciated patients placed in the lateral position, the underlying sciatic nerve can be damaged by direct pressure on the buttock at the point where it exits from the pelvis [8]. Lateral position with the good lung down is contraindicated in patients with pulmonary hemorrhage or lung abscesses.

While venous air embolism has been described in association with a wide variety of surgical procedures and positions, it remains the most feared complication of the operative sitting position [9]. Monitoring for this complication includes placement of a right atrial catheter. If a patient has a condition that precludes appropriate monitoring or treatment, all parties should consider whether it is advisable to continue with the sitting position. Patients with any heart defects should have prior cardiac evaluation and approval before any procedure in which they are to assume a sitting position. A history of treated hydrocephalus with a ventriculo-atrial shunt requires consideration that air may be aspirated via a patent VA shunt from the ventricle and deposited directly into the heart. A history of cervical myelopathy requires an evaluation to determine if positioning will cause worsening of the condition. Most authorities consider relative contraindications to the sitting position to include: Patent VA shunt, right atrial pressure in excess of left atrial pressure, patent foramen ovale, platy-orthodeoxia (a condition in which there is a right-to-left shunting of the blood at the atrial level only with assumption of the upright position), and cerebral ischemia when upright and awake [10]. Relative contraindications may also include extremes of age, uncontrolled hypertension, and chronic obstructive pulmonary disease.

Patient Interview

Arguably, the single best preanesthesia evaluation tool for the anesthesiologist assessing the ability of the neurosurgical patient to assume and maintain the requisite position is the patient interview. Two valuable questions are first, "How do you sleep at night and what position do you sleep in?" The second question is "Do you have a position you cannot sleep in, is painful or wakes you up?" Additionally, always make sure that the side and the level of the patient's symptomatology agrees with the history and physical examination and radiographic findings noted in the patient's record and the scheduled surgery. The patient should physically indicate which side is symptomatic. If the patient sleeps in the position required for the surgery, there is probably little to fear from its use. If the patient indicates he cannot assume or maintain the position during their sleep, further investigation into the advisability of that specific position is warranted. Note should be taken of any deficits the patient notes when they wake up such as numb and tingly arms fingers, etc.

Does the patient have any limitations of their movements? Stiff shoulders may make positioning for prone position difficult. Various directional limitations should be noted and considered in the positioning process.

Whether the patient has experienced any vision problems should also be discussed as well as the patient's current medications. Recent use of erectile dysfunction medications in association with prolonged prone position in the presence of large fluid shifts should be discussed with the surgeon.

Lastly, the patient interview, the operation scheduled, and the patient's chart all should agree on the following: (1) the correct side, (2) the patient and their physical findings are specific for that side, (3) the stability of the neck and the integrity of the spinal cord are consistent with laryngoscopic endotracheal intubation, and (4) the patient demonstrates neck movement consistent with intubation without symptomatology. Any disagreement must be resolved prior to proceeding with the anesthetic (Fig. 4.1).

Preoperative Tests When Indicated

Selective preoperative tests (i.e., tests ordered after consideration of specific information obtained from sources such as medical records, patient interview, physical examination, and the type or invasiveness of the planned procedure and anesthesia) may assist the anesthesiologist in making decisions about the process of perioperative assessment and management. Preoperative tests to aid in the preanesthesia evaluation of neurosurgical patients for the ability to assume and maintain the desired position should be requested after consideration of specific information obtained.

Other Consultations When Appropriate

Probably the single most important consultation involves agreement on the correct side and level of the pathology to be addressed. This can be most simply accomplished by asking the patient to demonstrate the side of their body that is producing symptoms. If this is not in agreement with the scheduled procedure, consultation

Fig. 4.1 Results of the patient interview

During the Patient Interview

- The patient must physically indicate which side is symptomatic.
- A simple left or right response is not sufficient
- The side indicated must agree with:
    - The "history and physical" and radiographic findings in the patient's record
    - The scheduled surgery
- The stability of the neck and the integrity of the spinal cord are consistent with laryngoscopic endotracheal intubation
- The patient demonstrates neck movement consistent with intubation without symptomatology

with the neurosurgeon is immediately indicated. Certainly, confusion as to side can be complicated by issues such as central cord syndrome, but all parties must be in agreement as to side and location of pathology prior to initiating anesthesia.

Physical examination findings not noted in history and physical or determination of additional pathology such as cervical spine findings should be discussed with the surgeon along with their possible anesthesia implications.

If patients are found to have ipsilateral metastatic pathology involving the brain and chest, consultation with pulmonary medicine may be indicated.

Basic Elements of a Directed Preanesthetic Physical Examination

A directed preanesthetic physical examination for the ability of a neurosurgical patient to assume and maintain the position required for the specific procedure should include having the patient assume the position prior to the surgery under the vision of the anesthesiologist and have the patient comment on the sustainability of maintaining that position.

Evaluation of the cervical spine is a critical element in the preoperative anesthesia workup of neurosurgical patients. This patient population is particularly predisposed to harbor an accompanying cervical condition, given the relatively high incidence of tandem degenerative disease (e.g., concomitant cervical and lumbar stenosis), poly-traumatism (e.g., intracranial hemorrhages and spinal fractures), metastatic masses (associated intracranial and spinal metastases), and mixed neurological syndromes (e.g., Syrinx and Chiari malformation). If cervical instability or neural element compression are present before surgery, patient positioning and/or intubation maneuvers may cause enough mechanical stressors that can result in worsening postoperative neurological deficits. The anesthesiologist and the neurosurgeon should be sensitive to the clinical signs and symptoms hinting at a cervical pathology that may be worsened by laryngoscopic intubation. Management of the airway in all cases of cervical pathology whether involving instability or not should be agreed between anesthesia and neurosurgery.

The cervical spine assessment is accomplished by moving the head in all planes and noting any discomfort. The head is also flexed, extended, and rotated Fig. 4.2. Any indication of a potential difficult airway is noted. Simple push-pull with the arms and hand grips are assessed. Ability to raise the arms above the head is also noted. Flexion and extension of the feet and movement of the knees are also assessed. The ocular movements are assessed along with tongue movement, swallowing, and speech noted.

Cervical Stability

In considering spinal stability at the cervical level, from both a mechanical and a pathological perspective, two separate regions can be identified. The *upper* cervical spine provides most of the rotatory movements of the neck at the atlanto-axial junction (C1–2). It also majorly contributes to the cervical flexion/extension at the occipito-cervical joint. The *lower* or subaxial cervical spine (C3–7) is responsible for flexion/extension as well, mostly between C5 and C7 where the highest incidence of degenerative disease is encountered. Orotracheal intubation produces movement in the cervical spine. During orotracheal intubation, the least movement was obtained by the use of in-line stabilization by an assistant [11].

Ligaments mainly maintain stability of the upper cervical spine, especially at the *atlanto-occipital* joint (Fig. 4.3). Most important of these are the tectorial membrane and alar ligaments. While the alar ligaments connect the dens of C2 to the occipital condyles, the tectorial membrane is considered to be a rostral continuation of the posterior longitudinal ligament, which spans the ventral wall of the foramen magnum and the posterior aspect of the dens and C2–3 vertebral bodies. Counterintuitively, the ligaments connecting the atlas to the occiput (anterior atlanto-occipital membrane, which is the extension of the anterior longitudinal ligament, and posterior atlanto-

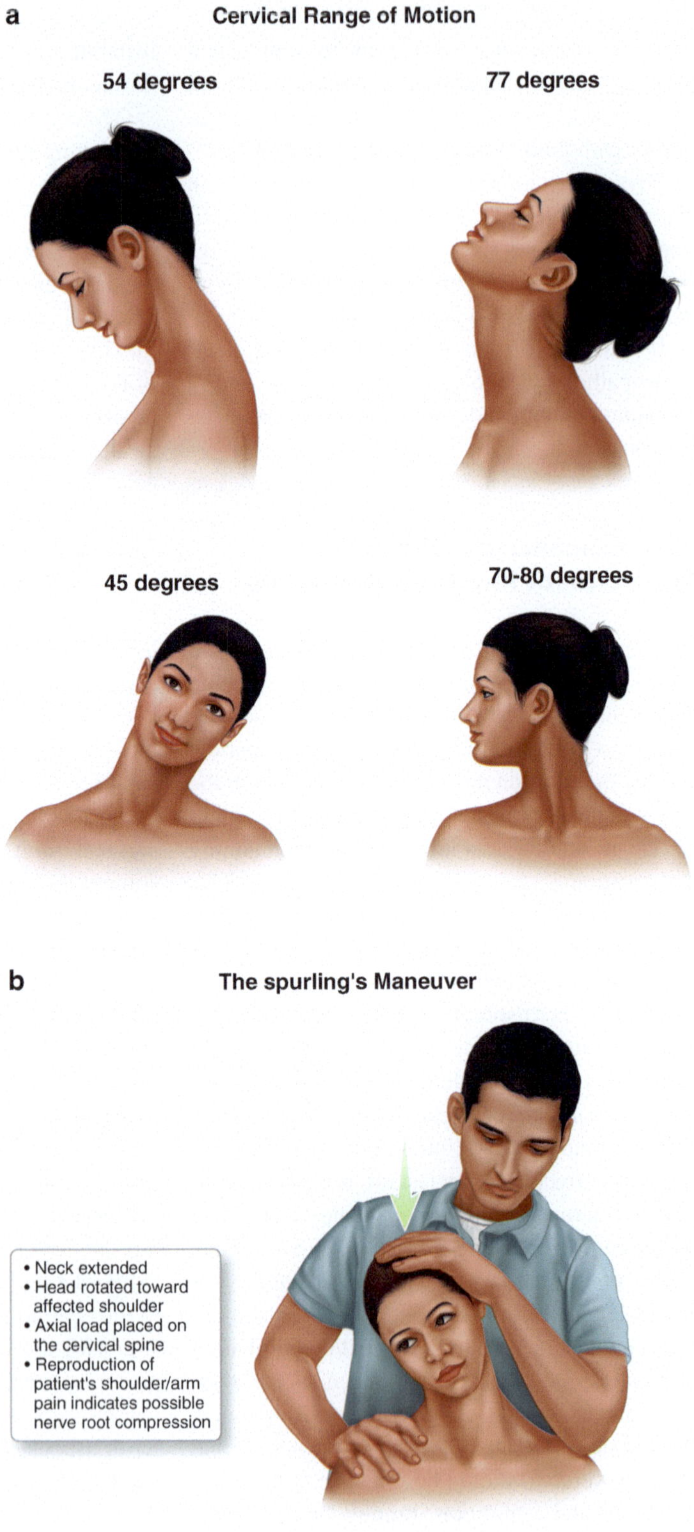

Fig. 4.2 Radicular symptoms are frequently dynamic and it is prudent, whenever there is no contraindication otherwise, to evaluate them with the cervical range of motion (**a**) and with the Spurling maneuver (**b**)

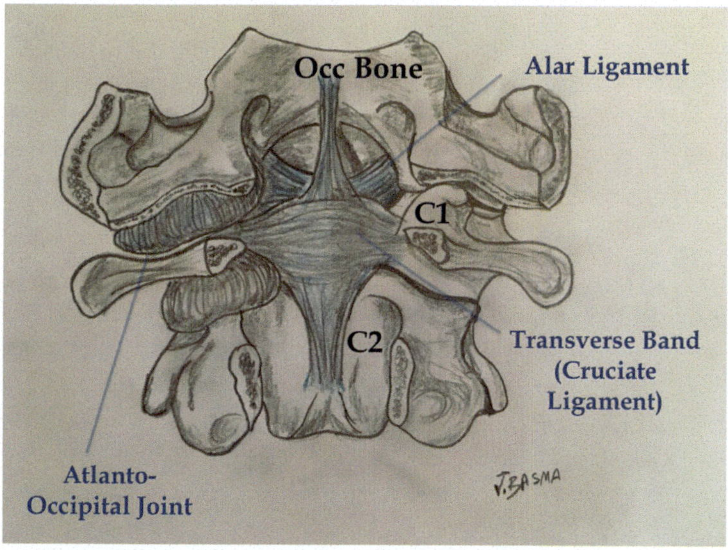

Fig. 4.3 Dorsal internal view of the occipito-cervical region showing the alar and cruciate ligaments. The transverse ligament is the horizontal segment of the cruciate ligament. It locks the odontoid process of the axis posteriorly. The tectorial membrane (not shown) drapes over these structures as a continuation of the posterior longitudinal ligament. The atlanto-occipital joint is between the occipital condyle and the articular surface of the atlas. C1: Atlas, C2: Axis, Occ Bone: Occipital Bone

occipital membrane) play a less crucial role in atlanto-axial stability [12]. In adults, the basion-dental interval should be less than 8.5 mm on CT or less than 12 mm on X-rays and the atlanto-occipital interval (AOI) less than 1.4–2 mm. Otherwise, an atlanto-occipital dislocation should be suspected [13]. Attention should be made however in the neurosurgical population to the occipital condyle and joints, noticeably in those undergoing current or previous skull base or upper cervical surgeries requiring a trans-condylar approach. It is believed that one half to two thirds of the occipital condyle can be drilled without disturbing stability [14].

At the *atlanto-axial* joint, the interlocking structure of the dens against C1 and the foramen magnum prevents hyper-flexion injuries (Fig. 4.3). This configuration is held in place posteriorly by the strong transverse ligament (TAL, or transverse component of the cruciate ligament) [12]. For instance, integrity of the TAL is the most important factor to consider in atlanto-axial subluxation or in C1 fractures. It can be directly assessed on cervical magnetic resonance imaging, or using the atlanto-dental interval (>3 mm in adults is abnormal) and the rule of Spence on plain radiographs or CT scans [15]. A fracture through the neck of the dens of C2 usually confers more instability and risk of non-union than the other odontoid fractures. Integrity of the disc space between C2–3 is also important to consider in the stability of C2 fractures (e.g., Hangman fracture or bilateral C2 pars fractures, and tear-drop hyper-flexion vertebral body fractures) [16].

Stability of the subaxial spine (C3–7) follows more closely Deni's three column model of the spine, which was initially described for thoraco-lumbar spine fractures (Fig. 4.4). The anterior column of the spine includes the anterior half of the disc and anterior vertebral body, the annulus pulposus, and the anterior longitudinal ligament. The posterior half of the disc and vertebral body, the posterior longitudinal ligament, and the pedicles form the middle column. The posterior column encompasses the posterior arch (lamina, lateral masses, facets), supraspinous and interspinous ligaments, facet joints and capsules, and ligamentum flavum. Disruption of two or more columns results in spinal instability [17]. Along the same trend, the Spine Trauma Study Group

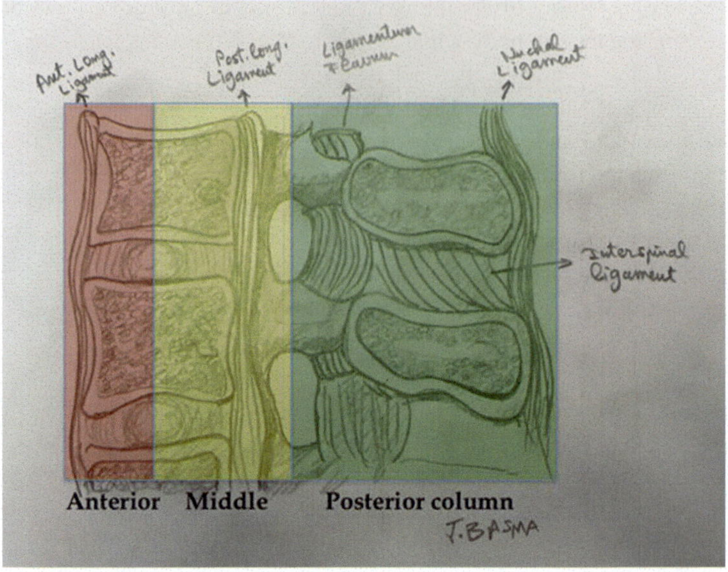

Fig. 4.4 The anterior, middle, and posterior stability columns of the subaxial spine (C3–7). Adapted from Denis' thoraco-lumbar model 17

Subaxial Cervical Spine Injury classification (SLIC) was adapted from the thoraco-lumbar classification (TLICS). It is intended to predict spinal instability, indications for surgical intervention and long-term prognosis. It includes three major components: morphology of fracture (compression/burst/rotation), integrity of disco-ligamentous complex (intact, intermediate, or disrupted), and neurologic status (intact function, root injury, complete and incomplete spinal cord injuries) [18].

Significant cervical spinal stenosis from degenerative disease is defined as cervical canal <10 mm, loss of CSF intensity around the spinal cord, myelomalacia, and increased medullary T2 signal. The Torg and Pavlov method uses the ratio of the diameter of the cervical canal to the width of the cervical body. A ratio of <0.8 on the lateral view is an indication for cervical stenosis. In cases of degenerative disease, there is no true mechanical instability. However, given the stenotic canal and compressed spinal cord, exaggerated movements, especially with hyperextension such as during intubation and surgical positioning, increase the risk of traumatic injury and contusion of the spinal cord (e.g., central cord syndrome and worsening neurological deficits) [19].

Evaluation of Cervical Instability and Neural Compression

Although cervical pathology can occur in asymptomatic patients, a thorough clinical evaluation prior to positioning and intubation is a good screening tool to evaluate for most serious cervical instabilities and neural stenosis/compression. Patient's medical history may reveal a previous neck trauma, neck surgery, or systemic predisposing factors, such as rheumatoid arthritis, Down syndrome, diffuse spinal degenerative disease (e.g., lumbar stenosis, see below). The clinical examination should focus on two groups of signs and symptoms: those related to (1) structural instability or (2) neural compression. Nerve root compression from disc herniation, osteophyte formation, or bony fragments results in clinical radiculopathy, which typically produces lower motor neuron findings in the related myotome. Paresthetic pain and/or numbness may involve the associated dermatome. Radicular symptoms are frequently dynamic, and it is prudent, whenever there is no contraindication otherwise, to evaluate them with different cervical range of motion (rotation, flexion/extension, Spurling maneuver). Spinal cord compression, on the other hand, results in myelopathy and upper motor neuron findings. These typically include hyperreflexia (Hoffman, Babinski, clonus, exaggerated deep tendon reflexes), neurogenic bladder, spastic and ataxic gait. Also encountered are sensory level loss (bilateral or unilateral, e.g., Brown-Séquard syndrome) and bilateral finger and hand weakness/tingling (central cord syndrome). The cervical spine should be examined in its normal range of motion to assess for dynamic pathologies. Dynamic clinical findings can include worsening pain, alignment deformity, radicular or myelopathic findings. If a non-diagnosed cervical pathology is highly suspected prior to surgery, the anesthesiologist and the neurosurgeon should have a low threshold for further imaging workup. Depending on the findings, AP and lateral X-rays can help evaluate the general alignment and overt fractures of the spine. Flexion/extension X-rays help assess cervical spine stability. Computed tomography shows the bony structures in detail, and the magnetic resonance imaging the ligamentous, disc, and neural elements. Diagnosing a serious cervical instability or compression may lead to postponing the current elective surgery and prioritizing addressing the cervical spine first.

Incidence of Cervical Stenosis Accompanying Lumbar Stenosis

Tandem stenosis of both the cervical and lumbar spine is not uncommon in the aging population. Based on previous studies, the reported incidence ranges between 5 and 25% [20–25]. The incidence varies depending on the definition of significant cervical stenosis—radiologic, clinical, or surgical. It is not clear whether congenital spinal stenosis is a predisposing factor for combined cervical and lumbar stenosis [21]. Lumbar surgery for degenerative stenosis is a common neurosurgical procedure and consideration of an accompanying cervical pathology should be done preoperatively (Fig. 4.5). The symptomatology may be vague, and findings attributable to one spinal region commonly overshadow the other. The clinical picture can be complex and can encompass a spectrum of signs and symptoms related to either cervical stenosis (myelopathy, radiculopathy) or lumbar stenosis (radicular pain, neurogenic claudication). In some cases, a triad of complex clinical findings is exhibited: intermittent neurogenic claudication, mixed upper and lower neuron findings, and complex gait disturbances (pseudo-diabetic proprioceptive gait from degeneration of posterior column, proximal lower extremity weakness, and flexed posture with compensatory neck hyperextension to relieve back and leg pain and facilitate straight gaze) [22]. If there is an undiagnosed cervical pathology in a patient undergoing a lumbar decompression, there is a risk of spinal cord or nerve root injury during hyperextension for intubation or positioning. It is usually recommended to surgically address the clinically more prominent cervical pathology prior to intervening on the lumbar spine. However, there have been reports of postoperative worsening neurological deficits (including cauda equina) from severe lumbar stenosis after surgery for cervical decompression in a prolonged supine position [26]. Patients should be rigorously questioned on their symptoms after specific prolonged positions prior to surgery (axial pain, radicular pain, weakness/numbness/tingling, etc.).

Evaluation for Intrinsic Cervical Spinal Cord Pathologies

Intrinsic spinal cord pathology (tumors, vascular malformations, cavernomas, syrinx, etc.) is relatively rare and is not typically associated with spinal instability. Symptomatology also frequently involves upper motor neuron findings and varying degrees of radicular symptoms. Depending on the location of the lesion, different spinal cord syndromes can be encountered (Brown-Séquard, posterior column, anterior spinal cord); nonetheless, central cord syndrome is more frequently associated with traumatic compression and degenerative stenosis of the cervical spine. Syringomyelia is defined by a cystic collection in the spinal cord close to the central canal, which is not lined by ependyma

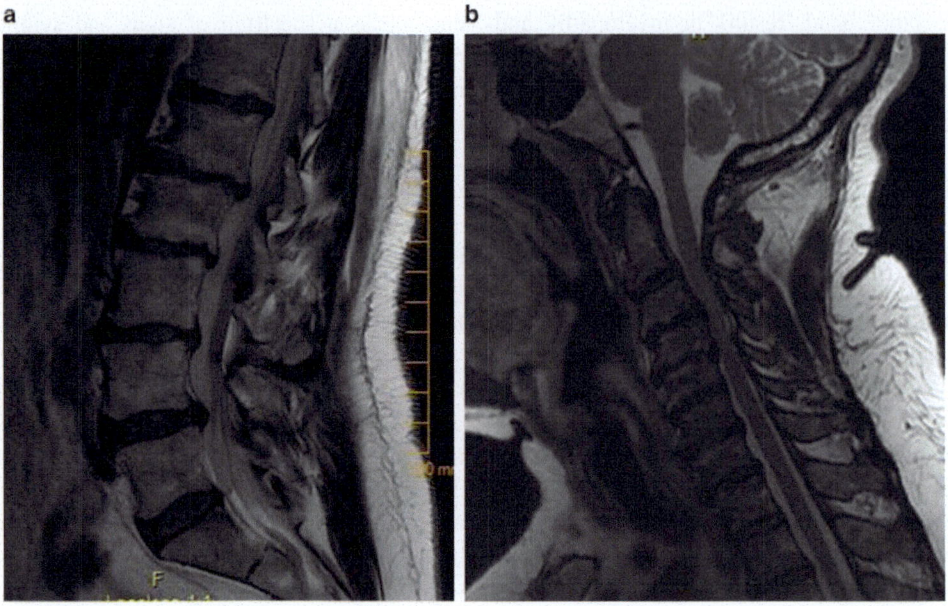

Fig. 4.5 Concomitant lumbar and cervical degenerative disease. A patient was referred to our neurosurgical department for surgical management of her lumbar stenosis resulting in lower back and lower extremity radicular pain (**a**). On exam she was also found to be myelopathic and a new MRI of her cervical spine revealed significant stenosis requiring an earlier cervical intervention (**b**)

(as opposed to hyromyelia). In fact, it results from a dissection of the ependymal lining of the central canal and accumulation of CSF within the cord itself. It can either be congenital (Arnold-Chiari malformation, scoliosis, spina bifida) or acquired (trauma, tumor, hemorrhage, arachnoiditis, meningitis). Clinically, syringomyelia is commonly associated with paresthetic pain (neck, arms). Because it affects the regional decussating thermo-algic fibers close to the central canal, it typically results in a cape-like distribution of pain and temperature sensation loss. Suspecting syringomyelia prior to patient positioning should warrant further investigation and diagnostic testing if needed [27].

References

1. Committee on Standards and Practice Parameters. Practice for preanesthesia evaluation an updated report by the society of anesthesiologists task force on preanesthesia evaluation. Anesthesiology. 2012;116(1):8.
2. Shih P, Slimack N, Roy A, Fessler R, Koski T. Abdominal complications following posterior spinal fusion in patients with previous abdominal surgeries. Neurosurg Focus. 2011;31(4):e16–21.
3. Grisell M, Place H. Face tissue pressure in prone positioning. Spine. 2008;33(26):2938–41.
4. Leibovitch I, Casson RLC, Selva D. Ischemic orbital compartment syndrome as complication of spinal surgery in the prone position. Ophthalmology. 2006;113(1):105–8.
5. Stambough J, Dolan D, Werner R, Godfrey E. Ophthalmologic complications associated with prone positioning in spine surgery. J Am Acad Orthop Surg. 2007;15(3):156–65.
6. Singer M, Salim S. Bilateral acute angle-closure glaucoma as a complication of facedown spine surgery. Spine J. 2010;10:e7–9.
7. Kwee MM, Ho YH, Rozen WM. The prone position during surgery and its complications: a systematic review and evidence-based guidelines. Int Surg. 2015;100(2):292–303.
8. Anderton J, Keen R, Neave R. Positioning in the surgical patient. London: Butterworths; 1988.
9. Porter J, Pidgeon C, Cunningham A. The sitting position in neurosurgery: a critical appraisal. Br J Anesth. 1999;82(1):117–28.
10. Black S, Cucchiara RF. Tumor surgery. In: Cucchiara RF, Black S, Michenfelder JD, editors. Clinical neuroanesthesia. 2nd ed. New York: Churchill Livingstone; 1998. p. 351.

11. Weinlander CM, Coombs DW, Plume SK. Myocardial ischemia due to obstruction of aortocoronary bypass graft by intraoperative positioning. Anesth Analg. 1985;64:933–6.
12. Dickman CA, Crawford NR, Brantley AGU, Sonntag VKH, Koeneman JB. In vitro cervical spine biomechanical testing. BNI Quarterly. 1993;9:17–26.
13. Rojas CA, Bertozzi JC, Martinez CR, Whitlow J. Reassessment of the craniocervical junction: normal values on CT. Am J Neuroradiol. 2007;28:1819–23.
14. Rhoton AL Jr. The far lateral approach and its transcondylar, supracondylar, and paracondylar extensions. Neurosurgery. 2000;87:555–85.
15. Dickamn CA, Greene KA, Sonntag VK. Injuries involving the transverse atlantal ligament: classification and treatment guidelines based upon experience with 39 injuries. Neurosurgery. 1996;38:44–50.
16. Levine AM, Edwards CC. The management of traumatic spondylolisthesis of the axis. J Bone Joint Surg. 1985;67A:217–26.
17. Denis F. The three column spine and its significance in the classification of acute thoracolumbar spinal injuries. Spine. 1983;8:817–31.
18. Vaccaro AR, Hulbert RJ, Patel AA, Fisher C, Dvorak M, Lehman RA Jr, et al. The subaxial cervical spine injury classification system: a novel approach to recognize the importance of morphology, neurology, and integrity of the disco-ligamentous complex. Spine. 2007;32:2365–74.
19. Torg JS, Naranja RJ, Pavlov H, Galinat BJ, Warren R, Stine RA. The relationship of developmental narrowing of the cervical spinal canal to reversible and irreversible injury of the cervical spinal cord in football players. J Bone Joint Surg. 1996;78A:1308–14.
20. Okada E, Matsumoto M, Ichihara D, Chiba K, Toyama Y, Fujiwara H, et al. Aging of the cervical spine in healthy volunteers: a 10-year longitudinal magnetic resonance imaging study. Spine (Phila Pa 1976). 2009;34:706–12.
21. Lee SH, Kim KT, Suk KS, Lee JH, Shin JH, So DH, et al. Asymptomatic cervical cord compression in lumbar spinal stenosis patients: a whole spine magnetic resonance imaging study. Spine (Phila Pa 1976). 2010;35:2057–63.
22. Dagi TF, Tarkington MA, Leech JJ. Tandem lumbar and cervical stenosis: natural history, prognostic indicices, and results after surgical decompression. J Neurosurg. 1987;66:842–9.
23. Teng P, Papatheodorou C. Combined cervical and lumbar spondylosis. Arch Neurol. 1964;10:298–307.
24. Boden SD, McCowin PR, Davis DO, Dina TS, Mark AS, Wiesel S. Abnormal magnetic resonance scans of the cervical spine in asymptomatic subjects. J Bone Joint Surg Am. 1990;72(8):1178–84.
25. Epstein NE, Epstein JA, Carras R, Murthy VS, Hyman RA. Coexisting cervical and lumbar spinal stenosis: diagnosis and management. Neurosurgery. 1984;15:489–96.
26. Caron TH, Gordon RB. Combined (tandem) lumbar and cervical stenosis. Semin Spine Surg. 2007;19:44–6.
27. Heiss JD, Oldfield EH. Pathophysiology and treatment of syringomyelia. Contemp Neurosurg. 2003;25:1–8.
28. Wroski M, Ferber J, Wroski J. Acute tension pneumocephalus as a complication of surgical procedures of the posterior cranial fossa in prone position. Neurol Neurochir Pol. 1987;21:167–70.

Organization of the Operating Room for Neurosurgical Procedures

5

Jaafar Basma and Daniel Hoit

Introduction and General Principles

Organizing the operating room is a crucial step in any neurosurgical procedure. Conceptualization of the operating room design prior to positioning and skin incision has tremendous consequences on the progression of surgery. Initial misplacements or entanglements can cause delays, physical and psychological discomfort, or even preventable adverse events. The organization of the operating room should be viewed as an extension of the surgical approach. It follows the surgical principles of order, rhythm, and unrestrained view. When applied to the conceptual planning and physical arrangement of the operating room, these surgical axioms coincide with the seven basic principles of interior design [1].

1. *Unity:* The operating room organization should be guided by a sense of harmony and uniformity. It should direct the surgical devices, instruments, and the operating team towards one common goal that is the patient's safety and the successful outcome of the surgery.
2. *Balance:* Surgical instruments, tables, and devices should be arranged in an ordered fashion to prevent entanglements, obstructions, and discomfort. Open spaces should be more or less symmetric and balanced around the patient to allow freedom of movement for the surgeon and the operating room staff.
3. *Rhythm:* Physical arrangement of the operating room should enable a smooth flow of movement for the staff and the surgical equipment. For this reason, wheeled devices and articulating arms are very helpful in creating a dynamic space, which can be tailored for each surgical approach. Contamination-controlled airflow systems are employed to minimize the concentration of airborne pollutant particles and constantly regulate temperature and humidity.
4. *Emphasis:* The patient is always the focal point of the entire room organization. More specifically, the pathology as a target of the surgical approach should be the geometrical focal point from which all other lines are drawn and extrapolated. This creates a more targeted perspective and reinforces the principle of unity in the routine coordination between the surgical staff.
5. *Contrast:* Lighting in surgery is of utmost importance and constant contrast should be maintained in both the macro- and microsurgical stages of the operation.

J. Basma (✉)
University of Tennessee Health Sciences Center, Memphis, TN, USA
e-mail: jbasma@uthsc.edu;

D. Hoit
Department of Neurosurgery, Semmes-Murphey Brain and Spine Institute, University of Tennessee Health Sciences Center, Memphis, TN, USA
e-mail: dhoit@semmes-murphey.com

A. Arthur et al. (eds.), *Perioperative Considerations and Positioning for Neurosurgical Procedures*,
https://doi.org/10.1007/978-3-319-72679-3_5

Different instruments and devices are colored and tagged to maximize visualization, spatial transitions, and easy exchange between the operating staff.

6. *Scale and proportion:* Operating rooms used for aneurysm surgery are supposed to be spacious to fit all the modern required technological tools. The size of surgical devices and instruments usually follows their respective functional importance. Choosing specific devices for a specific operating room is important in dictating space flexibility and maneuverability.
7. *Details:* Never to be undermined, the smallest structure in the operating room can have crucial effects on the flow of surgery. Specific elements should be checked and re-adjusted daily by the operating staff to prevent unexpected difficulties or complications.

History of Operating Room Organization

Early operating rooms of the enlightenment era were designed following the basic plans of anatomical class theaters. The operating room or "theater" had a very simple organization consisting of a raised table in the center, surrounded by elevated rows of seats to allow students to observe the different steps of surgery. A major modifier was the introduction of antisepsis by Lister in 1867, then aseptic restrictions and the autoclave by von Bergmann in Berlin and the German surgeon Gustav Neuber. William Halsted and Charles McBurney in the United States further advanced these protocols [2]. Asepsis created an insurmountable separation between the sterile surgical field and the surrounding space. The surgeon's area was confined to a strictly aseptic zone and more assistants and equipment were needed for anesthesia and instrument handling. During the late nineteenth and early twentieth centuries, endotracheal intubation techniques and general anesthetics evolved through the efforts of Trendelenburg, Macewen, Rosenberg, Kuhn, Magill, Miller, and Macintosh. These developments added a large mandatory space for the anesthesia staff, machine, and carts. Ventilation systems in modern operating theaters were also promoted to an efficiency of 80–95% in removing airborne particles > or = 5 μm. Laminar airflow systems with HEPA filters, which can remove airborne particles of 0.3 μm and above with 99.97% efficiency have been developed and are widely used in neurosurgical and other implant procedures. HEPA filters were commercialized in the 1950s and they have resulted in significant further reduction of surgical site infections [3].

Technological advancements and the introduction of different surgical devices have complicated the organization of the operating room. Cushing and Bovie introduced the monopolar coagulator. Cushing, who forever changed the history of neurosurgery, was known for using a headlamp and being surrounded by observing students. In 1938, Dandy described clipping of an intracranial aneurysm for the first time. Different sets of instruments had to be invented to serve the purpose of the emerging field of vascular neurosurgery. In the late 1960s, Yasargil revolutionized and popularized the microsurgical techniques for aneurysm surgery. The introduction of the microscope to the operating theater was a major advancement, which improved the outcome of brain aneurysms, including those previously deemed inoperable. The operating microscope is a large device that provides better visualization. Its placement has become a key element in any aneurysm surgery. Many microsurgical instruments were invented and added to the previous inventory of necessary surgical tables and trays. Malis introduced the bipolar coagulator in the 1950s, which was further popularized by Yasargil. This instrument has increased the safety and precision of electrocoagulation, in combination with its dissecting capability using the recoil mechanism of its forceps. Fluoroscopic angiography was merged with the microscope, allowing immediate assessment of aneurysm filling and patency of the normal surrounding vasculature. Frameless stereotaxy has also made the organization of the operating room more difficult given its sizeable equipment. Advent of innumerable spine hardware and instrumentation techniques has also significantly influenced the way operating room organization and patient positioning are performed. Several operating tables were developed to accommodate particular nuances for spine surgery, including Jackson tables (which can be open or flat), Wilson frames, radiolucent head attachments, and retractors. Spinal implants require an extremely high degree of asepsis to avoid surgical infections. Navigation devices now include C-arm X-ray fluoroscopy, O-arm tomographic machines and frameless stereotaxy, and their placement in the operating room should be well prepared prior to sterile draping.

Technology continues to fascinate the progress of neurosurgical techniques and strategies. Nowadays, endovascular means can be merged with microsurgery in the same hybrid operative theater to perform combined endovascular and surgical treatments of brain aneurysms and arterio-venous malformations. New techniques in endoscopic neurosurgery continue to expand in spine, skull base, and intraventricular pathology. The endoscope brought its own set of equipment, devices, and instruments, which must be considered in every modern neurosurgical operating room. The first robot-assisted surgical intervention was performed in 1985, and robotic technology has been widely incorporated in the disciplines of urology, cardiac surgery, orthopedics, general surgery, and gynecology. Robotic surgery is believed to provide higher precision, three-dimensional orientation, and stability with less ergonomic constraints on the surgeon through a smaller area of exposure [4, 5]. In neurosurgery, robotics has been gaining grounds through the emergence of computer-assisted and stereotactic technologies [6, 7]. Robotic microscopes were merged with frameless registration technique [8]. Robotic techniques are also gaining popularity in spine surgery including assisting in pedicle screw placement to reduce exposure to radiation and increase the accuracy of screw placement [9, 10].

Basic Scheme

Operating room organization is tailored to the specific planned neurosurgical procedure and required patient's positioning. Different nuances apply to the basic scheme for a craniotomy compared to a spinal surgery. In cranial cases, the anesthesiologist's access to the head may be more difficult. Close attention should be made to implant asepsis in spinal surgeries. In general, the patient's table is placed in the center of the operating room to maximize head position beneath the overhead lights and the central ventilation system. Usually, the anesthesia machine with attendant respirator and the anesthetic devices are close to the center of the room. Although mobile, they are kept in most cases in a specific constant location for practical reasons. The operating table can rotate (90–180°) in relation to the anesthesiologist depending on the side of the pathology and the desired surgical approach. Checking the correct side of the surgery in the preoperative holding, before positioning, at the time of time-out, and before skin incision cannot be overemphasized. The microscope is moved in towards the head of the patient and is positioned in a way that its articulating arm can be manipulated and adjusted by the surgeon. In our facilities, an extra eyepiece is placed for teaching purposes. The microscope is angled in a way to accommodate the comfortable positioning of the assistant surgeon (Fig. 5.1).

The electrical unit(s) supplying the monopolar and the bipolar coagulators, the drill engine, and the suction cannulas can be placed separately, or carried by surgical booms, which can rotate in conjunction with the operating table. These instruments are most commonly placed on the side of the patient's feet, but can be positioned elsewhere in the room depending on space availability. The tables supporting the surgical instruments are often arranged in an L fashion at the side of the patient opposite to anesthesia, generally away from the door for sterility concerns. A "Mayo table" carrying the most important instrument for each specific stage of the surgery is advanced and placed above the patient's chest close to the operative field. Aneurysm clips should be laid out in a separate space in an organized fashion to allow easy access and selection when needed. Video monitors should be readily available throughout the surgery, mainly during the microscopic stage, so that the scrub technician

a b

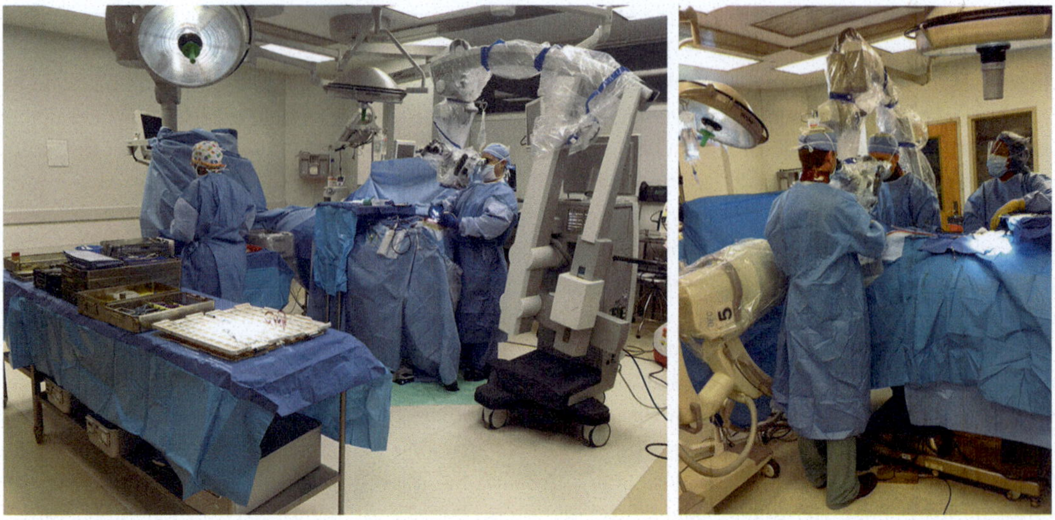

Fig. 5.1 (**a**) Basic operating room organization for a craniotomy surgery in our center. The microscope should have enough space around the patient's head. The anesthesia equipment is located at the side of the operating table and is separated from the surgical field by a sterile drape. The instrument tables are organized in an L-shaped fashion to allow more room for the scrub nurse and assistants. (**b**) Organization of the operating room for a spine procedure, showing the opposing positions of the fluoroscopic machine and the microscope

can follow and anticipate the surgical steps. Also, monitors provide a feedback to the anesthesiologist and the circulating nurse to facilitate communication between the surgical personnel. There are three types of monitors in our institutions: imaging, microscope related, and educational monitors. They can be immediately connected to the microscope, carried by articulating arms from the ceiling of the room, or attached to the room walls.

When needed, navigation devices are placed in a way to optimize both capturing of 3D coordinates by the navigation probe and visualization of the imaging monitor by the surgeon during the procedure. While the navigation "camera" is located towards the patient's head, the navigation screen is at the side of the feet in line of sight with the surgeon. Neurological monitoring devices, when used, such as SSEP and EEG are usually placed in the widest empty corner of the operating room and their cables should be freely connected to the patient without obstructions or kinks. Intraoperative troubleshooting can thus be easily carried out if necessary. The circulating nurse usually has a fixed station in a constant corner of the room with computer(s) accessing the medical chart at all times. Surgical supplies, which are immediately needed during surgery (such as sutures, cotton materials), are placed in accessible cabinets. Their location should be consistent and they are frequently checked following inventory lists to allow constant availability. A C-arm can be called in to perform an intraoperative angiogram if the room is not hybrid or already equipped with angiographic devices.

Operating Table and Head Holder

The operating table supports the patient during the surgical procedure and lies at the center of the room. Many different table systems exist, but the common functions should include stability, flexibility, and safety. Before positioning, and using a simple wheeling system, the operating table can be turned to change the patient's orientation in the room, depending on the side of the pathology and the desired position. Orientation of the operating table should optimize the benefit provided by the laminar airflow in filtrating airborne particles. The table can be adjusted for patient's positioning in different directions (up/down, reflex, Trendelenburg, tilt, back up/down, etc.). The operating tables do not have any shock-absorbing features. Securing the Mayfield head holder and the navigation probe should be performed after the table is placed in its planned position. Moving the table with such instrumentation exposes the head to jiggling motion that can dislodge the headrest or compromise the accuracy of navigation. The patient's pressure points are padded and all the lines and cables should be well inspected and secured prior to surgery. In cranial surgery, the head should be elevated above the level of the right atrium to enhance venous drainage. The head holder should be firmly secured and inspected and the neck must not be twisted or under tension. Cranial and supine approaches can be performed in the supine, lateral, and prone positions, which will be described separately in the following chapters. In spinal procedures, positioning should further take into account fluoroscopic visualization for both localization and hardware placement. Furthermore, limb positioning can be sometimes more problematic, and care must be taken to avoid iatrogenic peripheral neuropathies and plexopathies.

Intraoperatively, the table can still offer some degree of movement to maximize the surgeon's visibility and maneuverability. However, during the entirety of the procedure the operating table should be locked to provide the optimal stability and safety to the patient. The cranial three-point fixation device attaches the patient's head to the table, and is adjusted based on the angle of the surgical approach. Head fixation should also be planned in accordance with the general room organization. For instance, the navigation tracker, which attaches to the head holder, should not be obstructed from the main navigation arm, and should not hinder the surgical view after draping. A brain retractor can be attached to the head holder or directly to the Table. A "Layla bar" can also be attached to the operating table to allow retraction of soft tissue. The Fukushima retractor can be attached to the Mayfield head holder itself. Attention must be made to avoid leaning against the retractor or moving the table or the microscope while the retractors are still applied to the brain. Self-retaining retractors were also developed in spine surgery (examples include the Mcculloch lumbar retractor, the Trimline cervical retractor, the Greenberg retractor) and should be considered during positioning planning. For instance, in minimally invasive spinal surgery, the muscle can be retracted using a tube, which is usually attached through a flexible arm to the ipsilateral side of the bed. Tubular retractors have also been developed for brain surgery.

Operating Microscope

The introduction of the microscope to aneurysm surgery has had a great impact on patients' outcome. Given its size and its central position at the side of the patient's head, the organization of the operating room in the 1960s had to adapt to accommodate this permanent new comer. The microscope provides better illumination, magnification, and most importantly telescopic and stereoscopic vision. Most modern microscopes use a counterweight-balanced system with a heavy base and a flexible articulating arm. This allows "floating" movements in the three-dimensional space, in a 360° fashion. The surgeon thus can gain a great margin of maneuverability that he exploits to move his visual and working angles around the pathology [11]. A button on the hand switch or a mouthpiece can initiate these movements. The microscope's orientation in surgery should then take into account these special features and ensure their optimal functioning.

The heavy part of the microscope is usually pushed forward towards the head of the patient in line with the surgical approach. The base of the microscope should be at a suitable distance to allow free three-dimensional movements of its articulating arm (Fig. 5.2a). Modern microscopes have monitors on the side to allow scrub techs to follow the surgery and the circulating staff to follow the surgical steps. Wall monitors are available for observers, including in three-dimensional technology, which is extremely useful for the

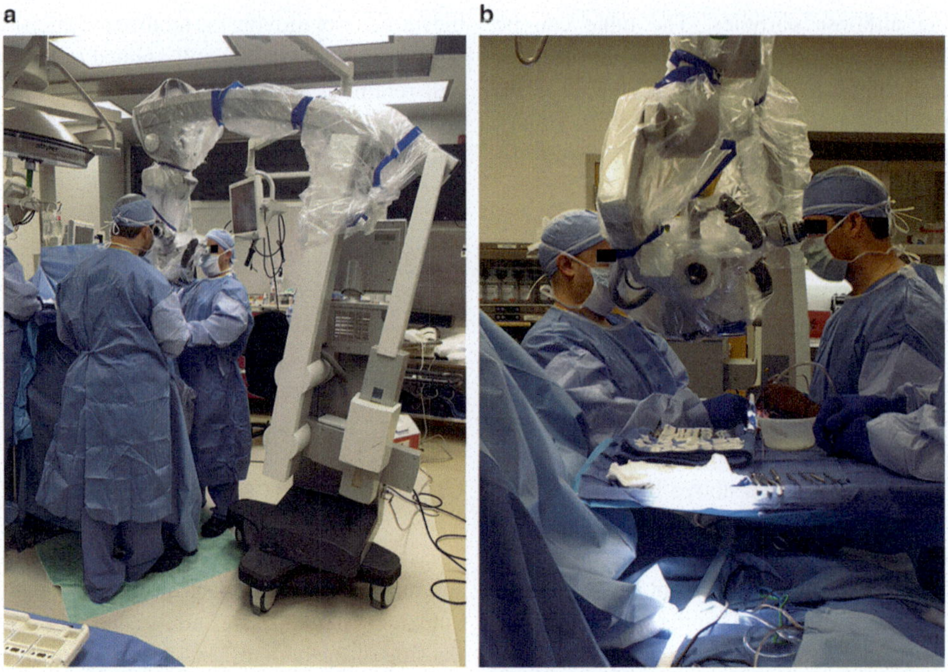

Fig. 5.2 (**a**) Positioning of the standing lead surgeon, assisting surgeon, and the microscope. (**b**) This setup allows both the surgeon and the assisting surgeon to work simultaneously under the microscope

observing medical students, residents, and fellows. Besides their learning benefits, these monitors facilitate communication between the surgeon, the anesthesiologist, the scrub technician, and the circulating nurse. Video monitors should be accessible to the circulating nurses to adjust for light intensity, focus speed, and fluorescence imaging. Surgeries can be recorded for future analysis or for research purposes (Fig. 5.3).

Many microscopes are equipped with additional features, which are very helpful in aneurysm surgery. For instance, fluorescent imagery can assess the aneurysm obliteration and patency of surrounding vessels after clipping of the aneurysm. Some microscopes can also be connected to the navigation system and the surgeon can thus orient himself around the pathology by immediately correlating the surgical view to preoperative imaging.

Head-mounted loupes and lights are very helpful in spinal surgery, mainly for the ligamentous and bony stages of the procedure. Nonetheless, the microscope remains necessary for the parts of surgery where neural elements are being manipulated or dissected (spinal and nerve root decompression, intradural surgery), or when the surgeon needs a tubular stereoscopic vision through a small skin incision (minimally invasive spine surgery, microdiscectomy). The microscope positioning should take into account the lead and assistant surgeons' comfort, and the neighboring navigation devices (fluoroscopy, frameless stereotaxy) and operating tables.

Surgeon's Positioning

The primary surgeon's space within the operative field should be unrestricted. A comfortable position during surgery is mandatory. Adequate freedom of movement is important to adjust the surgical working angle. While some surgeons prefer to operate in a sitting position, with or without an armrest, other surgeons feel more at ease standing to accommodate for an assistant surgeon. In the latter case, the organization of the room and the angulation of the microscope are adjusted to provide extra space for the other

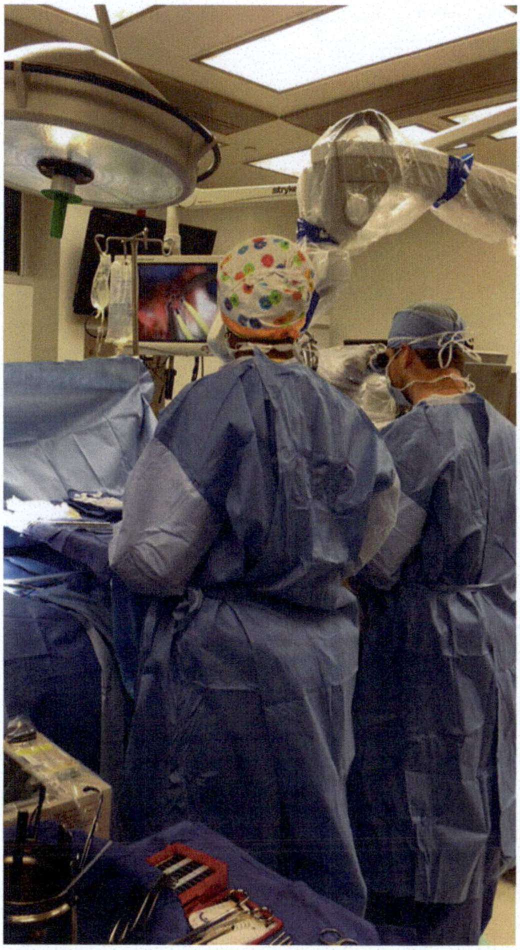

Fig. 5.3 Well-placed monitors permit the scrub nurse or technician to closely follow the microsurgical steps of the procedure

surgeon to work comfortably [11, 12]. The foot pedals and their communications to the surgical instruments are checked prior to the beginning of the surgery and the circulating nurse should always be available to correct their positions.

In our institution, we prefer the standing position using the microscope to accommodate for an assistant surgeon. We believe that this positioning has a much more effective teaching value in an academic setting than alternating the operating surgeon role in a sitting position. Face to face allows more involved interaction and more hands on work by the resident. Residents gain early exposure to the microscopic field during their junior years and their skills develop in a faster fashion. The primary operator side is usually reserved for senior residents. Experienced surgeons may be on the assistant side, and depending on the difficulty of the surgical steps, the attending and the senior residents can alternate roles. However, the assistant role from the opposite side is more difficult because the working angle is not immediately in line with the target. The reach of suction is also more restricted and the angle of the microscope usually creates for a height disadvantage. The additional bipolar and suction tubing can also create increased entanglements. We were able to deal with these issues in our experience by continuously adapting the microscope angle for both surgeons (often the microscope has to be moved away), by using stools and separate trajectories for suction tubing and bipolar cables (Fig. 5.2).

Anesthesia Space

The anesthesia space is constant in the operating room and consists of the anesthesia machine, the anesthesia cart, electronic monitors, and an automated blood pressure measuring machine. Because the surgeon has to stand on the side of the patient's head during cranial surgery, the anesthesia space is usually to the side, and in some centers it can be towards the feet. The anesthesiologist should have permanent access to the endotracheal tube. Lumbar and extraventricular drains are usually attached to poles close to the anesthesiologist. These drains can be opened and closed, and their levels adjusted, based on feedback from the surgeon. In spinal procedures, including the cervical spine, the anesthesiologist is usually positioned on the side of the patient's head. Spinal traction may be adjusted from behind the sterile drape if necessary (Fig. 5.4).

Lighting

Lighting during surgery is crucial. Overhead light intensity and configuration vary between different operating rooms. Overhead lights are important during the initial phases of craniotomy

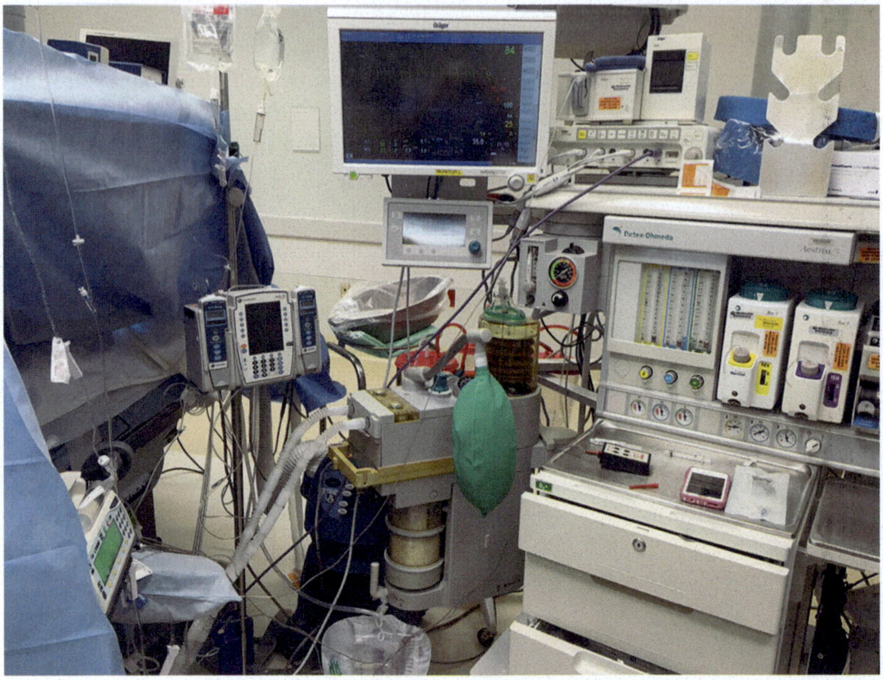

Fig. 5.4 The anesthesia space is on the other side of the sterile field with its full equipment and monitors

for aneurysm surgery. Position of overhead light arms can vary in configuration and intensity from operating room to another. Often times, the organization of the remainder of the operating room, including equipment booms, anesthesia gas lines and positioning of monitors, doors, sub-sterile rooms are derived from the position of the overhead lighting. Choosing the right operating room to perform aneurysm surgery is purpose driven and starts by choosing the room with the appropriate orientation of its headlights. Articulating lighting arms can be used, which are usually flexible and their position can be adjusted throughout the surgery using disposable sterile handles. They also have a focusing technology to allow concentration of light on the areas of interest of the surgical field. Over headlights should be carefully adjusted prior to draping, as their position changes with the patient's orientation, to prevent intraoperative discomfort and lack of illumination. In some instances, headlights can be employed which can be easily mounted and connected to portable batteries. The room itself should also be well illuminated to allow ease of movement for all the operating personnel. Following the principle of contrast and emphasis, the room's lights can be dimmed after initializing the microscope to maximize the surgeon's visibility and focus.

Instrument Tables

The importance of organizing the surgical instruments in their trays and on the table cannot be underemphasized. Instruments are arranged in specific trays after being autoclaved based on their specific functions in different surgical procedures. Examples include basic craniotomy trays, microinstruments, separate anterior cervical, posterior cervical and lumbar trays with their specific retractor systems, etc. All instruments should be laid out on two different tables in an organized fashion in terms of their function, size, and expected chronological use in surgery. A "Mayo" table can be advanced to above the patient's chest close to the operating field to allow a closer distance to the surgeon and more

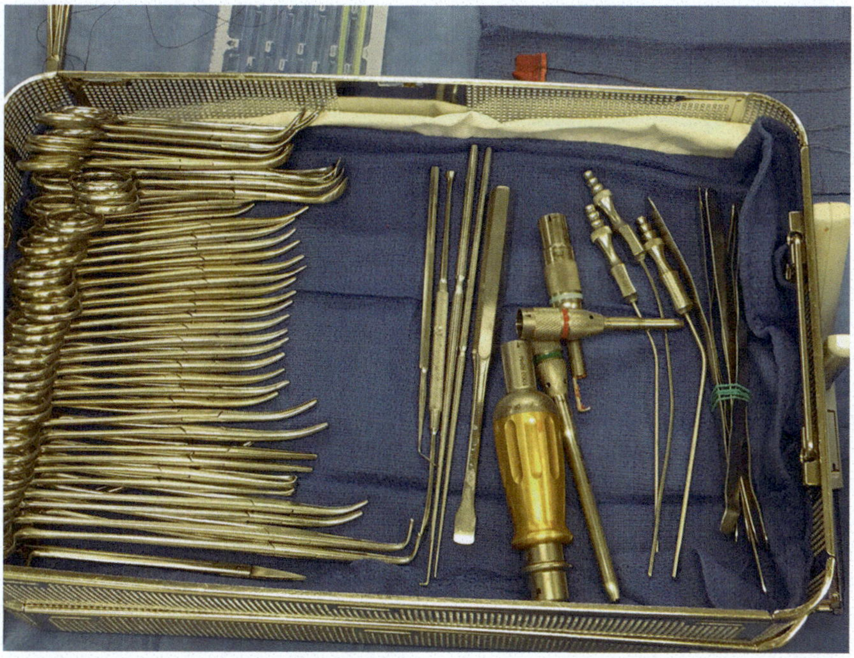

Fig. 5.5 Basic instrument tray for a craniotomy procedure

immediate handing of instruments. Instruments on this table can be changed depending on the different surgical steps and should always be organized in a way to predict their use by the surgeon for maximal efficiency. Hardware and respective tools for spinal instrumentation should be opened shortly before their use to minimize the risk of contamination. Their trays are most commonly provided, organized, and regularly checked by the vendor (Fig. 5.5).

Suction tubing and electrocoagulation and drill cables should be appropriately connected with the least possible entanglements to allow freedom and efficiency of movement. It is of utmost importance that the suction apparatus is working at full desired function during the entire surgery, and it should always be checked and fixed as necessary by the circulating nurse.

Basic Surgical Devices: Bovie, Bipolar, Suction Cannulas, Drill, and Pedals

The suction cannula, along with the drill system, the bipolar and the monopolar electrical generator (s) are usually placed on the surgical boom on the side of the patient's feet. Since the boom has an articulating arm, its position in the room can be adjusted following the patient's orientation. The tubes and the cords are usually plugged just after draping, and the instrument functioning is checked prior to skin incision. These devices should be accessible at all times for the circulating nurse to adjust their settings and troubleshoot them in cases of malfunction. The suction pump can be regulated at different pressure settings following the level of dissection being carried out.

The suction is ideally connected to multiple cannulas, which can offer immediate alternatives if one cannula stops working. A potent larger caliber suction apparatus should immediately be available in the surgical field to control the blood flow and guide the surgeon to the bleeding source. The power setting of the electrosurgical units can also be adjusted (monopolar and bipolar coagulation are usually set at 30–35 in the bony and muscular stages of cranial procedures, and 35–45 in spine cases). Bipolar electrocoagulation is usually set at lower levels close to critical neurovascular structures [10–25].

Airflow Regulation and Prevention of Surgical Infections

Airborne particles including dust, skin scales, respiratory aerosols, and textile fibers may settle on the surgical instruments and wound, and result in surgical site infection. The contamination-controlled airflow system (heating, ventilation, air-conditioning system (HVAC)) is devised to minimize such morbidity. It reduces the amount of air particles through several synergistic mechanisms, including air distribution (particle dilution and airflow movement), room pressurization (which creates an infiltration barrier) and filtration. Optimized ventilation (recommended at 15–20 exchanges per hour) allows dilution of gaseous pollutants and airborne particles and microbes [3]. It is recommended that airflow is maintained in a *laminar* pattern, wherein air travels in parallel lines causing the contaminants to be constantly and smoothly directed towards the exhaust outlets to prevent them from landing on the surgical site. High efficiency particulate air (HEPA) is a filter that is defined by the United States Department of Energy as being capable of removing 99.97% of particles that have a size of 0.3 μm or above. Laminar airflow through HEPA filters has significantly reduced the risk of surgical site infection. Modern devices can be ceiling mounted (vertical flow), wall-mounted (horizontal flow), or combined [13, 14].

Patient's position should maximize the advantage offered by the airflow system to prevent particle settling on the surgical site. Laminar flow should be circulating above the patient and the instruments, i.e., the sterile field. As modern neurosurgical procedures (both spinal and cranial) are evolving, we are seeing a tremendous increase in operating and neurovascular suite traffic. Vendors, students, residents, monitoring technicians, nurses, and anesthesia staff are all crowding into confined areas with ongoing interventions. Optimal traffic position should be where the laminar air is leaving the sterile fields towards its filtering ducts. This position should be assigned and constantly checked by the circulating nurse (Fig. 5.6).

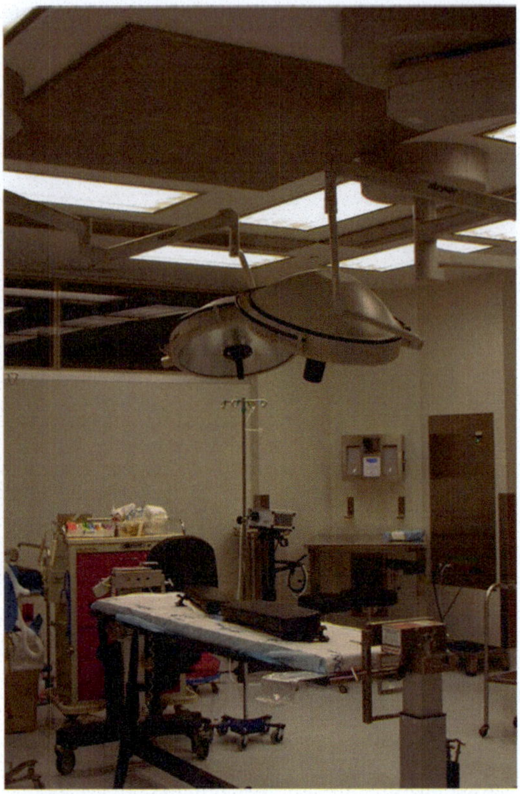

Fig. 5.6 The laminar airflow system in the roof of the operating room should be just above the operating table. The overhead lights are mounted on articulating arms in the same area

Surgical site infections are preventable complications that result in increasing morbidity and a considerable economic burden. The world health organization developed evidence-based global guidelines for the prevention of SSI, which were developed by international experts on the basis of predetermined research questions and associated systematic literature review [15]. Topics include preoperative bathing, decolonization with mupirocin in patients with known nasal carriage of S. aureus, surgical antibiotic prophylaxis performed before incision (within 120 min), use of alcohol-based and Chlorhexidine solutions antiseptic solutions for surgical site skin preparation, nutritional support, preoperative oxygenation (80% FI-O_2 intraoperatively and 2–6 h in case of general anesthesia), maintaining normothermia (use of warming devices), use of protocols for intensive blood glucose control, maintaining normovolemia, use of sterile drapes and gowns, etc.

Neuro-Imaging and Neuro-Navigation Devices

Each operating room should have special monitors to display the preoperative imaging studies, such as cerebral angiograms, computed tomography, and magnetic resonance. Specific angiographic or tomographic reconstruction images are selected preoperatively and exposed on the monitor for quick intraoperative analysis. These imaging studies should be available for the surgeon to review at any time during the procedure. By correlating intraoperative findings with preoperative imaging studies, the surgeon can tailor the approach and surgical plans.

Neuro-navigation technology allowed the integration of preoperative images in the three-dimensional space of the patient's head. The system typically includes an articulating piece attached to a tracker and fixed on the head holder. The tracker communicates with a receiver or "camera" which is mounted on an articulating arm connected to a wheeled base. This arm should be on the side of and in line with the patient's head, with no obstruction between the two. Usually, the head's space coordinates are registered prior to draping and accuracy is checked before and after draping. The stealth technology can also be connected to the microscope allowing the surgeon to focus on a point of interest in the surgical field and correlate it to preoperative imaging (Fig. 5.7). Surgical cameras can also be mounted to create an "augmented reality" when the view is merged with preoperative angiographs [16]. This is one good example of how much technology has complicated the organization of the operating room in our modern era. The surgeon must be cognizant about all the different tools and devices and plan their optimal placements prior to commencement of the surgery.

Neuro-Monitoring

Because the patient is anesthetized, a neurological exam cannot be obtained to evaluate the effects of different surgical steps, such as temporary or permanent clipping, on the patient's neurologic function. Many neuro-monitoring modalities are now available to provide patient's

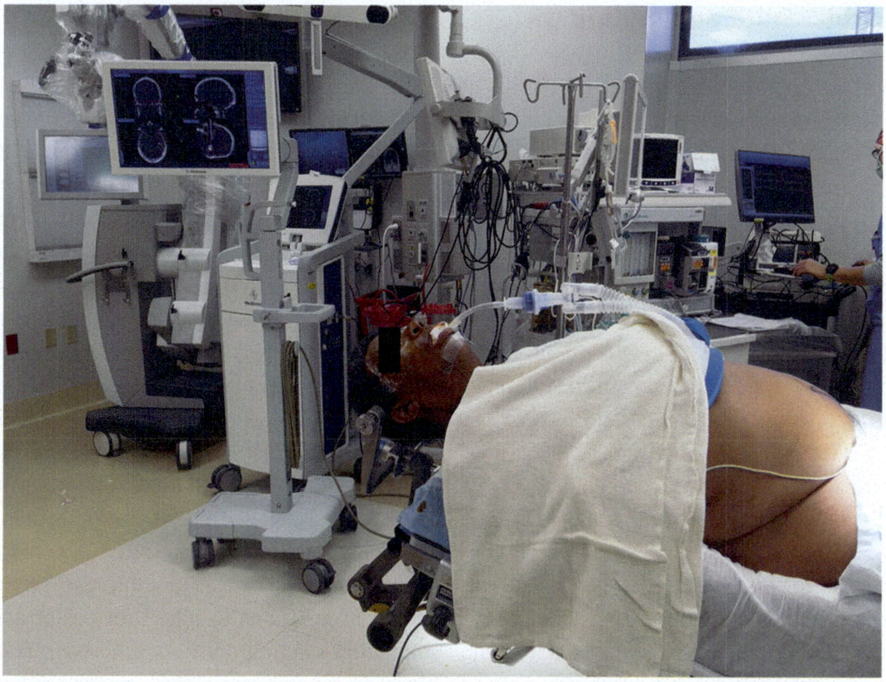

Fig. 5.7 Placement of the navigation device in a trans-sphenoidal surgery for a pituitary tumor

physiological feedback. These include but are not limited to somatosensory evoked potentials (SSEPs), transcranial motor evoked potentials (TcMEPs), brainstem auditory evoked potentials (BAEPs), and EEG [17]. Changes in electrophysiological parameters and their reversibility were correlated with patient's neurological outcome [18].

An experienced technician places the electrodes on the patient and connects them to a monitor after intubation. During positioning, the wires must be free of entanglements and accessible for troubleshooting during the procedure. A baseline recording is checked prior and after positioning. During surgery, the monitoring technician should communicate with the surgeon and the anesthesiologist with clear audible voice, so that plans for troubleshooting or surgical or anesthetic readjustments made. The monitoring wires are connected to their special monitors, which are placed in a relatively distant and spacious area, so that the monitoring equipment does not obstruct the visual and physical flow of the surgery.

Intraoperative Angiography, Endovascular Suite, and "hybrid OR"

Some modern operating rooms are "hybrid" in that they harbor endovascular angiographic technologies alongside with the standard operating room appliances [19, 20]. Nevertheless, an intraoperative or postoperative angiography can always be performed in the operating rooms lacking the hybrid design. Some patients may have undergone a cerebral angiography prior to surgery and a vascular access sheath left in place. Alternatively, arterial access can still be obtained in a sterile fashion in the operating room. A wheeled C-arm or O-arm X-ray machine can be rolled in the operating room. It can be draped in a sterile way; however, other equipment such as the microscope and navigation devices should be moved to the side. Although it is difficult to manipulate the specific angles of X-ray shots, an experienced dually trained surgeon can adjust the incidence to obtain the most pertinent needed X-rays. In our center, the neurovascular suite is in proximity to the operating room. Given the availability of fluorescent angiography, the time and effort required moving the microscope and the X-ray machine and the imperfections of intraoperative images, we prefer to perform a formal postoperative angiogram and a DYNA CT scan at the angio-suite immediately after the surgery. The operating tables are kept open and sterile and the anesthesia space ready in case the aneurysm has to be re-operated.

The angiogram suite retains its own particularities in relation to positioning and overall room organization. The digital subtraction angiography unit may employ a one plane or a bi-plane C-arms, which movement should be unhindered. The flat screens must offer optimal visualization for the interventionist, who in turn has to be well shielded from the X-ray emission. Because most angiograms and endovascular interventions are done nowadays through femoral access, the patient is always in the supine position. The anesthesiologist is usually stationed on the left side of the patient and has constant access to the ETT, venous and arterial lines, and extraventricular or lumbar drains.

Modern techniques in micro neurosurgery and endovascular intervention offer the possibility for combined treatments of complex cerebrovascular disease [19–21]. These include combined bypass and endovascular trapping for large complex aneurysms, AVM embolization followed by surgical resection, coil embolization followed by surgical evacuation of hematoma after aneurysm rupture, treatment of complex dural fistulas and management of intraoperative complications. However, given the time and constraints required for patient transportation a new model for a "hybrid" operating room has emerged in several centers [19, 20]. A neuroangiographic digital subtraction angiography (DSA) unit with a ceiling mounted C-arm is installed. The C-arm can be moved the corner of the operating room to allow adequate working space around the cranial operating field. The operating table can be rotated in different positions to allow for easier anesthesia induction, angiography, or microsurgical procedure. Ceiling mounted flat screens are located on one or two sides of the operating room.

Doppler Probes

Besides fluorescent microscopic angiography and digital subtraction angiography, Doppler probes can be used intraoperatively to check arterial flow in the aneurysm and the surrounding vasculature. From a logistic perspective, these are usually very easy to mount and operate. When needed, a sterile probe is opened and hooked to a small Doppler machine, which can be manipulated and adjusted by the circulating nurse. The machine can then be turned off and set on standby at the side of the table.

Storage, Supplies, and Trash Management

The operating room is equipped with storage cabinets where immediate surgical supplies are available at all time during surgery. These include but are not limited to, cotton materials, coagulation catalysts (surgicel, thrombin, gelfoam), sutures (small diameter threads should be immediately accessible especially if a bypass procedure is required)… Disposable instruments can be quickly replaced from a local stock, and sterile trays can be obtained from the central supply. Appropriate blood should be prepared in the room in case transfusions are required. Diuretic medications (Furosemide, Mannitol) can be ordered and used to help with brain relaxation when needed. Case cart system utilizes a perpetual inventory that is continuously updated according to the surgeon's utilization patterns. Preferred instruments, equipment, and supplies are noted for each case type and surgeon. This system has significantly helped in reducing costs related to operating room supplies.

To prevent retained foreign bodies, the circulating nurse and the scrub technician follow a counting protocol for cottonoids, gauze, and needles. The operating personnel, including the surgeon, should be mindful of this protocol to avoid unnecessary risks and surgical stoppage time. Counts are done before and after usage of the supplies and confirmed multiple times.

Sterility is mandatory in neurosurgery. The surgical field usually drains to a bag connected to a suction cannula to avert pooling of blood and resected tissue. The scrub technician and the surgeon constantly clear the field of instruments and supplies. Instruments are consistently cleaned to clear them from contaminating blood and tissue and optimize their functions. The circulating nurse collects the trash and falling instruments and directs them to their proper disposals. Attention should always be made to the airflow ventilation and filtration system in the operating room to avoid obstructing the air ducts and interfering with the laminar flow.

Operating room organization and management has tremendous effects on decreasing cost and optimizing patient and working personnel satisfaction. Focus on reducing wasted time should be maintained and it can be performed through parallel processing and task distribution, exploiting technological devices (e.g., exchangeable operating room table tops) and continuous standardization. Recycling and employing reusable devices whenever appropriate coupled with efficiency in room cleaning and turnover have resulted in significant cost reduction [22, 23].

Communication and Teamwork

An experienced team of surgeons, anesthesiologists, nurses, and scrub technicians is necessary to optimize the operating room organization and surgical outcome. Experience is gained with practice and continued education of the operating personnel. A routine must be established from the moment the surgery is booked to when the patient leaves the room. Checklists and redundant verifications assure that the smallest details are not neglected. Chronological steps are anticipated and prepared in an orderly fashion to avoid time wasting. Tasks are consistently divided between team members to optimize confidence, responsibility, and communication. Supervised students and new employees are progressively integrated in the team to ensure enough practice and experience is gained prior to operating independently.

Communication is a key element for the success of any surgery. The questions, requests, and updates should be clearly stated to ensure reciprocal understanding. With experience, the operating staff can communicate faster with body language, anticipation of steps, and recollection of similar previous scenarios. For this reason, monitors are very helpful in providing visualization of the microsurgical part of the surgery. Professionalism, mutual respect, and a friendly behavior are important to avoid unnecessary disputes and passive aggressive reactions. While the surgeon occupies a leadership position, he should be receptive to warnings, observations, and suggestions from his trusted and experienced team members. Organization of the operating room and healthy teamwork go hand in hand to guarantee surgical rhythm, order, and proficiency [12].

Patient Safety and Checklists

Adverse events in surgery can be attributed to human error and failures in communication [24]. Implementation of checklists is aimed at reducing such complications, and thus optimizing patient safety. The World Health Organization has devised a surgical safety checklist, which can be divided into three sections: Sign In (before induction of anesthesia), Time Out (before skin incision), and Sign Out (before the patient leaves the operating room). It targets "critical actions," which if missed, can lead to never events, can be life threatening, or actions that are frequently missed but contribute to preventable high-risk events. Implementation of this checklist was found to result in a significant drop of surgery-related morbidity and mortality (from 11 to 7% and from 1.5 to 0.8%, respectively). Recommendations focus on confirming patient's identity and side of the surgery, reviewing anesthesia machine and medication checklists, instruments checklists, allergies, airway evaluation, administering prophylactic antibiotic, monitoring sterility, and completion of instrument, sponge, and needle counts [25].

In the context of patient positioning and the operating room organization, it is mandatory to emphasize safety related to fall, electrical, and fire hazards. The patient must be well strapped and the head holder well secured. The operating room is designed to sustain the electrical demands of multiple devices (surgical tools, anesthesia devices, imaging and monitoring equipment, etc.). Surgery must be halted and adjustments made when the electrical overload alarm goes off. Special attention must be made to irrigation, which can increase the electrical hazards. Fire can be initiated by different sources of ignition (Bovie, microscope light) and promoted by flammable materials (oxygen-rich environment in anesthesia, wound preparation solutions, drapes, etc.). Safety measures do not only apply to the patient, but also to the surgeon and to the operating personnel. Surgeons are advised to wear eye protection shields. Hands-free zones are designated for the exchange of needles. All operating room personnel are urged to use lead X-ray aprons and protective screens. The large amount of crossing cords, lines, and wires increases the risk of falls, especially when the floor is wet from surgical irrigation. Organization of the operating room and its different devices should consider all these factors among others to maximize safety [26].

Conclusion

Maximizing patients and staff safety, minimizing risks of adverse events and optimizing the successful outcome of surgery begin with proper operating room organization. Understanding the functioning of different surgical and positioning devices, along with their respective spatial orientations, is mandatory. Safety, instruments, and counting checklists must be implemented consistently. Effective communication techniques in a respectful environment guarantee cooperation and continued learning among the surgical and anesthesia personnel.

References

1. Ballast DK. Interior construction and detailing for designers and architects. New York: Professional Publications, Inc; 2013.
2. Essex-Lopresti M. Operating theatre design. Lancet. 1999;20:1007–10.

3. Fernstrom A, Goldblatt M. Aerobiology and its role in the transmission of infectious diseases. J Pathog. 2013;2013:493–960.
4. Marano A, Choi YY, Hyung WJ, Kim YM, Kim J, Noh SH. Robotic versus laparoscopic versus open gastrectomy: a meta- analysis. J Gastric Cancer. 2013;13:136–48.
5. Carpentier A, Louimel D, Aupacie B, Reliand J. Computer-assisted cardiac surgery. Lancet. 1999; 353:379–80.
6. Kwoh YS, Hou J, Jonckheere EA, Hayathi S. A robot with improved absolute positioning accuracy for stereotactic brain surgery. IEEE Trans Biomed Eng. 1988;35:153–60.
7. Kelly PJ, Alker GJ, Goerss S. Computer assisted stereotactic laser microsurgery for the treatment of intracranial neoplasms. Neurosurgery. 1982;10:324–31.
8. Marinov M, Roberts D. Interactive image-guided cranial neurosurgery using the SurgiScope. Bulg Neurosurg. 1996;4:9–18.
9. Devito DP, Kaplan L, Dietl R, Pfeiffer M, Horne D, Silber-stein B, et al. Clinical acceptance and accuracy assessment of spinal implants guided with SpineAssist surgical robot: retrospective study. Spine. 2010;35:2109–15.
10. Kantelhardt SR, Martinez R, Baerwinkel S, Burger R, Giese A, Rohde V. Perioperative course and accuracy of screw po-sitioning in conventional, open robotic-guided and percutaneous robotic-guided, pedicle screw placement. Eur Spine J. 2011;20:860–8.
11. Yasargil MG. Microneurosurgery. New York: Thieme Stratton Inc; 1984.
12. Lehecka M, Laakso A, Hernesniemi J. Helsinki microneurosurgery basics and tricks. Helsinki; 2014.
13. Diab-Elschahawi M, Berger J, Blacky A, Kimberger O, Oguz R, Kuelpmann R, et al. Impact of different-sized laminar air flow versus no laminar air flow on bacterial counts in the operating room during orthopedic surgery. Am J Infect Control. 2011;39:25–9.
14. Chow TT, Yang XY. Ventilation performance in operating against airborne infection: review of research activities and practical guidance. J Hosp Infect. 2004;56:85–92.
15. Allegranzi B, Bischoff P, de Jonge S, Kubilay NZ, Zayed B, Gomes SM, et al. New WHO recommendations on preoperative measures for surgical site infection prevention: an evidence-based global perspective. Lancet Infect Dis. 2016;16:276–87.
16. Kersten-Oertel M, Gerard I, Drouin S, Mok K, Sirhan D, Sinclair D, et al. Augmented reality in neurovascular surgery: feasibility and first uses in the operating room. Int J Comput Assist Radiol Surg. 2015;10(11):1823–36.
17. Skinner SA, Cohen BA, Morledge DE, McAuliffe JJ, Hastings JD, Yingling CD, et al. Practice guidelines for the supervising professional: intraoperative neurophysiological monitoring. J Clin Monit Comput. 2014;28:103–11.
18. Sahaya K, Pandey AS, Thompson BG, Bush BR, Minecan DN. Intraoperative monitoring for intracranial aneurysms: the Michigan experience. J Clin Neurophysiol. 2014;31(6):563–7.
19. Murayama Y, Arakawa H, Ishibashi T, Kawamura D, Ebara M, Irie K, et al. Combined surgical and endovascular treatment of complex cerebrovascular diseases in the hybrid operating room. J Neurointerv Surg. 2013;5(5):489–93.
20. Hacein-Bey L, Connolly ES Jr, Mayer SA, Young WL, Pile-Spellman J, Solomon RA. Complex intracranial aneurysms: combined operative and endovascular approaches. Neurosurgery. 1998;43(6):1304–12.
21. Spetzler RF, Kalani MY, Nakaji P. Neurovascular surgery. New York: Thieme; 2015.
22. Krupka DC, Sandberg WS. Operating room design and its impact on operating room economics. Curr Opin Anaesthesiol. 2006;19(2):185–91.
23. Park KW, Dickerson C. Can efficient supply management in the operating room save millions? Curr Opin Anaesthesiol. 2009;22(2):242–8.
24. de Vries EN, Ramrattan MA, Smorenburg SM, Gouma DJ, Boermeester MA. The incidence and nature of in-hospital adverse events: a systematic review. Qual Saf Health Care. 2008;17:216–23.
25. Mahajan RP. The WHO surgical checklist. Best Pract Res Clin Anaesthesiol. 2011;25:161–8.
26. Donaldson LJ. The quest for safer surgery. Surgeon. 2007;5:324–6.

6 Overall Positioning Considerations for Intracranial Procedures

Adam Arthur

Patients undergoing cranial neurosurgical procedures expect and deserve an expert team that will see them safely through one of the most dangerous and anxiety provoking days of their lives. The team that provides this service and the manner in which it will be done vary greatly from institution to institution and from day to day. While good results can be obtained under a variety of different circumstances, there are some uniform truths that we may observe.

At one extreme on this spectrum are the cases where positioning is not difficult or greatly important. When the pathology of interest lies on the cranial convexity and is therefore easily surgically accessible, the positioning of the patient is straightforward. This is true of most emergent cranial procedures. The team generally can expect that the bed will not be tilted a great deal, and operative times are usually shorter. In these cases, patients are generally positioned supine and the operating table can be left flat. Simple padding of pressure points is sufficient.

On the other extreme, there are cases where the pathology is deep and surgical exposure, operating and closure is expected to take more time and effort. Sometimes these cases involve minimally invasive approaches to safely allow operating at a depth through a smaller opening. On other occasions, these cases require extensive skull base approaches or delicate microsurgical work. These cases require more planning and positioning becomes a significant and critical endeavor.

At greater depths from the skin surface, brain retraction becomes an important consideration. The surgeon must consider how to facilitate the egress of spinal fluid to facilitate operations in the subarachnoid space. Brain retraction should be minimized or avoided and proper positioning often allows gravity to assist in opening a safe and adequate surgical corridor. With any turning of the neck, the surgical team must avoid compression of the jugular veins and concomitant bleeding. Exposure and control of vascular structures is almost always a consideration for these surgeries, multiplying the concerns that must be taken into account.

For these cases often the operating table may need to be tilted over a greater range of angles which makes it more difficult to ensure that pressure is distributed evenly over the surface of the patient's body. Longer cases also increase the stress on the operating surgeon, who must consider the biomechanics of positioning themselves and their assistants in addition to the patient. The dexterity and stamina that is required of surgeons for these procedures are certainly significant, but hard-won experience and careful planning are arguable of greater importance.

A. Arthur (✉)
Semmes-Murphey Neurological and Spine Clinic, University of Tennessee Health Sciences Center, Memphis, TN, USA
e-mail: aarthur@semmes-murphey.com

A. Arthur et al. (eds.), *Perioperative Considerations and Positioning for Neurosurgical Procedures*, https://doi.org/10.1007/978-3-319-72679-3_6

While surgeons usually have some degree of control over their own approach to an operation and over who might be available to assist, the same cannot always be said for all aspects of operating room care. Under budgetary pressure, hospitals usually cannot provide everything a surgeon might want for positioning and operating on complex cranial cases. Surgeons rarely have complete control over what anesthesia providers will present. Busy operating rooms are increasingly staffed by an array of different professionals, with differing amounts of training and experience. Nowadays many surgeons do not know who will arrive to provide anesthesia for a given patient. Even when the surgeon can choose their anesthesia personnel for the start of a case, these personnel often change several times during a single craniotomy.

Under these circumstances, the responsibility for patient positioning and for any complications related to positioning is not always clearly delineated. In a busy operative environment, anesthesia providers may not always examine patients carefully during the postoperative period. Pressure ulcers and other complications are not often immediately apparent in the operating or recovery rooms. If a positioning-related complication does occur, who is responsible for discussing this with the patient and their family? Who is responsible for ensuring that the patient understands what has occurred and that they receive the best treatment for it? While it is beyond the scope of this work to mandate specific policies in these areas, they are certainly due careful consideration.

The following chapters review cranial neurosurgical positioning considerations and provide specific guidance and illustrations. It is hoped that this material is of use to doctors, nurses, technologists, and others who seek to perform safe cranial neurosurgical procedures.

Intracranial Procedures in the Supine, Semi-Sitting, and Sitting Positions

7

Jaafar Basma, Vincent Nguyen, and Jeffrey Sorenson

Introduction

Surgical positioning is the first decisive step of any neurosurgical procedure. When done well, it can create a direct angle of approach, maximize the surgical view and obviate brain retraction. Indifference sets the stage for unnecessary struggle and danger from position-related complications and adverse effects on surgeon ergonomics. The supine setting offers the most natural position for the human body while also permitting a wide variety of cranial approaches. It is ideal for avoiding dependency of the globes, pressure on the abdomen, and unnatural strain on the neck and limbs. Normal cervical range of motion allows the head to be rotated, flexed, or extended to further optimize the operative angle for each approach. The supine position is commonly used in anterior and anterolateral approaches such as the pterional and its variations, orbital, bifrontal, subfrontal, and interhemispheric. It is standard for trauma craniotomies as well as transnasal and transoral approaches to the sella, anterior fossa floor, and clivus. Less commonly, it is adapted to other skull base approaches such as pretemporal, petrosal, and retrosigmoid. The supine position also allows for patient comfort and ease of intraoperative communication during awake craniotomies. The sitting position, a variant of supine, allows for excellent venous drainage of the brain, cerebrospinal fluid (CSF) drainage, and gravity-assisted retraction of the brain. Approaches enhanced by these advantages include the supracerebellar-infratentorial, suboccipital, occipital-interhemispheric, and the combined occipital supra-infratentorial. The brain relaxation achieved through decreased venous congestion and improved CSF outflow also facilitates opening the parietal and occipital sulci [1]. As described by Yasargil, lesions posterior to the interauricular line are well suited to attack via the sitting position [1]. These include lesions of the fourth ventricle, vermis, foramen magnum, pineal region, cerebellopontine angle, tentorium, and tectum of the midbrain [1, 2]. In this chapter, we will review the fundamental aspects of the supine and sitting positions, and their variations for common neurosurgical approaches.

J. Basma (✉) · V. Nguyen
University of Tennessee Health Sciences Center, Memphis, TN, USA
e-mail: jbasma@uthsc.edu; vnguyen@uthsc.edu

J. Sorenson
University of Tennessee Health Sciences Center, Memphis, TN, USA

Semmes-Murphey Clinic, Memphis, TN, USA
e-mail: jsorenson@semmes-murphey.com

A. Arthur et al. (eds.), *Perioperative Considerations and Positioning for Neurosurgical Procedures*,
https://doi.org/10.1007/978-3-319-72679-3_7

General Setup

Supine Position

In our institution, we typically place the patient supine on a Skytron Jackson table before the induction of anesthesia. The table is appropriately cushioned to avoid pressure sores of the dorsal-dependent areas of the body. The head is elevated above the level of the right atrium of the heart to maximize venous drainage and avoid unnecessary intracranial venous congestion or bleeding. This is usually accomplished through head positioning, flexing the upper half of the operating table to elevate the back, or tilting the whole table (reverse Trendelenburg). For simple supine cases, the head may be positioned on a loose foam headrest placed directly on the operating table. To increase working space, the head of the operating table can be detached and replaced by a secured horseshoe-shaped headrest. These simple headrests allow for intraoperative repositioning of the head to alter the surgical perspective, but care must be taken not to disrupt the sterile drapes or the endotracheal tube. Although such headrests are effective in many cases, they do not secure the head enough to permit significant table rotation. Rigid fixation and additional control of the head can be achieved with devices such as the Mayfield three-pin fixation head holder, which offers excellent stability and versatility for delicate cranial procedures and frameless stereotaxy. During application, the pins are secured with appropriate force away from the surgical field on opposite sides of the head, perpendicular to the skull to avoid slipping. Thin squamosal temporal bone and thin bone over aerated sinuses should also be avoided. If the scalp is difficult to close, one must consider the possibility that a pin has slipped. A radiolucent head holder should be used if intraoperative magnetic resonance imaging or angiography is planned. This type of frame allows the head to be precisely rotated, flexed, extended, or tilted to facilitate a variety of approaches. Neurological complications may arise from extreme, or sometimes ordinary neck positions in certain patients. In the preoperative area, the patient should be asked to move their neck into the planned operative position to check for symptoms such as neck pain, radiculopathy, or myelopathy. If neck mobility is limited or significant rotation of the head is desired, then optimal positioning may require the use of a shoulder roll or rotation of the table. In some cases, neck immobility may necessitate conversion to a lateral position.

The upper extremities are usually placed on arm boards on the sides of the body with the palms facing the thighs (army position). Arm boards should form an angle of less than 60–90° of abduction from the torso to avoid axillary or subclavian vascular injuries and brachial plexopathies. The arms should be well padded, especially at the cubital tunnel. Excessive extension or supination should be avoided to prevent ulnar neuropathy. The arms can also be tucked-in against the torso with a sheet secured under the patient's body or the bed's mattress. If the ipsilateral shoulder is elevated, then the ipsilateral arm should be placed over the body towards the opposite side. The legs should be slightly flexed with pillows placed under the knees to relax the sciatic nerve, with the lateral aspect of the knee free of any compression to avoid peroneal neuropathy. The legs are elevated to prevent venous stasis (table in "reflex" positioning, or lawn chair position).

The heels should be padded with foam to mitigate against pressure ulcers. We place sequential compression devices on the calves for deep venous thrombosis prophylaxis. The body of the patient is secured with safety straps and silk tape to prevent its movement during table tilting. These straps should be appropriately padded, and under enough tension to resist shifting, but not so much that abdominal pressure is elevated or ventilation is restricted. For transsphenoidal and other skull base cases, the abdomen is prepped and exposed to allow for harvesting of a fat graft. Venous and arterial lines, sphygmomanometer hoses, and the oximeter cable should remain accessible to the anesthesiologist for troubleshooting.

The navigation captor device is connected to the Mayfield head holder after final positioning is completed. Minor modifications of the head may be performed without invalidating the registration if its relationship with the captor remains unchanged. However, we advise rechecking accuracy after any changes in head positioning are made since inadvertent manipulation can move the joints that secure the device, necessitating a repeat registration. The captor should be positioned within the line of sight of the navigation camera, but it should not impair access to the surgical field or make contact with the surgeon. Frameless stereotaxic navigation helps in planning an optimal skin incision and may occasionally influence a surgeon to alter the head position after registration.

Sitting Position

First introduced by French surgeon Thierry de Martel in 1913 and by Frazier in the USA in 1928, the sitting position in neurosurgery has classically been utilized for approaches to the posterior fossa and cervical spine [1]. The position capitalizes on gravity-assisted brain retraction and improved venous drainage due to reduced thoracic outlet pressure for improved visualization of the operative field [3]. It was also appreciated for easy access to the airway and observation of the face during surgery. It has fallen out of favor in many centers for its association with perceived catastrophic complications, most importantly venous air embolism.

After induction in the supine position, surgical, positioning, and anesthetic adjuncts are applied to the patient. Compressive garments or sleeves can be employed to decrease venous pooling in the lower extremities [2]. Precordial Doppler, transesophageal echocardiogram, arterial lines for blood pressure measurement, and central venous lines for medication administration and aspiration of air are placed based on the preferences of the surgical and anesthesia teams [4]. Typically, the Mayfield head holder is more easily applied while still supine. The patient is gradually transitioned from supine to sitting to avoid hemodynamic compromise [5]. Once the patient has reached the sitting position, the head holder is fastened anteriorly to a Mayfield cross bar adapter that is secured to the table [3]. The legs are elevated to increase central venous pressure and avoid hypotension, with flexion at the hips and knees to improve venous return [4, 6]. Arterial monitoring should be referenced to the head level for accurate measurement of cerebral perfusion pressures. The patient sits essentially upright on the operating table, with variations in the final position of the head as deemed appropriate for individual cases.

Variations of the sitting position include the "praying" or "forward somersault" position endorsed by Hernesniemi [2]. Here, the upper torso and head are bent forward and downward. This allows the surgeon to rest his hands on the patient's shoulders and back to reduce fatigue during surgery. This position also improves visualization of deeper structures in the posterior fossa, as the tentorium reaches a nearly horizontal position with about 30° of forward bending of the head [2] (Fig. 7.1a, b).

Complications

Supine Position

Compared to other positions in neurosurgery, the supine position has fewer adverse respiratory and hemodynamic effects. Nonetheless, the functional residual capacity decreases by about 25–30% compared to the upright position; and ventilation is more dependent on the abdominal muscles and the diaphragm. In elderly, obese, and pregnant patients, the closing capacity may exceed the functional residual capacity and lead to hypoxemia. Increasing PEEP may help solve the ventilation/perfusion mismatch, and the lawn chair position relaxes the abdominal muscles while improving peripheral venous return. Air embolism is the most feared cardiopulmonary complication of the supine or sitting position, as elevation of the head can lead to negative venous pressures that promote intake of air through venous structures around the brain and within the skull. Cardiac Doppler and end tidal CO_2 monitoring facilitate early recognition of this

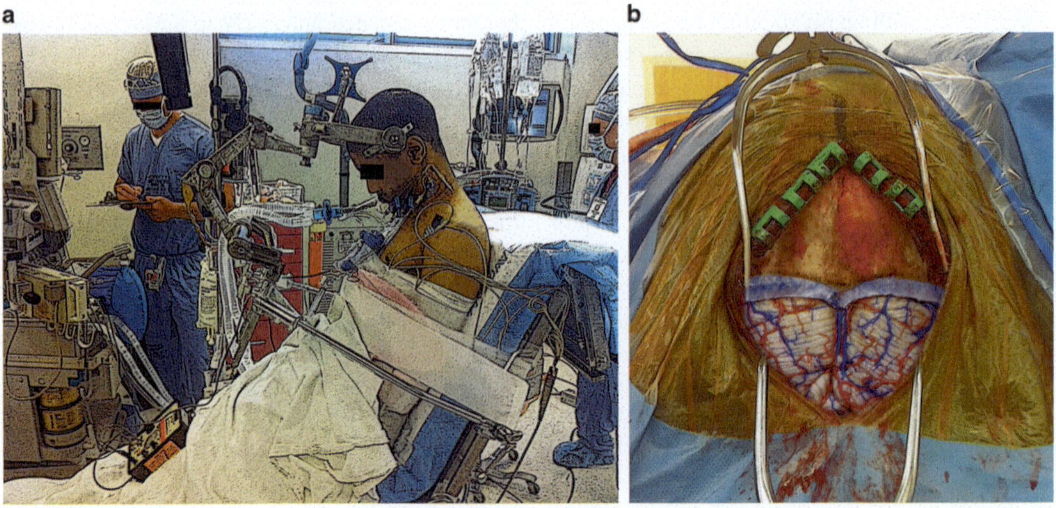

Fig. 7.1 (**a**) General setup for a craniotomy in the sitting position. Note the head flexion in this case to help bring the angle of the tentorium in line with the floor. The edge of the bed and the headrest can be used as an armrest to minimize surgeon's fatigue. (**b**) Artistic rendering of an operative photograph showing the location of the transverse sinuses and cerebellum. This position allows gravity-dependent retraction of the cerebellum, which widens the infratentorial corridor during a supracerebellar-infratentorial approach

complication. Aspiration of air from a central venous catheter in the right atrium, irrigation, and lowering the head to eliminate negative venous pressure are all potentially life-saving measures [7–10].

Neuropathies are among the more common complications of the supine position. Injuries related to intraoperative compression of the ulnar nerve at the medial condyle of the humerus may be further exacerbated by ischemia and hypoxia. Ideally, the forearm is supinated and slightly flexed to minimize stretching the nerve at the elbow. Brachial plexus neuropathies are also possible. To avoid lower plexus injuries, the arms should not be abducted more than 60–90°. Excessive traction of the shoulder with tape can lead to stretch injuries of the upper plexus. External rotation and posterior displacement of the arm should also be avoided.

The vertebral arteries must follow the transverse foramina of the cervical vertebrae as they are rotated, so extreme rotation of the head can cause impairment of flow, intimal dissection, thrombosis, or occlusion. The jugular veins may also be occluded from extreme neck positioning, which can lead to cerebral venous hypertension and related complications such as cerebral edema and hemorrhage. Patients with underlying cervical instability or stenosis are more susceptible to neurological injury with extreme or inattentive neck positioning [10].

Pressure sores, pressure alopecia, and skin breakdown in the areas of the occiput, heels, and sacrum are possible after prolonged surgeries. Backache is not infrequent and is caused by the combination of paraspinal muscle relaxation by the anesthetics and reversal of the lumbar lordosis due to lying flat, which together lead to increased ligamentous tension and pain.

Sitting Position

The sitting position has been associated with serious complications, most importantly venous air embolism [11]. With exposure of non-collapsible cerebral dural venous sinuses, the negative venous pressure gradient created by the sitting position facilitates atmospheric air entry into the head [12]. The lower venous pressures provided in the sitting position also make dural sinus violations less evident as there may not be as much bleeding. Most reported series of venous air embolism do not report significant untoward consequences, likely because of aggressive measures taken both from a surgical and anesthetic perspective once changes in adjunct modalities to detect air emboli are seen. Bone edges are waxed, the surgical field is flooded with irrigation, intermittent jugular venous compression is applied to improve detection of any violated venous structures with subsequent repair if possible, and aggressive hemodynamic support with fluids and/or vasopressors ensues by the neurosurgical and anesthesia teams [6, 12]. Ischemic complications have also occurred when blood pressure monitors are not referenced to the head. A blood pressure cuff on the leg may cause the anesthesiologist to severely overestimate cerebral perfusion.

Other theoretical disadvantages of the sitting position include that of supratentorial tension pneumocephalus. Lunsford proposed the "inverted pop bottle" analogy—where air bubbles rise to the top of a container as CSF and blood pour down—to explain how this phenomenon can occur, particularly in situations with increased CSF drainage through a ventriculostomy [5].

A recent large series of 1792 cases from the Mayo Clinic demonstrates a significantly higher incidence of complications in intradural compared to extradural sitting cervical spine cases. Specifically, tension pneumocephalus in their series occurred in intradural sitting cervical spine and suboccipital craniotomy cases, lending credence to Lunsford's theory. Their series demonstrated an overall low complication rate, with the highest risk seen in suboccipital craniotomy or craniectomy cases. With appropriate technological adjuncts, they demonstrate the safe modern use of the sitting position for attacking various pathologies [3].

Other rare complications have been reported with the sitting position. Subdural, epidural, and even remote intraparenchymal hematoma formation have been reported [1, 3]. Postoperative quadriplegia, most likely due to excess neck flexion, can be minimized by allowing for adequate distance between the chin and neck, and by preoperative screening for myelopathy or abnormal imaging findings. Macroglossia and recurrent laryngeal nerve palsies leading to postoperative airway compromise and hypoxia or hypercapnia can be minimized by using smaller diameter transesophageal echo probes and endotracheal tubes, and withdrawing these devices to the extent that their tips also serve as bite blocks in the final positioning [5]. Peripheral neuropathy, most often involving the common peroneal or sciatic nerves, is avoided with proper padding at the neck of the fibula and avoidance of thigh hyperflexion [3, 5].

Contraindications to the sitting position include significant atherosclerotic cerebrovascular disease, particularly if a patient is determined to be symptomatic in the sitting position preoperatively [2]. Severe cervical stenosis should raise alarm in avoiding excess neck flexion—a consideration for both the sitting and prone positions. Cardiac pathologies involving increased right- to left-sided shunting such as a patent foramen ovale, or the presence of a patent ventriculoatrial shunt should lead to discussing alternative approaches given the risk of systemic air embolism.

Rationale for Approach-Guided Positioning: Basic Mechanics and Nuances

The ideal neurosurgical approach provides wide exposure and requires minimal brain manipulation. Following the dictum of Yasargil, fissures, sulci, and cisterns can be dissected and surrounding bony structures drilled to reach deep-seated pathology while sparing normal brain tissue [1]. Therefore, the main goal of head positioning is to enhance the surgeon's ability to follow these natural operative corridors. The following aspects should always be kept in mind when positioning the patient: (1) mechanics of head and neck rotation, (2) surgical *perspectives* of natural anatomical corridors, (3) gravity-assisted retraction, and (4) ergonomic working angles. We will discuss these factors in general and then expand upon nuances of the supine position in several common neurosurgical approaches. Note that these factors are tailored to each patient, pathology and approach, and their modifications are guided by the surgeon's judgment and experience.

Head, Neck, and Body Mechanics

The supine position includes a wide range of possible body and head positions and can therefore accommodate a variety of cranial approaches.

The *head* may be in the neutral position—facing straight up—or it can be rotated in three planes. In the supine position, the axial and sagittal planes of the head are vertical, while its coronal plane is horizontal. (1) In the vertical sagittal plane, the head can be flexed or extended. Flexion elevates the head and facilitates exposure of the posterior parietal and occipital areas during the sitting and semi-sitting position. Conversely, extension promotes gravity retraction of the frontal lobes and improved access to the under surface of the brain, which is particularly useful in aneurysm and anterior skull base surgery. (2) The head can be rotated in its axial plane to match a natural operative corridor, or to bring the surface of the presumed craniotomy to the highest point, which helps maximize the surgeon's view and working space for superficial lesions. Contralateral rotation is often helpful for temporal, trans-sylvian, orbito-zygomatic, and lateral approaches [13]. (3) In the horizontal coronal plane, the head can be tilted right or left, which may help to level the surface of the craniotomy or widen the working space between the head and the shoulder. The surgeon should keep in mind that neck extension with tilting will likely exacerbate any preexisting cervical stenosis—central or foraminal.

Body positioning increases the effective range of head rotations—relative to the floor—beyond what can be safely or comfortably achieved from neck movements alone. Shoulder rolls can assist with head rotation in the axial plane and provide a "semi-lateral" or "oblique" setting when necessary, especially if the neck is not sufficiently mobile. The body can also be rotated ("airplaned") right or left, allowing further intraoperative head rotation. The torso and head can be elevated relative to the rest of the body to achieve a semi-sitting position, thus increasing the effective range of head rotation in the sagittal plane (Fig. 7.2). Reflex or lawn chair positions augment venous drainage and relax the abdominal musculature for easier ventilation. Similarly, the body can be placed into the reverse Trendelenburg position to obtain these advantages, but care must be taken to prevent the body from sliding inferiorly, which may result in untoward cervical traction or pin-related scalp lacerations. Therefore, only modest degrees of reverse Trendelenburg positioning are typically employed. The Trendelenburg position could be used to further expose the basal areas of the brain through gravity-assisted retraction of the frontal lobes, but the concomitant increase in venous pressure makes this position unappealing except for the case of an intraoperative air embolism.

Body positioning is particularly helpful for patients with limited neck mobility due to neurological complaints, fusion, or degenerative changes. If the neck is completely fused, such as in many patients with ankylosing spondylitis, then all head rotation must be accomplished via body rotation. Even in asymptomatic patients, excessive manipulation of the head and neck may cause vascular and neurological injuries. The vertebral arteries may be compromised by extreme ipsilateral rotation or hyperflexion, leading to spinal cord or brainstem ischemia. For this reason, and especially in patients with degenerative or atherosclerotic disease, a couple of fingerbreadths should be maintained in the thyromental space during neck flexion, and neck rotation of more than 45–60° should be avoided.

Surgical Perspectives to Anatomical Corridors

Patient's positioning is largely dictated by the desired surgical approach. Ideally, the surgeon should have an unfettered view and working channel extending from the skin to a deep-seated target, created by opening natural brain corridors

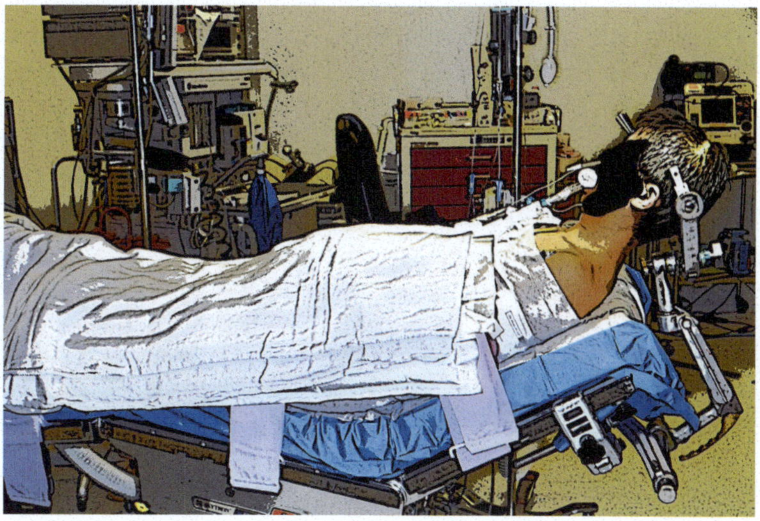

Fig. 7.2 Setup for a semi-sitting position during an interhemispheric approach. Note the head elevation and flexion

while avoiding injury to surrounding normal brain tissue. Neurosurgical approaches typically provide cone-shaped visual and working spaces that are larger on the surface and progressively narrow towards their deep apex. The optimal surgical cone is one with a wide base and a short neck, providing a wide variety of possible perspectives and a short distance to the target [14]. This is a particularly important concept in skull base surgery that has helped to inspire many of its classical approaches such as the petrosal, which shortens the distance to the cerebellopontine angle compared to the retrosigmoid approach. The fronto-temporal orbito-zygomatic approach (FTOZ) also provides a shorter working distance and wider surgical cone compared to a standard pterional craniotomy, but it also offers multiple anatomical corridors through which a lesion can be attacked. In order to take full advantage of this approach, however, the patient must be positioned in such a way that permits a wide variety of viewing angles—typically with the malar eminence at the highest point [15, 16].

When tackling superficial or lobar intra-axial lesions that do not require dissection through a fissure or cistern, it is often optimal to rotate the skull so that the highest point is closest to the lesion. In this case, the craniotomy surface is positioned in a plane roughly parallel to the floor, and the microscope is facing straight down at the lesion. The surgical ergonomics are advantageous as the surgeon's hands can easily rest on the head and a comfortable posture can be maintained. This rule does not necessarily apply if the lesion is deep-seated or if the approach requires a view that aligns with a natural corridor, such as the sylvian fissure, the transfacial sinonasal corridors, subfrontal space, interhemispheric fissure, or the pretemporal corridor. In these cases, the optimal head rotation must account for the anatomical orientation of these corridors. For instance, if a trans-sylvian approach is used, the head may be rotated to the contralateral side to bring the cisternal plane of the distal fissure into a perpendicular direction with the floor and thus in line with the microscopic view (Fig. 7.3). Of course, in many operations the perspective that is optimal for opening a fissure and obtaining initial exposure may not be the best perspective for attacking the lesion. In these cases, the surgeon should consider an "in-between" head placement that can be optimized for different phases of the operation with modest adjustments of the table or microscope. Thus, positioning for a posterior communicating artery aneurysm is typically different than for an anterior communicating artery aneurysm, even though both operations may initially gain exposure through a sylvian fissure dissection [17].

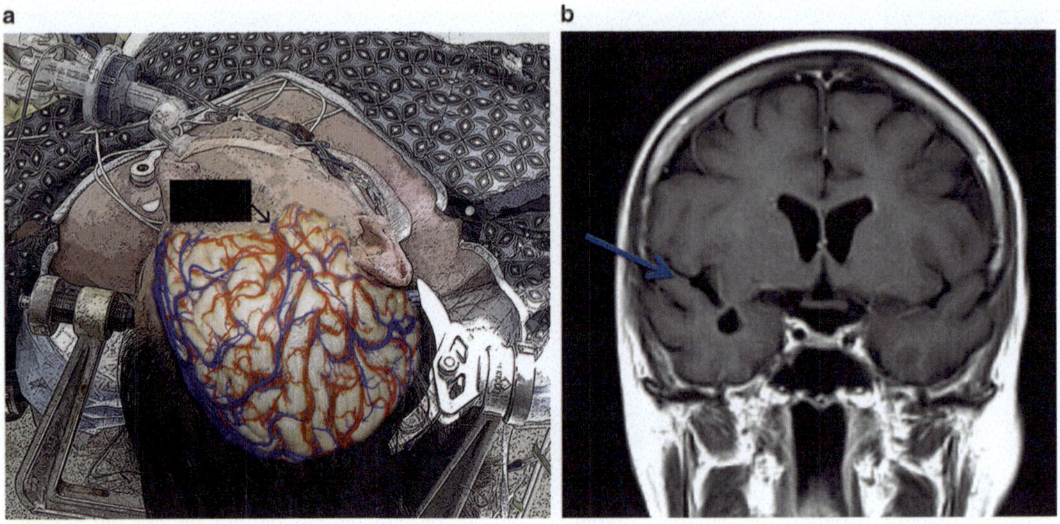

Fig. 7.3 (**a**) Artistic rendering of an operative photograph showing the head positioning for pterional trans-sylvian approach. Contralateral rotation and placing the malar eminence at the highest point of the head, aligns the surgeon's perspective with the sphenoid wing and the sylvian fissure (arrow). (**b**) Gadolinium-enhanced T1 sequence magnetic resonance imaging in the coronal view showing the trans-sylvian corridor to a medial temporal lesion inferior to the limen insulae

Gravity-Dependent Retraction

Rigid brain retraction can be helpful to open narrow surgical corridors to deep brain structures, but it may cause contact abrasions, ischemia, and cerebral edema. In an effort to avoid complications, the surgeon should strive to minimize brain retraction using modern techniques of neurosurgery, such as cerebrospinal fluid drainage, bone drilling, dynamic retraction with handheld instruments, and most importantly, strategic head positioning [13]. Head positioning should exploit "gravity-assisted retraction" by placing the dependent brain inferior to the surgical corridor so that it falls away [18, 19]. Placing the craniotomy at the most superior point, as described above, allows for gravity-dependent retraction, though cerebral edema may still result in brain extrusion. In the anterior interhemispheric approaches, the head can be rotated parallel to the floor, which promotes gravity retraction of the frontal lobe to widen the operative corridor with minimal or no retraction. Gravity retraction is often helpful in the subfrontal or pterional approaches, in which the neck is extended to permit the frontal lobe to fall away from the anterior skull base (Fig. 7.4). In the sitting position, the cerebellum will sag from the tentorium, further opening the natural corridor for the supracerebellar-infratentorial approach [18] (Fig. 7.1b). Blood and cerebrospinal fluid are naturally cleared from the surgical field, providing an optimized view of the pineal region

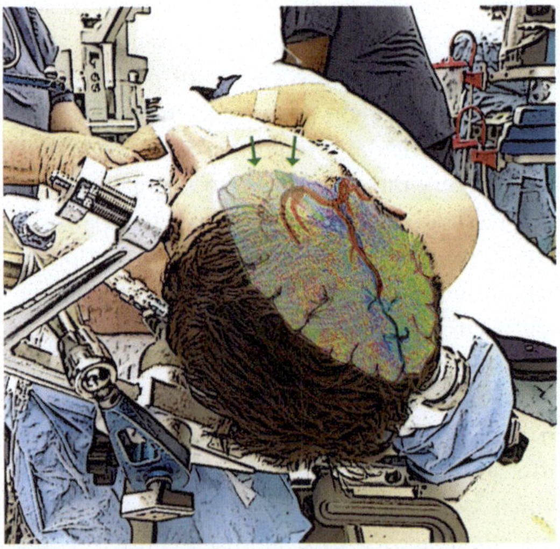

Fig. 7.4 Head extension allows gravity-assisted retraction of the frontal lobe and increased exposure of the circle of Willis

with good brain relaxation [20]. Gravity retraction has been shown to decrease blood loss, postoperative cerebral edema, and operative duration [18]. Therefore, head positioning should promote gravity retraction if possible.

Ergonomic Working Angles

Surgeon comfort is a very important factor to consider in choosing the optimal patient positioning. Whether sitting or standing, the shoulders should be relaxed, and the arms resting comfortably. The surgeon's spine should be as neutral as possible. A suboptimal working angle into the operative corridor may result in increased brain manipulation and operative time. Moreover, an uncomfortable posture may discourage the surgeon from taking the necessary time to perform a meticulous dissection. If an assistant surgeon is involved, then the head position and orientation of the microscope should account for the comfort of both surgeons, which may be different from the optimal position for a single surgeon. For instance, in the pterional approach, instead of directing the microscopic visual angle in line with the sylvian fissure, as is the case for a single surgeon in the sitting position, the eyepieces are perpendicular to the fissure when two surgeons are standing across from each other.

The Pterional Approach (Yasargil)

The pterional approach was devised by Yasargil to exploit the natural dissection planes of the sylvian fissure, the sphenoid wing, and the orbital roof. The approach is centered on the pterion, which overlies the sylvian fissure and the sphenoid wing. The surgical corridor between the frontal and temporal lobes is expanded by drilling the sphenoid wing and opening the proximal sylvian fissure to provide access to the deep structures in the basal areas of the brain—mainly the circle of Willis and the parasellar area [1]. This provides a working area shaped like a pyramid, with its apex near the anterior clinoid process (Fig. 7.3).

The head holder is traditionally attached with one pin behind the ipsilateral ear above the mastoid and two contralateral pins above the superior temporal line to minimize the risk of bleeding, fracture of squamosal temporal bone and instability. Alternatively, the two pins may be placed above or behind the ipsilateral ear while the contralateral pin is on the forehead lateral to the mid-pupillary line. Proper positioning of the head allows the mobilized frontal and temporal lobes to drop away from the skull base, necessitating less retraction. Yasargil advocates turning the head to the opposite side about 30° to align the surgical perspective with the sylvian fissure and the sphenoid wing, with a direct view of the anterior clinoid process and suprasellar area. The head is also elevated, and extended with the vertex down about 20°, to bring the malar eminence to the highest point of the surgical field. This inclination will bring the basal parts of the brain into more direct view and allows gravity retraction of the frontal lobe [1]. Some surgeons also tilt the head away (lateral torsion) to further open the space between the head and the shoulder and allow further "horizontalization" of the fronto-temporal craniotomy.

The preferred head orientation varies between surgeons. Rhoton summarized the basic head movements in the pterional approach as follows: (1) elevation of the head, (2) contralateral rotation, (3) neck extension, and (4) lateral neck extension (head tilt) [21]. Contralateral rotation (20° by Rhoton, 30° by Yasargil) with lateral neck extension (head tilt) places the sylvian fissure on the convexity parallel to the surgeon's view. Excessive rotation makes the temporal lobe fall over the frontal lobe, which can make splitting the sylvian fissure more difficult. Further rotation also deepens the proximal part of the sylvian fissure, which has a different orientation than its distal segment [21]. Spetzler has recommended 60° of head rotation for anterior communicating aneurysms (ACOMM), 45° for middle cerebral artery (MCA) aneurysms, and 20–35° for posterior communicating (PCOMM) or basilar aneurysms [22] (Fig. 7.5). The training and practice of the senior author has followed a similar scheme. Although neck exten-

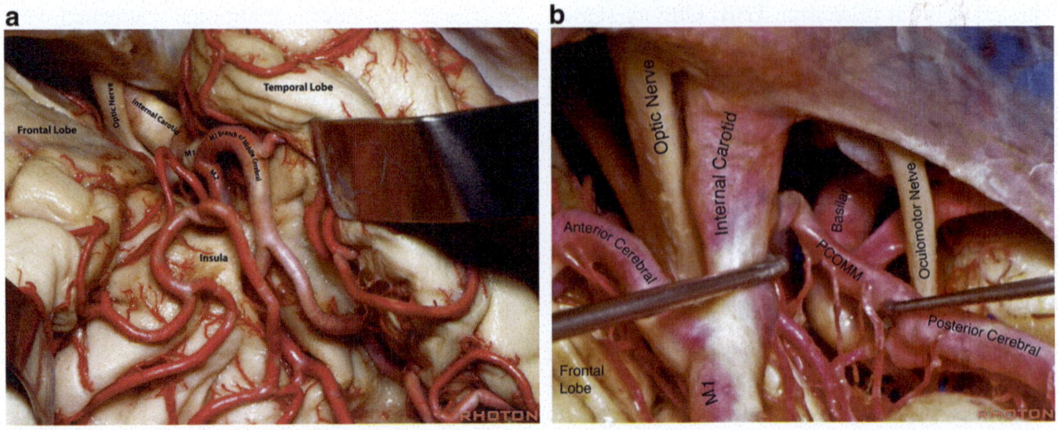

Fig. 7.5 (**a**) Increased head rotation with a lateral perspective to the sylvian fissure shows the branches of the middle cerebral artery well, but not the proximal circle of Willis. (**b**) The circle of Willis (including the posterior communicating artery and the basilar apex) is seen through the proximal sylvian fissure from an anterolateral perspective, with less head rotation

sion is helpful in a pterional exposure as described above, excessive extension may place the orbital roof and ridge further into the line of sight, and the anterior clinoid process deeper into the surgical view. In one cadaveric and clinical study, optimal head orientation was measured for various anterior circulation aneurysms. The authors concluded that proximal aneurysms (ophthalmic, posterior communicating) require less extension to keep the orbital roof out of the surgical view [17].

We believe that head orientation should be individualized for each patient and pathology, as should bone drilling and cerebrospinal fluid diversion. Three-dimensional angiographic reconstructions can be helpful in assessing the geometry of aneurysms and their associated vessels. Often, the vascular anatomy is rotated or otherwise altered from normal. This information is often useful in planning an approach and head position that provides the best surgical view and angle of attack.

Fronto-Temporal Orbito-Zygomatic Approach (FTOZ) and Supraorbital Modification

The FTOZ approach is an extension of the pterional craniotomy to include the orbital roof, superolateral orbital rim, and the zygomatic prominence. This creates a significant increase in surgical exposure, adding excellent pretemporal and subtemporal corridors while enlarging the subfrontal corridor. This approach is particularly helpful for lesions located at the orbital apex, parasellar region and cavernous sinus, interpeduncular fossa and basilar tip, and anterior and middle fossa floor (Fig. 7.5b). The malar eminence is typically positioned at the most superior point in the surgical field to allow relatively straightforward access to all of the surgical corridors that this versatile approach provides. To achieve this position, the head is rotated 30–60° to the contralateral side and the neck is slightly extended [15, 16]. A modified supraorbital orbito-zygomatic approach, or orbito-pterional approach has also been described [23]. Head positioning and rationale are typically the same as in the FTOZ approach, but only the orbital roof and ridge are removed.

Lateral Supraorbital and "Eye-Brow Incision" Approaches

The lateral supraorbital approach was described and widely used by Hernesniemi as a simple, less invasive, and faster alternative to the pterional approach [24]. It uses a more anterior, subfrontal corridor compared to the pterional approach. In a supine position, the head is elevated above the heart, rotated 15–45° to the opposite side and slightly tilted. As opposed to the "eye-brow incision" the skin is opened behind the hairline, but with a smaller and more anterior and frontal incision than with the pterional approach. The craniotomy flap is also smaller and more frontal than the pterional flap, but can be used for anterior fossa tumors, sella and anterior circulation aneurysms.

The supraorbital keyhole approach through an eye-brow incision was described as a minimally invasive ("Keyhole") substitute to the subfrontal and pterional approaches for addressing certain well-confined pathologies [25]. It employs a subfrontal corridor and is best suited for smaller straightforward midline lesions. Examples include anterior skull base meningiomas, craniopharyngiomas, and even anterior circulation aneurysms. The incision can be supraciliary, transciliary, or transpalpebral, and it is important to place it lateral to the supraorbital nerve to avoid its injury. The head is fixed in a three-pin holder with the two pins placed posteriorly on the ipsilateral side and the one pin on the contralateral frontal bone. Given the small corridor used in this approach, head positioning is crucial in accessing skull base lesions. The head is slightly extended to about 15–20°, allowing gravity retraction of the frontal lobe, and rotated about 15–45° to the contralateral side. Additional rotation is typically needed for midline lesions, such as olfactory groove meningiomas. It has been recommended to use 10–15° of rotation for suprasellar and medial temporal lobe lesions, 30° for planum sphenoidale pathologies, and 45° for the cribriform plate [26]. The bed can be further rotated for intraoperative adjustments as needed.

Pretemporal Approach

First described by Dolenc, the pretemporal approach combines the exposure provided by the pterional approach with that of the temporopolar and subtemporal approaches [27]. Extending the craniotomy to the temporal side facilitates extradural mobilization of the temporal pole and exposes the middle fossa floor from an anterolateral perspective. While most middle fossa approaches are approached in a lateral position, the pretemporal approach offers access to the Kawase rhombus in a supine position [28]. The pretemporal approach is particularly beneficial for access to the cavernous sinus and parasellar area, basilar artery and interpeduncular fossa, anterior tentorial incisura, Meckel's cave, petrous apex and orbito-sphenoid regions [29, 30]. Removing the anterior and posterior clinoid and opening the cavernous sinus, dividing the tentorial incisura, drilling Kawase's space, and mobilizing the temporal pole significantly enlarges the deep working area to the posterior fossa when accessed from the supratentorial space. Different degrees of orbito-zygomatic osteotomies can be performed to increase the superficial exposure. Head positioning is similar to that of a traditional pterional approach with elevation of the head, contralateral rotation of the head of 20–30° (Fig. 7.5), neck extension (which can be increased to 30° for basilar aneurysms) and lateral extension of the neck. The sphenoid ridge and the sylvian fissure remain at the center of the approach. After the sylvian fissure is split through a traditional pterional perspective, the table can then be adjusted to gain more pretemporal and subtemporal access.

Temporal and Subtemporal Approaches

The temporal approach is oriented more posteriorly and inferiorly than the pterional approach. It is designed to access the temporal lobe, particularly for tumors or anterior temporal lobectomy for epilepsy. The patient is placed supine with a shoulder roll placed ipsilaterally to help with head rotation. The head is extended and rotated about 45° to the opposite side. Two pins are placed at the level of the inion and the contralateral pin at the frontal bone anteriorly. Head positioning places the temporal lobe in an almost horizontal plane and tilting the head downwards allows the temporal pole to fall away from the greater sphenoid wing [21].

The subtemporal approach uses the intradural corridor under the temporal lobe to access the tentorial incisura, the crural and ambient cisterns, parasellar area, and the basilar and posterior cerebral arteries. This approach is typically performed through a lateral position, but a supine position with a shoulder roll may be used if the neck has sufficient mobility. The head is effectively rotated 90°, but also tilted slightly downward below the horizontal plane to optimize the subtemporal surgical corridor and minimize retraction. Retraction is a common cause of morbidity in this approach as it can easily produce cerebral contusions and cortical vein injuries [31].

Parieto-Occipital Approaches

Pathologies of the parieto-occipital region are most commonly approached in the prone, lateral, or sitting positioning. Occasionally, patients for which the prone position would provide the best exposure are precluded from this position by extreme obesity or difficulties with ventilation and oxygenation. In such cases, the supine position with a shoulder roll or a supine semi-sitting position might be used even though it may be suboptimal because of the limits of neck range of motion. As a basic principle, the cranial opening should be as close to perpendicular to the surgeon's line of sight as possible, even if it is not positioned at the highest point.

Midline Approaches

Bifrontal Craniotomy and Subfrontal Approach

The midline subfrontal approach evolved through the works of Durante (1885), Frazier (1913), and Cushing for the resection of anterior skull base, sellar, and suprasellar lesions. The approach can also be used for frontal tumors, traumatic and non-traumatic hematomas, hypothalamic and anterior third ventricular lesions (through the lamina terminalis), CSF leak repair, and anterior cerebral artery aneurysms [32, 33]. The head is slightly extended to about 15° to allow the frontal lobe to fall away with gravity and open the subfrontal corridor with minimal retraction. Depending on the location and extent of the pathology, a midline approach with bilateral exposure may be chosen with the head kept neutral. If a unilateral approach is chosen, the head can be turned to the opposite side by about 20°. For this approach, the Mayfield head pins should be placed more posteriorly, with the two pins in a vertical position, so they do not encroach upon the bicoronal skin incision (Fig. 7.6).

Anterior Interhemispheric Transcallosal Approach

The interhemispheric approach utilizes the surgical corridor between the cerebral hemispheres and the falx. This approach can be used to access the medial frontal lobe, the cingulate gyrus, and the distal pericallosal branches of the anterior cerebral artery [1]. The transcallosal approach allows access to the lateral and third ventricles. This approach is considered to follow the shortest distance to the third ventricle and is often used for colloid cysts and tumors of the third ventricle. The patient is positioned supine, which allows an assistant to

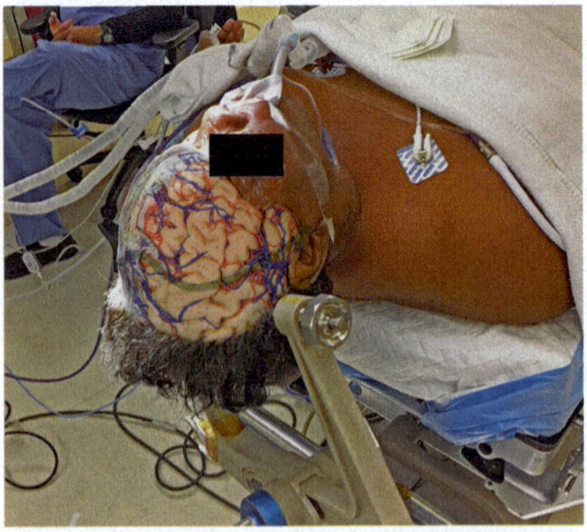

Fig. 7.6 Artistic rendering of an operative photograph showing the head positioning for a bicoronal approach

participate, or less frequently three-quarters lateral for a single surgeon with the advantage of gravity retraction of the dependent frontal lobe. The torso is elevated and the head is flexed to bring the vertex into a near horizontal plane. Midline approaches, such as this, expose the superior sagittal sinus and increase the risk of venous sinus injury with bleeding and air embolism. If an air embolism is suspected, copious irrigation should be used to flood the surgical field and any visible openings in the sinus should be occluded. The patient should be placed in a Trendelenburg position to increase venous pressure, and the anesthesiologist should attempt to aspirate the embolus through the central line placed in the right atrium.

Cranio-Facial Approaches

Transnasal and Trans-Sphenoidal Approaches

First described for the resection of pituitary adenomas by Schloffer, Cushing, and Hirsch, trans-sphenoidal surgery has evolved to include surrounding areas, including the clivus, anterior cranial fossa, and suprasellar areas. It can be performed either through a sublabial or transnasal routes, using either the microscope and/or the endoscope. Griffith and Veerapen introduced the transnasal approach in the 1980s. It is performed in the supine position with the head secured with either a three-pin or horseshoe head holder. For a right-handed surgeon, the endotracheal tube should emerge from the left corner of the mouth and the head is tilted about 30° to the left. The head is elevated relative to the heart with modest reverse Trendelenburg positioning to optimize venous drainage and decrease bleeding from multiple venous sinuses around the sella. The transnasal route to the sella typically forms an angle of about 20° with the maxilla. For sellar lesions, the head is usually neutral or slightly flexed. For infrasellar and clival lesions, 10–15° of neck flexion may be beneficial. Slight extension may be necessary for suprasellar and anterior fossa lesions (10–15°). The head is rotated to the right side (towards the surgeon) and tilted to the opposite side. This will place the patient's right nostril face to face with the surgeon to begin the exposure through the microscope [34, 35] (Fig. 7.7). Frameless stereotactic navigation of transnasal cases are typically performed with a magnetic system at our institution since it allows freedom to reposition the head. The abdomen is also typically prepped for these cases to allow a fat graft to be harvested if needed.

Transnasal approaches are increasingly performed with an endoscope, which decouples the surgeon's line of sight from the surgical corridor, since the video monitor can be placed in any ergonomic position. This relaxes many of the constraints discussed above for surgery through a microscope. Nonetheless, a supine position with the head slightly elevated is still desirable for anterior endoscopy [36].

Transoral Approaches

Transoral approaches are traditionally used to address midline craniovertebral junction lesions, between the lower clivus and C2 vertebral body [37, 38]. These mainly include extradural clival chordomas, chondrosarcomas, giant cell tumors, and rheumatoid or degenerative pannus. The approach provides direct access to the anterior cervico-medullary junction using the shortest route without requiring brain retraction. Important issues are manipulation and retraction of the tongue, healing of the soft palate and pharyngeal soft tissues, and achieving a watertight dural closure for intradural pathologies. Gardner-Wells tongs and traction may be employed to attempt reduction prior to surgical intervention, and traction may be maintained during surgery. Jaw opening should be evaluated prior to surgery because restricted movement may necessitate a more involved median labial mandibulo-glossotomy.

The patient is positioned supine with the head either stabilized with a Mayfield head holder or resting on a doughnut pad. The neck is slightly extended to bring the craniovertebral junction in

a b

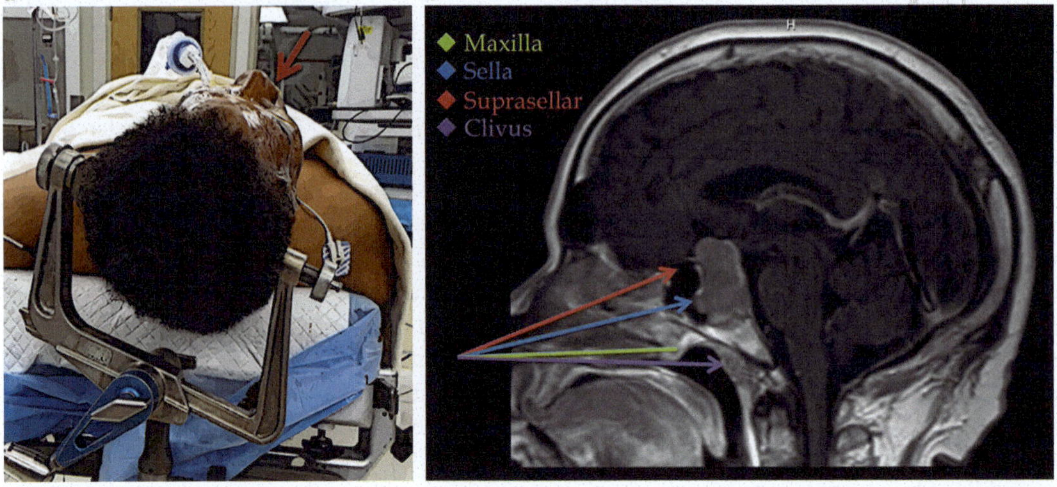

Fig. 7.7 (**a**) Head positioning for a right-sided transnasal approach. (**b**) Gadolinium-enhanced T1 sequence magnetic resonance imaging in the sagittal view showing a pituitary adenoma extending to the suprasellar space. Also shown are the angles of the maxilla and the microsurgical transnasal routes to the clivus and suprasellar regions. While extension may be needed for suprasellar lesions, more flexion is necessary for clival targets

line of sight of the surgeon. Oral intubation is typically used and topical steroids are administered to prevent tongue swelling. Many centers use the Spetzler-Sonntag transoral retractor system or the Crockard or Dingman mouth retractors. The retractor is fixed and secured to the operating table. The endotracheal tube is attached at the corner of the mouth to avoid excessive tongue compression and obstruction of the surgical view. Teeth guards are used with the retractor frame for protection. After closure, the patient can be turned prone to complete the posterior instrumentation and fusion if necessary.

Endoscopic approaches have been gradually replacing microscopic transoral approaches as they have the advantage of decoupling the surgeon's view from the surgical corridor [39]. This allows many of the operations that were traditionally done transorally to be done endoscopically through a transnasal approach without requiring splitting the soft palate or retracting the tongue, and with fewer constraints upon surgical positioning. An angled endoscope is often used for the best perspective.

Infratentorial Approaches

In addition to anterior endoscopic transclival approaches, the versatility of the supine position also allows lateral and posterior approaches to the posterior fossa. The choice of positioning can differ widely between surgical centers. Even the lateral supracerebellar-infratentorial approach, which is classically accomplished in the sitting or lateral positions, was described in the supine position with gravity-assisted retraction [40].

While we prefer to perform the retrosigmoid craniotomy in the lateral position, many surgeons feel more comfortable with a supine-oblique arrangement (Ojemann) [41]. The patient is placed supine with the ipsilateral shoulder elevated with a roll. The head is turned to the contralateral side as much as possible (more than 45°) until it is parallel to the floor. This will allow the cerebellum to fall away with gravity from the cerebellopontine cistern. It is also slightly flexed and tilted slightly towards the floor to widen the space between the head and the shoulder. Care must be taken to avoid excessive tension on the neck, and the head should be elevated above the level of the heart. The head holder is secured with two pins on the contralateral occipito-mastoid area and one pin in the ipsilateral frontal region. The shoulder is gently retracted with tape, if necessary, to prevent obstruction of the surgical view. The surgeon is usually sitting and positioned behind the patient's head with the chair at an optimal height so that a surgical perspective through the corridor between the cerebellum and the posterior petrous bone can be achieved. The table can be rotated during surgery to adjust the operative angle towards the cerebellopontine cistern and brainstem. The supine position can be used in this way if the patient has sufficient neck mobility; otherwise, a lateral position will be necessary. We prefer the lateral position in our academic center because it allows two standing surgeons to work opposite to each other at the same time.

The supine position can also be used for petrosal approaches, which entail a mastoidectomy to create a presigmoid working channel that can provide more direct access to cerebellopontine lesions. The degree of bone removal is typically tailored to the precise exposure that is needed, with the translabyrinthine variant being very common for tumors involving the internal auditory canal. The mastoid bone is at the center of the surgical field and its surface is typically positioned parallel to the floor [42]. The same considerations for the retrosigmoid approach apply.

The jugular foramen is usually approached through a combined distal cervical postauricular transtemporal approach, which is performed in the supine position. The head is turned to the opposite side, but a shoulder roll is usually not necessary. In order to allow adjustments for the different steps of this combined approach, the head is not fixated with pins. For example, further rotation is helpful as dissection is carried out towards the mastoid. Care must be taken to avoid compressing the contralateral jugular vein, especially in glomus jugulare tumors where it is dominant. The abdomen should also be exposed for a potential fat graft. For a preauricular transtemporal infratemporal fossa approach, the patient is also placed supine. The head is placed in a three-point Mayfield headrest and elevated, slightly extended and turned contralateral to the pathology [43, 44].

Asleep-Awake Craniotomies

Asleep-awake craniotomies are not commonly used in all neurosurgical centers. They are particularly indicated in addressing lesions located in or very close to eloquent brain cortex; or in epilepsy surgery, where localizing the seizure focus may be hindered by general anesthesia. Understanding the anatomy of eloquent areas is important in planning the surgical approach, patient's positioning and the steps of the awake procedure. Because the patient will have to communicate with the anesthesiologist or the neurologist during the awake phase, most of these craniotomies are done in a comfortable supine position [45–47].

Anesthesia is typically performed in three phases: asleep, awake, and sedation stages. During the asleep phase, the patient's airway is secured with LMA, and he is anesthetized with short-acting agents such as propofol and remifentanil. LMA is more suited for awake craniotomies to prevent coughing and agitation associated with endotracheal extubation at the beginning of the awake phase. Requisite local anesthetic infiltration of skin, galea, and pericranium, prior to pinning the head holder and to skin incision is necessary to maximize analgesia. Head positioning should allow constant access to the airway and to the laryngeal mask. The anesthesiologist should be able to easily remove the LMA before the awake procedure, and even to reinsert it if needed during the sedation phase. It should also permit the patient to see his examiner during the awake phase so that the anomia test can be performed. Patient's neck should be in the most comfortable position possible, his joints flexed and relaxed and his body well secured to the table. The drapes should not cover the patient's eyes, and adequate lighting should be provided under the drapes to minimize patient's anxiety.

Patient positioning during the awake phase can be problematic. The patient's comfort should be optimized, and continuous communication and reassurance maintained to prevent precarious movements. Table movements should be made slowly with the patient's eyes closed to avoid worsening of nausea. The patient should be continuously assisted with joint movements, temperature adjustments, and addressing his complaints to minimize any discomfort. Patient's ease is crucial for the smooth progression of surgery and of the cortical mapping procedure. Antiepileptic medications should be at therapeutic levels because the risk of seizure from cortical stimulation is higher in an awake patient. Wild movements from seizure activity can inflict neck trauma or scalp laceration from the head pins [47].

After the awake procedure is completed, sedation is necessary to avoid confusion and agitation while the patient is still in the Mayfield headrest. If the airway is lost, it is managed with correcting any obstructive position, including pulling the chin forward, especially in medication overdose. If endotracheal intubation is necessary, a fiberoptic approach may be employed, or the head should be removed from the Mayfield head holder for direct visualization. During the last phase, the patient should be adequately sedated to prevent confusion and agitation while avoiding medication overdose and possible loss of airway. If sleep doses of propofol are required, the LMA should be reinserted for the rest of the procedure [45].

Conclusion

The supine position is extremely versatile, allowing for a wide variety of neurosurgical approaches. Although the complexity and potential complications require additional attention to details, the sitting position remains useful for particular approaches to the posterior fossa. Optimal positioning should consider the desired surgical corridor, the patient's neck mobility, venous drainage, gravity retraction, and the surgeon's comfort. Increasing use of endoscopes and exoscopes that decouple the surgeon's line of sight from the surgical corridor will greatly reduce positioning constraints imposed by the surgeon's comfort, so that only patient-related factors will need to be considered.

References

1. Yasargil MG. Microneurosurgery. New York: Thieme Stratton Inc.; 1984.
2. Martin Lehecka AL, Hernesniemi J. Helsinki microneurosurgery basics and tricks. Helsinki: Druckerei Hohl GmbH & Co. KG; 2011.
3. Himes BT, Mallory GW, Abcejo AS, Pasternak J, Atkinson JLD, Meyer FB, et al. Contemporary analysis of the intraoperative and perioperative complications of neurosurgical procedures performed in the sitting position. J Neurosurg. 2017;127(1):182–8.
4. Gale T, Leslie K. Anaesthesia for neurosurgery in the sitting position. J Clin Neurosci. 2004;11(7):693–6.
5. Porter JM, Pidgeon C, Cunningham AJ. The sitting position in neurosurgery: a critical appraisal. Br J Anaesth. 1999;82(1):117–28.
6. Dilmen OK, Akcil EF, Tureci E, Tunali Y, Bahar M, Tanriverdi T, et al. Neurosurgery in the sitting position: retrospective analysis of 692 adult and pediatric cases. Turk Neurosurg. 2011;21(4):634–40.
7. Rozet I, Vavilala MS. Risks and benefits of patient positioning during neurosurgical care. Anesthesiol Clin. 2007;25(3):631–53. x.
8. Shapiro H, Drummond J. Neurosurgical anesthesia. In: Miller RD, editor. Anesthesia. 4th ed. New York, NY: Churchill Livingstone Inc.; 1994. p. 1897–946.
9. Clatterbuck R, Tamargo R. Surgical positioning and exposures for cranial procedures. In: Winn H, editor. Youmans neurological surgery. 5th ed. Philadelphia, Pennsylvania: Sounders Elsevier Inc; 2004. p. 623–45.
10. Toole JF. Effects of change of head, limb and body position on cephalic circulation. N Engl J Med. 1968;279(6):307–11.
11. Ammirati M, Lamki TT, Shaw AB, Forde B, Nakano I, Mani M. A streamlined protocol for the use of the semi-sitting position in neurosurgery: a report on 48 consecutive procedures. J Clin Neurosci. 2013;20(1):32–4.
12. Lindroos AC, Niiya T, Randell T, Romani R, Hernesniemi J, Niemi T. Sitting position for removal of pineal region lesions: the Helsinki experience. World Neurosurg. 2010;74(4–5):505–13.
13. Spetzler RF, Sanai N. The quiet revolution: retractorless surgery for complex vascular and skull base lesions. J Neurosurg. 2012;116(2):291–300.
14. Origitano TC, Anderson DE, Tarassoli Y, Reichman OH, al-Mefty O. Skull base approaches to complex cerebral aneurysms. Surg Neurol. 1993;40(4):339–46.

15. Lemole GM Jr, Henn JS, Zabramski JM, Spetzler RF. Modifications to the orbitozygomatic approach. Technical note. J Neurosurg. 2003;99(5):924–30.
16. Gonzalez LF, Crawford NR, Horgan MA, Deshmukh P, Zabramski JM, Spetzler RF. Working area and angle of attack in three cranial base approaches: pterional, orbitozygomatic, and maxillary extension of the orbitozygomatic approach. Neurosurgery. 2002;50(3):550–5. discussion 5–7.
17. Chaddad-Neto F, Doria-Netto HL, Campos-Filho JM, Ribas ES, Ribas GC, Oliveira E. Head positioning for anterior circulation aneurysms microsurgery. Arq Neuropsiquiatr. 2014;72(11):832–40.
18. Sanai N, Mirzadeh Z, Lawton MT. Supracerebellar-supratrochlear and infratentorial-infratrochlear approaches: gravity-dependent variations of the lateral approach over the cerebellum. Neurosurgery. 2010;66(6 Suppl Operative):264–74. discussion 74.
19. Ferroli P, Russo A, Albanese E, Tringali G, Broggi G. Gravity-aided trans-falcine removal of a contralateral subcortical ependymoma. Acta Neurochir. 2007;149(11):1147–50. discussion 50.
20. Engelhardt M, Folkers W, Brenke C, Scholz M, Harders A, Fidorra H, et al. Neurosurgical operations with the patient in sitting position: analysis of risk factors using transcranial Doppler sonography. Br J Anaesth. 2006;96(4):467–72.
21. Rhoton AL Jr. Operative techniques and instrumentation for neurosurgery. Neurosurgery. 2003;53(4):907–34. discussion 34.
22. Figueiredo EG, Deshmukh P, Zabramski JM, Preul MC, Crawford NR, Spetzler RF. The pterional-transsylvian approach: an analytical study. Neurosurgery. 2006;59(4 Suppl 2):ONS263–9. discussion ONS9.
23. Al-Mefty O. Supraorbital-pterional approach to skull base lesions. Neurosurgery. 1987;21(4):474–7.
24. Hernesniemi J, Ishii K, Niemela M, Smrcka M, Kivipelto L, Fujiki M, et al. Lateral supraorbital approach as an alternative to the classical pterional approach. Acta Neurochir Suppl. 2005;94:17–21.
25. Heros RC. The supraorbital "keyhole" approach. J Neurosurg. 2011;114(3):850–1. discussion 1.
26. Jallo GI, Bognar L. Eyebrow surgery: the supraciliary craniotomy: technical note. Neurosurgery. 2006;59(1 Suppl 1):ONSE157–8. discussion ONSE-8.
27. Dolenc VV, Skrap M, Sustersic J, Skrbec M, Morina A. A transcavernous-transsellar approach to the basilar tip aneurysms. Br J Neurosurg. 1987;1(2):251–9.
28. Tripathi M, Deo RC, Suri A, Srivastav V, Baby B, Kumar S, et al. Quantitative analysis of the Kawase versus the modified Dolenc-Kawase approach for middle cranial fossa lesions with variable anteroposterior extension. J Neurosurg. 2015;123(1):14–22.
29. Krisht AF, Kadri PA. Surgical clipping of complex basilar apex aneurysms: a strategy for successful outcome using the pretemporal transzygomatic transcavernous approach. Neurosurgery. 2005;56(2 Suppl):261–73. discussion 261–73.
30. Seoane E, Tedeschi H, de Oliveira E, Wen HT, Rhoton AL Jr. The pretemporal transcavernous approach to the interpeduncular and prepontine cisterns: microsurgical anatomy and technique application. Neurosurgery. 2000;46(4):891–8. discussion 8–9.
31. Drake CG. Bleeding aneurysms of the basilar artery. Direct surgical management in four cases. J Neurosurg. 1961;18:230–8.
32. Derome P. Spheno-ethmoidal tumors. Possibilities for exeresis and surgical repair. Neuro-Chirurgie. 1972;18(1):1–164.
33. Sekhar LN, Nanda A, Sen CN, Snyderman CN, Janecka IP. The extended frontal approach to tumors of the anterior, middle, and posterior skull base. J Neurosurg. 1992;76(2):198–206.
34. Funaki T, Matsushima T, Peris-Celda M, Valentine RJ, Joo W, Rhoton AL Jr. Focal transnasal approach to the upper, middle, and lower clivus. Neurosurgery. 2013;73(2 Suppl Operative):ons155–90. discussion ons90–1.
35. Campero A, Socolovsky M, Torino R, Martins C, Yasuda A, Rhoton AL Jr. Anatomical landmarks for positioning the head in preparation for the transsphenoidal approach: the spheno-sellar point. Br J Neurosurg. 2009;23(3):282–6.
36. Conger AR, Lucas J, Zada G, Schwartz TH, Cohen-Gadol AA. Endoscopic extended transsphenoidal resection of craniopharyngiomas: nuances of neurosurgical technique. Neurosurg Focus. 2014;37(4):E10.
37. Liu JK, Couldwell WT, Apfelbaum RI. Transoral approach and extended modifications for lesions of the ventral foramen magnum and craniovertebral junction. Skull Base. 2008;18(3):151–66.
38. Hsu W, Wolinsky JP, Gokaslan ZL, Sciubba DM. Transoral approaches to the cervical spine. Neurosurgery. 2010;66(3 Suppl):119–25.
39. Chan AK, Benet A, Ohya J, Zhang X, Vogel TD, Flis DW, et al. The endoscopic transoral approach to the craniovertebral junction: an anatomical study with a clinical example. Neurosurg Focus. 2016;40(2):E11.
40. Awad AJ, Zaidi HA, Albuquerque FC, Abla AA. Gravity-dependent supine position for the lateral supracerebellar Infratentorial approach: an alternative to the prone and sitting positions: operative nuance. Oper Neurosurg. 2016;12(4):317–25.
41. Ojemann RG. Retrosigmoid approach to acoustic neuroma (vestibular schwannoma). Neurosurgery. 2001;48(3):553–8.

42. Rhoton AL Jr. The temporal bone and transtemporal approaches. Neurosurgery. 2000;47(3 Suppl):S211–65.
43. Rhoton AL Jr. Jugular foramen. Neurosurgery. 2000;47(3 Suppl):S267–85.
44. Fisch U. Infratemporal fossa approach to tumours of the temporal bone and base of the skull. J Laryngol Otol. 1978;92(11):949–67.
45. Frost EA, Booij LH. Anesthesia in the patient for awake craniotomy. Curr Opin Anaesthesiol. 2007;20(4):331–5.
46. Piccioni F, Fanzio M. Management of anesthesia in awake craniotomy. Minerva Anestesiol. 2008;74(7–8):393–408.
47. Erickson KM, Cole DJ. Anesthetic considerations for awake craniotomy for epilepsy. Anesthesiol Clin. 2007;25(3):535–55. ix.

8 Intracranial Procedures in the Lateral Position

L. Madison Michael II and Douglas R. Taylor

Part I: Introduction

Neurological surgery is a vocation that requires detailed anatomical knowledge, diligent practice of technical surgical skill, and an understanding of the pathophysiology involved with a patient's disease process. Often overlooked, patient positioning plays a key role in ensuring the success of any operation. In order to facilitate tedious microsurgical movements around important neurovascular structures, it is crucial to position the patient in a way that optimizes the surgical approach. Additionally, we feel that an open line of communication with anesthesia is mandatory at all stages of the procedure. Appropriate patient positioning and multidisciplinary communication significantly increases the ability of the surgeon to safely perform the desired operation.

The lateral position in intracranial surgery is an important one that is used to approach a variety of lesions throughout the brain. Common surgical approaches that may require lateral positioning of the patient involve the middle fossa, retrosigmoid, posterior transpetrosal, and far lateral approaches. Surgical lesions necessitating these approaches may include—but are not limited to—vestibular schwannomas, vascular compression syndromes, meningiomas, brainstem cavernous malformation, and cerebral aneurysms. In addition, the lateral decubitus position can be used in operations involving the supratentorial region, such as the occipital transtentorial approach. There are many variations to the lateral decubitus position (LDP), and multiple modifications have been described including the park bench position, three-quarter prone position, and prone oblique position [1]. When preparing for such cases, it is important to become familiar with proper patient positioning in order to safely perform surgery by avoiding undue risk of positioning complications. Here, the lateral position for intracranial neurosurgery and relevant considerations are described.

L. Madison Michael II (✉)
Semmes-Murphey Clinic, Memphis, TN, USA

Department of Neurosurgery, University of Tennessee Health Science Center, Memphis, TN, USA
e-mail: mmichael@semmes-murphey.com

D. R. Taylor
Department of Neurosurgery, University of Tennessee Health Science Center, Memphis, TN, USA
e-mail: dtaylo16@uthsc.edu

A. Arthur et al. (eds.), *Perioperative Considerations and Positioning for Neurosurgical Procedures*,
https://doi.org/10.1007/978-3-319-72679-3_8

Part II: The Lateral Position for Intracranial Neurosurgery

When examining the lateral position for intracranial surgery, it is vital to take into account the anatomical characteristics and pathophysiological advantages or disadvantages of the patient. The patient should be positioned such that the operation may be performed in a comfortable posture while maximizing visualization of the operative field [1]. For example, unnecessary elevation in venous perfusion pressure, as well as airway pressure, should be avoided in order to allow desired brain relaxation [1]. The patient's head position may be adjusted at various angles, being careful not to use excessive force on the cervical vertebrae according to the patient's body habitus [1]. Furthermore, pressure points where the patient's skin is in contact with the operating table, as well as stretch on underlying nerves and nerve plexuses, should be taken into account [1].

With the exception of the lateral jackknife or flexed lateral positions that are not commonly required for cranial surgery, the lateral decubitus position does not appear to have a significant effect on most organ systems [2]. It is important however to understand the physiology of the cardiovascular and respiratory system in the lateral position in order to optimize the patient during surgery.

The use of general anesthesia alters the normal compensatory mechanisms of the body by depressing the carotid and aortic baroreceptors [2]. This becomes an issue when altering body position. The lateral position translates the mediastinum downward while the heart pivots in the same direction. Abrupt changes can obstruct venous return and impede cardiac output, leading to hypotension and possible cardiac collapse [2]. It is feasible that any intra-abdominal or thoracic mass may accentuate these risks, and both surgeons and anesthesiologists must be aware of their patient's total disease burden to avoid unnecessary complications. Additionally, the process of positioning should occur in a gentle, controlled manner with vital signs checked frequently [2]. When necessary, volume expansion as well as vasoactive drugs may be needed to increase cardiac output [2].

Concerning the respiratory system, after induction of anesthesia, the dependent lung areas become atelectatic [2]. While the total area of atelectasis remains relatively unchanged when the patient is positioned from supine to lateral, the total atelectatic area of the downward lung increases from 50 to 90% [2]. Positive end expiratory pressure can overcome this change.

Vital capacity appears to be decreased approximately 10% in the lateral decubitus position secondary to restricted movement of the downward ribs and subsequent impairment of the ipsilateral diaphragm [2]. Similarly, functional residual capacity is reduced in the dependent lung, especially after anesthesia induction [2]. At the same time, blood flow is increased to the downside lung [2]. In the awake patient, a shift in the ventilation/perfusion ratio occurs, which allows gravity to produce a vertical downward gradient that increases ventilation and blood flow, favoring the downside lung. In the anesthetized patient, however, a greater portion of the tidal volume is now delivered to the upside lung secondary to a decrease in the functional residual capacity and compliance of the dependent lung [2]. This leads to a mismatch in ventilation/perfusion such that the upper lung is well ventilated and poorly perfused while the lower lung is well perfused with diminished ventilation [2]. This is important to keep in mind with patients harboring unilateral lung disease because oxygenation occurs most consistently with the patient's unaffected lung in the downward position [2].

After a thorough assessment of a patient's medical history, a team approach is required to optimize the process of positioning the patient. The team includes the surgeon, the anesthesiologist, nurses, and surgical technicians. When the patient is brought into the operating room, they should undergo the standard anesthetic preparation for general endotracheal intubation, as well as obtain appropriate venous and arterial access. Lubrication is applied to the eyes to avoid corneal abrasion, sequential compression devices are applied to the lower extremities to avoid deep venous thrombosis, bite blocks are inserted into the mouth to avoid tongue injury, and a urinary catheter is inserted, if necessary. Subsequently, the attention of the operative team is turned to adequate positioning. The lateral decubitus position requires assistants for turning and positioning after intubation [3].

When appropriate, Mayfield headpins should be applied to the patient with pins located in the position that allows the long axis of the frame to be parallel to the floor. The pins, prepped with antibiotic ointment, should be placed in a "sweatband" orientation above the orbits and pinna according to the manufacturer [4]. They should be secured at approximately 60lbs of pressure in adults and 30–40lbs of pressure in pediatric patients [4, 5]. Care should also be taken to avoid the squamosal portion of the temporal bone and the frontal sinuses to decrease the risk of fracture [4, 5]. Conversely, if headpins are not used during the procedure, the patient's head may be placed on towels [6] or a foam headrest in order to prevent cervical strain. Simultaneously at this time, if nerve monitoring is required, appropriate positioning of the leads is performed.

Next, the patient is turned onto the opposite side respective to the surgical lesion. In the classic lateral decubitus (park bench) position, the patient's back is maintained at a 90° angle to the surgical table as seen in Fig. 8.1 [2]. The abdomen is free, decreasing intracranial venous engorgement, which may be seen in the prone position [2]. The patient's inferior leg is bent slightly to increase stability, while the superior leg is maintained in the straight position [2, 6]. An alternative modification to the park bench position is the semisupine position. In this position, the patient's thorax is allowed to roll dorsally about 40–50, (Fig. 8.2) [2]. Once the patient is secured appropriately to the operative table, the table can be rotated back and forth to achieve similar surgical trajectories as the standard park bench position, which may or may not be necessary depending on which area the surgeon is operating.

There are several options for maintaining the lateral position, including the use of a bean bag versus rigid fixation. A beanbag placed under and around the patient allows stabilization of the patient throughout the procedure by maintaining vacuum suction or deflation, (Fig. 8.1) [6]. This creates a firm boundary for the patient's torso [6]. A second option is the use of peg board fixation, which is the preferred method by the authors, (Fig. 8.3). Factors that favor using a peg board system are that no suction is required, patient size is less of an issue, and patient position changes intraoperatively are less likely [3].

Careful attention should be paid to padding the skin and bony prominences that come into contact with the operating table and fixation apparatuses. Pillows should be placed between the lower extremities to protect the bony

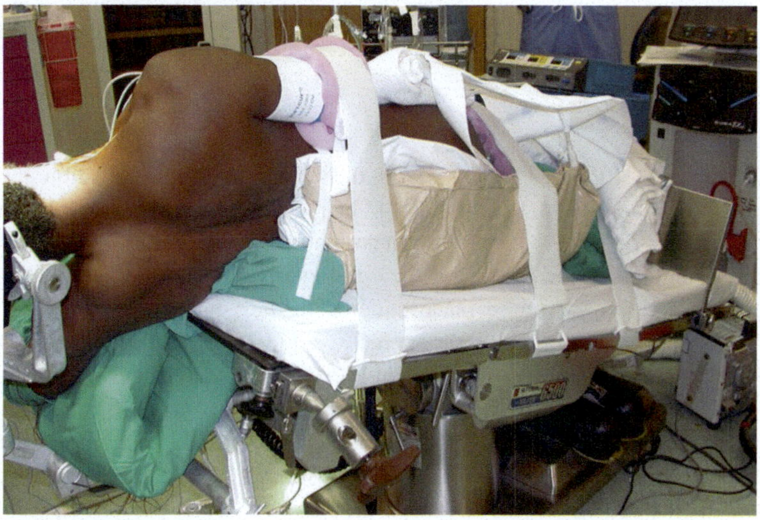

Fig. 8.1 The classic lateral decubitus (park bench) position. Notice the patient's back is maintained at a 90° angle to the surgical table. In this photo, also take note of the green axillary roll, deflated bean bag for maintaining the 90° body orientation, and three fixation points of well-padded Velcro straps to secure the patient to the operating table

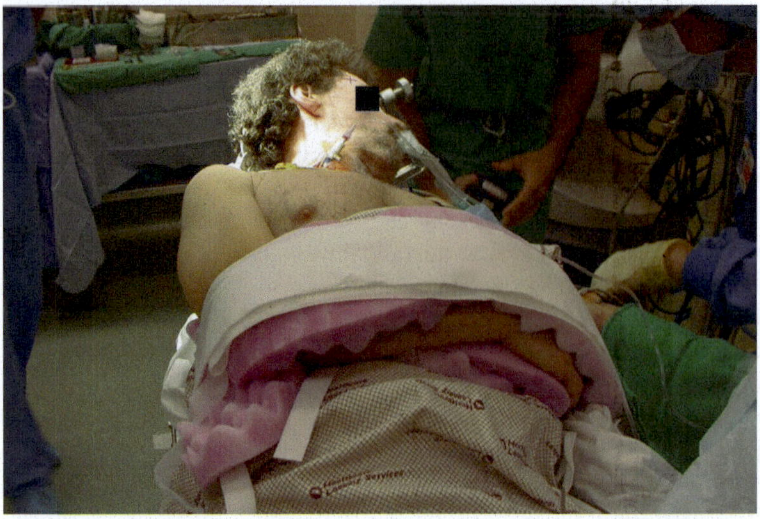

Fig. 8.2 The semisupine position. Here, the patient's thorax is allowed to roll dorsally about 40–50°

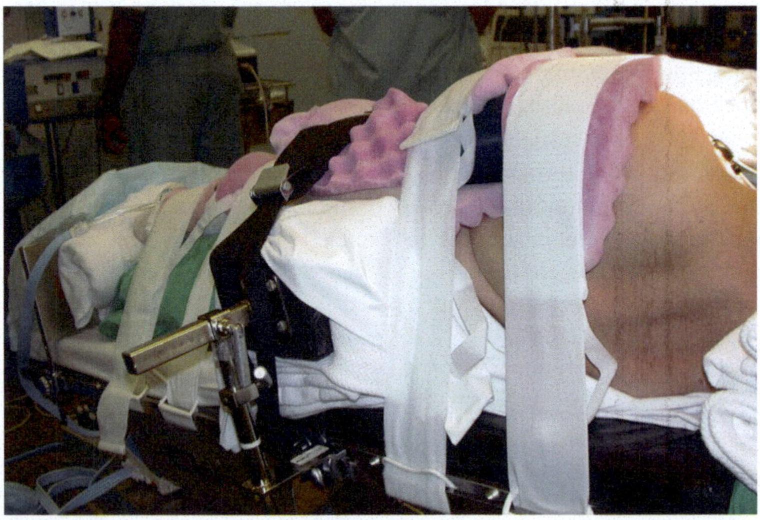

Fig. 8.3 The peg board is clasped onto the side of the operating table with a black cushion at the patient's back. Its use alleviates the suction required for the bean bag, easily accommodates patients of all sizes and decreases the likelihood of patient position changes intraoperatively when compared to the less rigid bean bag

prominences [6]. The lateral aspect of the knee or fibular head on the inferior leg should be padded with foam to avoid a compressive neuropathy of the common peroneal nerve [3, 6]. Additionally, an axillary roll should be place underneath the axilla of the down-facing, non-operative side in order to avoid injury to the brachial plexus [6]. Following this, the patient's legs, mid torso, and upper torso should be secured to the operating table with Velcro straps and/or tape, ensuring that foam padding is placed between the patient's skin and fixation apparatus. At least three points of fixation are recommended for maximal support. Additionally, a fourth strap may be placed to ensure maximal fixation. This is an important part of our practice and allows for maximal rotation of the patient without the fear of patient movement.

Once the patient's body is secured to the operating table, the patient's head—in Mayfield headpins—can be fixated to the operating table in its final operative position. Again, the subtle differences in head position should be catered toward the operation at hand. For example, when performing a microvascular decompression for trigeminal neuralgia or accessing ventral brainstem lesions, it is often better to angle the head gently toward the contralateral shoulder with the vertex tilted toward the floor, (Fig. 8.4) [7]. This increases the operative view by opening the angle between the operative site and the ipsilateral shoulder. However, for hemi-facial spasm or acoustic neuroma resection, it is often advantageous to keep the patient's sagittal suture parallel to the floor, (Fig. 8.5) [7]. Additionally, gentle flexion of the neck opens up the angle between the upper chest and the operative site, (Fig. 8.6) [7]. The occipital bone surface down to the foramen magnum becomes accessible at a shallow site, thus aiding execution of the craniotomy [1]. Once the head is positioned appropriately, if needed, image navigation is registered. The operation can then begin after sterile draping and a time-out procedure is performed.

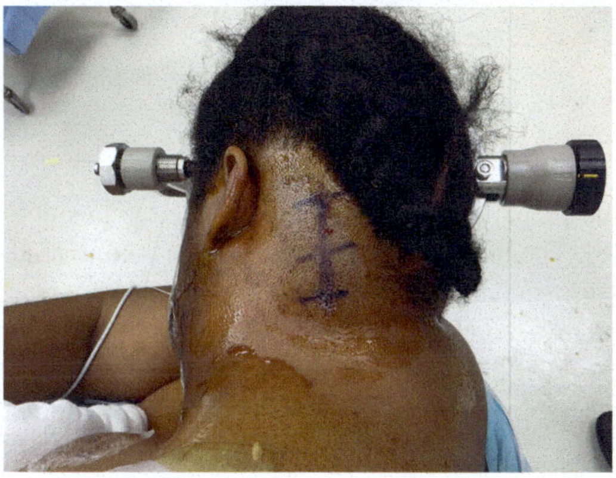

Fig. 8.4 A patient suffering from a metastasis ventral to the brainstem positioned for a minimally invasive far lateral approach with the head angled gently toward the contralateral shoulder with the vertex tilted toward the floor

It is not always necessary to use Mayfield headpins in the lateral position. Often at our institution, a padded, foam headrest or gel roll and folded blankets are fashioned to let the headrest comfortably during the operation as seen in Fig. 8.7. In this position, the headrest is taped into place to reduce movement of the head during the operation. One potential drawback that should be kept in mind when using this method is the decreased ability to fully airplane or rotate the bed, for risk of unwanted head movement.

Part III: Complications Specific to the Lateral Position

There are several well-recognized positioning-related complications associated with the lateral position, namely peripheral neuropathy and pressure ulcers. Other documented complications include postoperative visual loss (POVL) and acute postoperative sialadenitis. The risk of many of these complications is easily minimized with proper positioning technique.

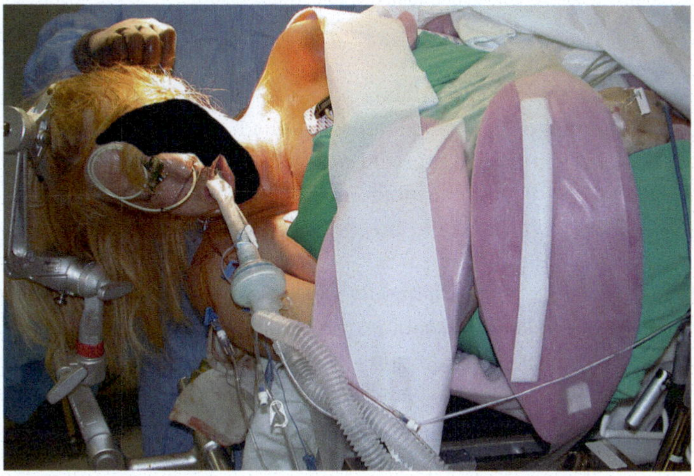

Fig. 8.5 A patient in the lateral position with sagittal suture parallel to the floor, often advantageous for hemi-facial spasm or acoustic neuroma resection

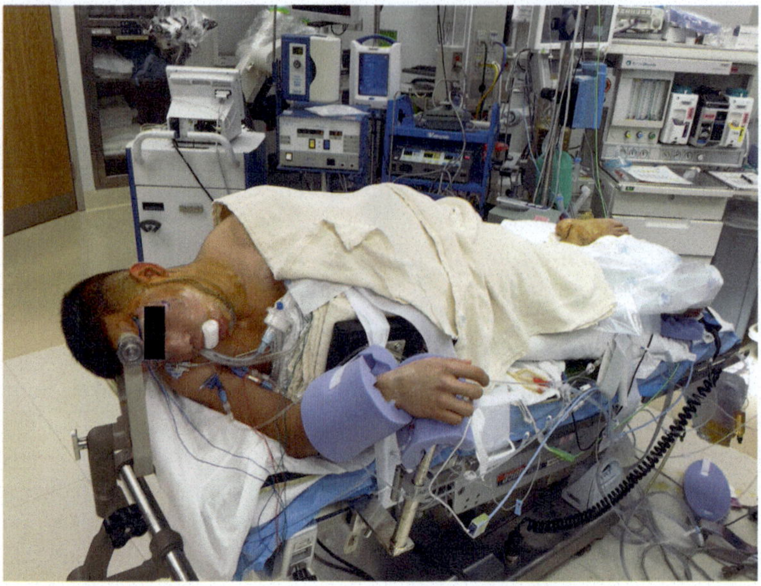

Fig. 8.6 A patient positioned laterally with gentle flexion of the neck in order to open up the angle between the upper chest and the operative site

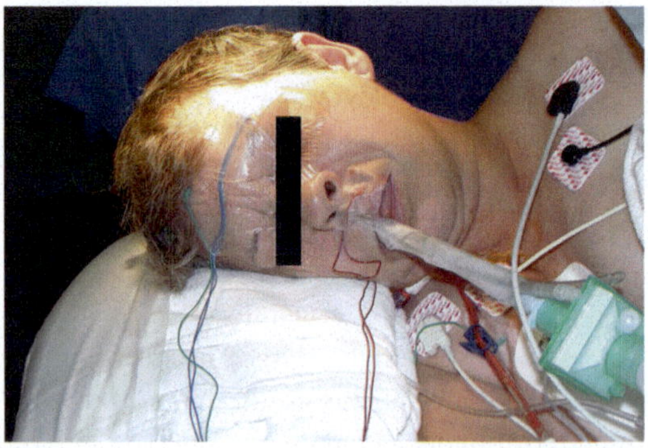

Fig. 8.7 A patient resting comfortably on a taped, padded, foam headrest, and folded blankets in preparation for a long operation

One commonly described position-related complication is peripheral neuropathy, which can be caused by prolonged pressure on a local body region. In the lateral position, the most likely effected nerves include the brachial plexus, the ulnar nerve, and the peroneal nerve. According to Jinnah et al., the most commonly reported complication of the lateral decubitus position is neuropraxia from excessive strain on the brachial plexus due to intraoperative traction with an incidence of 10–30%. Others have reported an incidence of 7.5% secondary to poor padding during the preparation of the lateral decubitus position [8]. The brachial plexus can become compressed with caudal traction on the downward shoulder relative to the healthy side [1]. Although the reported incidence of clinical neuropathy is considerable, persistent neurologic deficit is relatively rare [3]. Li et al. reviewed documented complications in the lateral decubitus position for arthroscopic shoulder surgery and found neuropathy involving one case of contralateral C7–T1 brachial plexus from unknown cervical ribs, three cases of the dorsal digital nerve of the thumb related to poor padding, as well as two musculocutaneous, two ulnar, and one axillary nerve neuropraxia without reported cause. Given the relatively superficial location of the ulnar nerve as it passes through the cubital tunnel on the medial humeral epicondyle, neuropathy may be caused by direct contact with the bed or fixating device [1]. Similarly, the common peroneal nerve travels superficially around the fibular head, making it liable to compressive injury [1].

Neurosurgical procedures in the lateral position can be lengthy at times. This elevates the possibility of developing pressure ulcers, if pressure points are not properly padded. Common anatomical prominences at risk include the greater trochanter of the femur and iliac crest [9]. Naruse et al. described an obstetric case in which a pressure ulcer developed on the intertrochanteric part of the right femur after suspended in the right lateral decubitus position for approximately 20 h [9]. Furuno et al. described development of stage I and II ulcers in the axilla (22 patients) and lateral thoracic region (12 patients) in a retrospective review of 71 patients with cerebellopontine angle lesions who had surgeries in the lateral position. Pressure ulcers located in the axilla and lateral chest may lead to postoperative pain and dyspnea [1]. The factors that were associated with ulcer development were operative time (mean duration of 11 h and 54 min) and increased body weight [1]. Prolonged tissue pressure combined with intraoperative hypotensive anesthesia can also lead to rhabdomyolysis or muscle necrosis, which may the result in renal failure [1, 9, 10].

As recommended, bony prominences are protected with foam pads. However, this is often neglected when taping the truncal regions, such as in positioning for lateral spine procedures, and can lead to skin abrasions [9]. Interestingly, Tatsumi et al. evaluated 56 awake volunteers in the lateral position with pressure sensors, as well as subjective Visual Analogue Scale (VAS) pain score analysis since the anesthetized patient is unable to communicate whether or not certain positions or straps are painful. The average tape pressure that was uncomfortable but tolerable was 9.2 lbs with a standard deviation of 1.2 [9]. While there is no formalized routine way to evaluate tape or strap pressure, proper padding underneath straps or tape with firm but not excessive tension is desired. Low resilience or viscoelastic foam should be used to pad all pressure points in order to diffuse pressure [1]. Another tactic for dispersing pressure in the upper torso and axilla is to rotate the trunk forward slightly. This was seen to reduce pressure in the axillary region by 59% [1].

In addition to adequate protection of anatomical pressure points, head fixation in the lateral position requires close attention. As indicated previously, it is important to have adequate venous drainage for improved brain relaxation, as well as for reduced bleeding, especially when working in the area of the posterior fossa [7]. Tilting the table in the reverse Trendelenberg direction allows for reduced venous engorgement in the operative field [6]. This is a maneuver that should be performed on every case and adjusted accordingly, depending on the degree of brain fullness at the time of surgery. Also, rotation and flexion or extension of the head may be utilized. It is important not to overstress the cervical vertebra in patients with cervical spondylosis to avoid creation of serious neurologic deficit [1]. Preoperative imaging of the cervical spine may alert the clinician of advanced spondylosis. Additionally, over-flexion of the neck may obstruct the patient's airway, leading to elevated airway pressure. Both impedance of venous drainage and airway can make brain relaxation difficult [1]. This may lead to unnecessary retraction, which can cause brain contusion and infarction [1]. Excessive flexion and rotation can also rarely lead to vertebral artery or salivary gland obstruction [1, 11, 12]. Furano et al. recommends a two-finger breadth space between the mandible and clavicle in order to ameliorate this risk [1].

Several studies indicate an association between the lateral decubitus position and an increase in intraocular pressure (IOP) of the dependent eye [13, 14]. Furthermore, head rotation in the lateral position from a high-to-low angle directed toward the floor has been implicated to increased IOP in the lower eye, compared with a supine posture [14, 15]. Interestingly, the dependent eye in the right lateral decubitus position (LDP) was found to be consistently higher than the left LDP, likely from a difference in blood flow pattern on neck vessels occurring from head rotation or neck flexion [14]. Increased intraocular pressure is a risk factor for intraoperative complications, such as anterior ischemic optic neuropathy, retinal artery occlusion, and deterioration of preoperative glaucoma [13, 15, 16]. While ischemic optic neuropathy is the most common cause of POVL, recent studies indicate that increase in IOP is not directly related to ischemic optic neuropathy [13, 17]. Additional risk factors for POVL include male sex, obesity, use of the Wilson spinal frame, longer anesthesia duration, greater blood loss, and lower percentage of colloid fluid administration [13, 14, 17]. Modifiable risk factors pertaining to the LDP in cranial surgery include decreasing operative time, minimizing blood loss, and adequate administration of colloid fluids.

An increase in IOP is thought to be secondary to change in body position, which alters the geometry of the neck vessels, shift body fluid, increase the choroidal vascular volume, and change episcleral venous pressure [13–15, 18]. Yamada et al. evaluated the use of sevoflurane versus propofol anesthetic in patients whose operation was performed in the LPD. While neither study group experienced POVL or other ophthalmic complication, IOP values in the LDP increased with sevoflurane but not propofol, which suggests an advantage to propofol in avoiding this complication during operations performed in the LDP. Lee et al. found that despite IOP lowering medications while in the lateral position, posture-induced IOP in the dependent eye were increased with the head tilted downward 30° when compared with the neutral of head-up position. Although this has not been specifically studied, it is surmised that in the reverse Trendelenburg or "head-up" table position, the degree of IOP elevation would be decreased despite downward head tilt.

Another rare complication of lateral positioning is acute swelling of the parotid gland, also known as anesthesia mumps or acute postoperative sialadenitis [19]. Anesthesia mumps can be unilateral or bilateral, is painless, and generally resolves spontaneously over hours to days [19]. Postaci et al. reports a case of a 35-year-old female who underwent an operation under general anesthesia in the LDP. Her head was maintained in a semisoft bandage head ring throughout the procedure. Following emergence from general anesthesia, it was noticed that she had developed swelling in the pre- and postauricular region extending to the angle of her mandible [19]. A portable ultrasound revealed parotid duct dilatation on the effected side, which disappeared 24 h postoperatively with administration of steroids and nonsteroidal anti-inflammatory drugs [19]. The authors attributed this case to compression and obstruction of Stenon's duct secondary to patient positioning [19]. Other causes are hypothesized to be related to systemic dehydration, drugs (such as atropine, succinylcholine, and morphine), retrograde airflow through Stenon's orifice during straining or coughing under anesthesia, and retention of secretions occluding the salivary ducts [19, 20]. These rare complications are likely to be minimized by using headpins instead of direct contact with a headrest for long neurosurgical procedures.

Many patients in the neurosurgical population have intracranial lesions secondary to metastatic disease. One unique problem that may occur in the lateral position is ipsilateral brain and thoracic lesions. In this situation, there is an increased risk of pulmonary or vascular compromise. Interestingly during a surgery, the patient can tolerate the lateral position well, and then have an intrathoracic mass either occlude the airway or compress a great vessel after rotating the table. For example, Fig. 8.8 depicts a patient with ipsilateral lesions in the right lung and right temporoparietal lobe. During this case, the thoracic tumor resulted in compression of the vena cava and the patient required 7 units of blood replacement during the course of the tumor removal. The importance of determining whether the patient can withstand the anticipated operative position is vital. Figure 8.9 illustrates a patient suffering from both an ipsilateral lung tumor with cortical metastasis. This patient noted that they could not sleep with their left side down. In fact, the patient slept best with their head elevated 30°. Given this information, we positioned the table accordingly with a slight turn of the head to the left and the operation proceeded without issue. The bottom line is that all patients with preexisting ipsilateral pathology need to be assessed for potential complications remote to the surgical site and surgeons should be aware of these prior to the operation.

There have been case reports of unusual complications associated with the LDP. However, when investigated, the patients involved had an underlying anatomical or genetic variant that contributed to the complication. For example, one case of hypotension arose in a patient in the

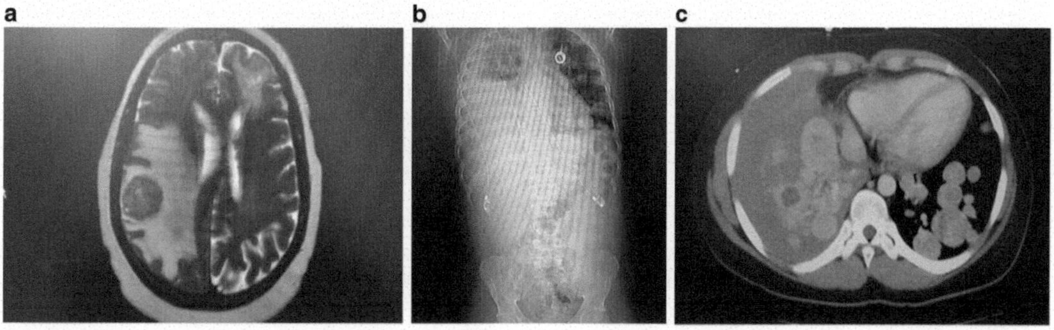

Fig. 8.8 (**a**) An axial T2-weighted MRI of the brain depicting a right supratentorial mass with associated edema. (**b**) A plain film X-ray depicting an ipsilateral right-sided lung mass. (**c**) An axial contrasted CT showing the patient's large right-sided lung mass 20

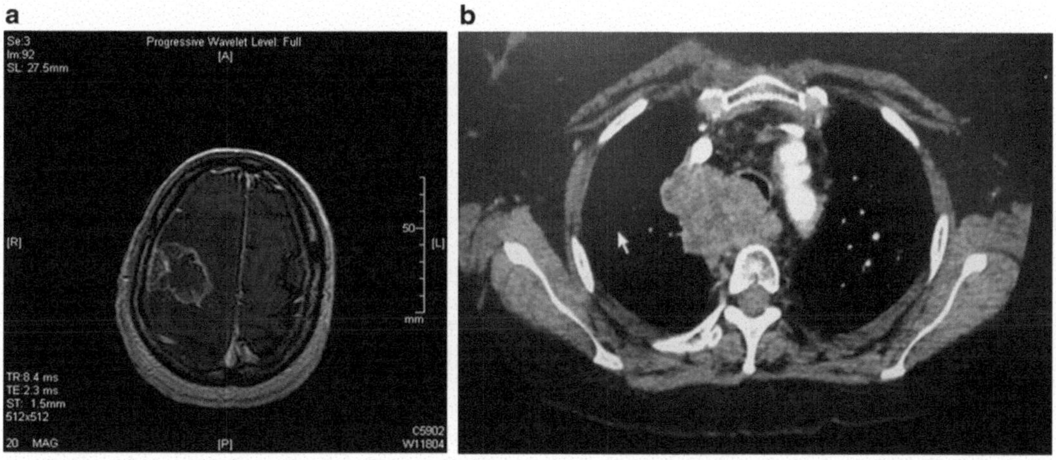

Fig. 8.9 (**a**) An axial T1-weighted MRI with contrast of the brain showing a large right frontoparietal ring-enhancing brain mass. (**b**) A contrasted CT of the chest depicting a right-sided thoracic mass

right LDP who had an abnormally narrow inferior vena cava [21]. Another case describes postoperative foot drop occurring contralateral to the lateral decubitus position in a patient diagnosed with hereditary neuropathy [22].

Part IV: Conclusion

Proper positioning of the patient enhances visualization of the surgical field and facilitates a successful operation. Becoming aware of potential adverse events associated with poor positioning and developing strategies to avoid them are crucial and necessary for all operating room staff. By using a team of well-informed and well-trained neurosurgeons, anesthetists, nurses, and technologists, neurosurgical patients can be positioned such that surgical exposure is maximized and complications minimized.

References

1. Furuno Y, Sasajima H, Goto Y, Taniyama I, Aita K, Owada K, et al. Strategies to prevent positioning-related complications associated with the lateral suboccipital approach. J Neurol Surg B Skull Base. 2014;75(1):35–40.

2. Noel W, Lawson DJMJ. Positioning in anesthesia and surgery. 3rd ed.; 1997.
3. Li X, Eichinger JK, Hartshorn T, Zhou H, Matzkin EG, Warner JP. A comparison of the lateral decubitus and beach-chair positions for shoulder surgery: advantages and complications. J Am Acad Orthop Surg. 2015;23(1):18–28.
4. Greenberg MS. Handbook of neurosurgery. Stuttgart, NY: Thieme; 2010.
5. Vitali AM, Steinbok P. Depressed skull fracture and epidural hematoma from head fixation with pins for craniotomy in children. Childs Nerv Syst. 2008;24(8):917–23. discussion 25.
6. Jinnah AH, Mannava S, Plate JF, Stone AV, Freehill MT. Basic shoulder arthroscopy: lateral decubitus patient positioning. Arthrosc Tech. 2016; 5(5):e1069–e75.
7. Rhoton AL. Rhoton cranial anatomy and surgical approaches. In: Apuzzo MLJ, editor. . Philadelphia, PA: LWW; 2003. p. 746.
8. Ellman H. Arthroscopic subacromial decompression: analysis of one- to three-year results. Arthroscopy. 1987;3(3):173–81.
9. Naruse S, Uchizaki S, Mimura S, Taniguchi M, Akinaga C, Sato S. Pressure ulcer caused by long-term keeping of the same body position during epidural labour analgesia. Masui. 2016;65(6):643–5.
10. Dakwar E, Rifkin SI, Volcan IJ, Goodrich JA, Uribe JS. Rhabdomyolysis and acute renal failure following minimally invasive spine surgery: report of 5 cases. J Neurosurg Spine. 2011;14(6):785–8.
11. Kim LJ, Klopfenstein JD, Feiz-Erfan I, Zubay GP, Spetzler RF. Postoperative acute sialadenitis after skull base surgery. Skull Base. 2008;18(2):129–34.
12. Singha SK, Chatterjee N. Postoperative sialadenitis following retromastoid suboccipital craniectomy for posterior fossa tumor. J Anesth. 2009;23(4):591–3.
13. Yamada MH, Takazawa T, Iriuchijima N, Horiuchi T, Saito S. Changes in intraocular pressure during surgery in the lateral decubitus position under sevoflurane and propofol anesthesia. J Clin Monit Comput. 2016;30(6):869–74.
14. Seo H, Yoo C, Lee TE, Lin S, Kim YY. Head position and intraocular pressure in the lateral decubitus position. Optom Vis Sci. 2015;92(1):95–101.
15. Lee TE, Yoo C, Lin SC, Kim YY. Effect of different head positions in lateral decubitus posture on intraocular pressure in treated patients with open-angle glaucoma. Am J Ophthalmol. 2015;160(5):929–36. e4.
16. Roth S. Perioperative visual loss: what do we know, what can we do? Br J Anaesth. 2009;103(Suppl 1):i31–40.
17. Lee LA. Perioperative visual loss and anesthetic management. Curr Opin Anaesthesiol. 2013;26(3):375–81.
18. Hwang JW, Jeon YT, Kim JH, Oh YS, Park HP. The effect of the lateral decubitus position on the intraocular pressure in anesthetized patients undergoing lung surgery. Acta Anaesthesiol Scand. 2006;50(8):988–92.
19. Postaci A, Aytac I, Oztekin CV, Dikmen B. Acute unilateral parotid gland swelling after lateral decubitus position under general anesthesia. Saudi J Anaesth. 2012;6(3):295–7.
20. Narang D, Trikha A, Chandralekha C. Anesthesia mumps and morbid obesity. Acta Anaesthesiol Belg. 2010;61(2):83–5.
21. Hutton MJ, Swamy G, Shinkaruk K, Duttchen K. Hypotension in the right lateral position secondary to inferior vena cava abnormality. A&A Case Rep. 2015;5(6):103–5.
22. Morgan KJ, Figueroa JJ. An unusual postoperative neuropathy: foot drop contralateral to the lateral decubitus position. A&A Case Rep. 2016;7(5):115–7.

9 Intracranial Procedures in the Prone Position

Mirza Pojskic and Kenan I. Arnautovic

Introduction

The ideal positioning of a patient involves balancing surgical comfort and optimal lesion exposure against the risks related to the patient's position [1]. The prone position is commonly used for approaches to the posterior fossa and suboccipital regions, for posterior approaches to the spine, and for approaches to posterior parietal and occipital regions as well as the pineal region. Because of the relatively higher complication rate of the sitting and semi-sitting positions, specifically due to venous air embolism, the prone position and its modifications (Concorde, arm-down Concorde, and semi-prone) are becoming more important in everyday surgical practice. Semi-prone, also known as the three-quarter prone or lateral oblique position, is discussed in Chap. 7 (Intracranial Procedures in the Lateral Position).

M. Pojskic
Department of Neurosurgery, Philipps University Marburg, Marburg, Germany

Department of Neurosurgery, Semmes-Murphey Clinic, University of Tennessee, Memphis, TN, USA

K. I. Arnautovic (✉)
Department of Neurosurgery, Semmes-Murphey Clinic, University of Tennessee, Memphis, TN, USA

Physiology of the Prone Position

The prone position is logistically a somewhat demanding position because of the challenges associated with providing adequate oxygenation, ensuring adequate ventilation, maintaining hemodynamics, and securing intravenous lines and the tracheal tube. Access to the patient's airway is poor, and pressure sores, vascular compression, brachial plexus injuries, air embolism, blindness, and/or quadriplegia can potentially occur [1]. Turning the patient prone from the supine position may increase intra-abdominal pressure, decrease venous return to the heart, and increase systemic and pulmonary vascular resistance. With either the head-up tilt or with the patient kneeling with flexed lower legs, venous blood pools in the lower part of the body, decreasing venous return and causing hypotension. For operations in the prone position, the patient is placed in a reverse Trendelenburg position of approximately 15° to promote venous drainage. Data suggest that the left ventricular ejection fraction and cardiac index may decrease, potentially causing hemodynamic instability. Oxygenation and oxygen delivery, however, may improve with prone positioning because of the improved matching of ventilation and perfusion, which occurs for three reasons. First, perfusion of the entire lungs improves. Secondly, the increase in intra-abdominal pressure decreases chest wall compliance, which, under positive-

A. Arthur et al. (eds.), *Perioperative Considerations and Positioning for Neurosurgical Procedures*,
https://doi.org/10.1007/978-3-319-72679-3_9

pressure ventilation, improves ventilation of the dependent zones of the lung. Thirdly, previously atelectatic dorsal zones of the lungs may open [1, 2]. When moving a patient into the prone position, an almost universal finding is a decrease in cardiac index (CI), up to an average of 24% [2, 3]. This was mainly as a result of decreasing stroke volume with little change in heart rate. Of the three factors involved in cardiac output (preload, afterload, and contractility), it seems likely that decreased preload was most to blame—compression of the inferior vena cava (IVC) reducing venous return to the heart. When the IVC is obstructed, blood uses a collateral return route—the vertebral wall venous plexuses [3].

The characteristic challenges with prone position include disconnection of pulse oximetry, the arterial line, and the tracheal tube, leading to hypoventilation, desaturation, hemodynamic instability, and altered anesthetic depth. To prevent complications from anesthesia, pulse oximetry and the arterial line could be left connected during the turn from supine to prone. Monitoring invasive blood pressure is especially important in patients with heart or lung disease and in trauma patients. For uncomplicated elective surgeries, when invasive blood pressure monitoring is not used, standard ASA monitoring could be applied [1, 4].

Influence of the Prone Position on Intracranial Pressure

It has been repeatedly observed that intracranial pressure (ICP) is lower in patients with supratentorial lesions operated on in the supine position than in those with infratentorial lesions operated on in the prone position [5].

Space-occupying lesions in the small infratentorial compartment induce higher ICP when compared with space-occupying lesions in the greater supratentorial compartment because the volume-pressure curve switches to the left. Rasmussen and Cold conducted two studies of ICP measurement during surgery with patients in the prone position, one regarding patients who underwent surgery for infratentorial lesions and one of those undergoing surgery for occipital lobe lesions. In both studies, ICP and jugular bulb pressure were significantly higher in patients in the prone position compared to those in the lateral and supine positions. The high levels of ICP during intracranial surgery with patients in the prone position (average of 18.3 mmHg for occipital lesions and 21.0 for infratentorial lesions) are associated with high jugular venous pressure (14.3 mmHg for occipital lesions and 12.1 mmHg for infratentorial lesions). The prone position also increases ICP and decreases cerebral perfusion pressure in patients with subarachnoid hemorrhage and acute respiratory distress syndrome [6]. Subdural ICP measurement can be used as a guide to prevent cerebral swelling after the dura is opened. Thresholds at which moderate cerebral swelling occurs are identical in supratentorial and infratentorial surgery. At an ICP below 5–7 mmHg, swelling rarely occurs. Above 13 mmHg, some degree of swelling is likely, and at 26 mmHg, pronounced swelling occurs. Therefore, when the ICP value reaches 13 mmHg, therapeutic measures to reduce it should be initiated [7].

The elevation of abdominal pressure leads to elevation of ICP. Transfer of pressure through the central venous system or by the cerebrospinal fluid (CSF) has been proposed as an explanation [8]. For this reason, laparoscopy should be used cautiously in patients with a baseline elevated ICP or head trauma, as intracranial pressure significantly increases with abdominal insufflation [9]. Prone position modifications that may reduce the ICP are placing the patient on the open frame Jackson table or on Wilson frame to allow for abdominal excursion along with how much this decreases the ICP.

Mechanical ventilation in the prone position and the use of positive end-expiratory pressure (PEEP) are frequently used techniques that improve oxygenation in patients at risk of respiratory failure [10]. Prone positioning can increase intracranial pressure (ICP) in patients with intracranial pathology by impairing jugular venous outflow [11]. PEEP can increase ICP and decrease mean arterial pressure, both resulting in decreased cerebral perfusion pressure (CPP) [12] by increasing central venous pressure and by impeding cerebral venous return to the right atrium. Consequently, in acutely brain-injured patients, ventilation goals are often in conflict with ICP control strategies [13, 14].

Recent study shows that in patients without head injury, ICP may increase in prone position, whereas the effect due to PEEP of 8 cm H_2O is negligible. TCD-derived formulae and optic nerve sheath diameter (ONSD) ultrasound measurement can be safe and easy techniques to non-invasively detect ICP, but ONSD seems to have the best performance in the detection of changes of body position [13].

The Full Prone Position: Technique and General Considerations

For purpose of this chapter, we will show the standard positioning for patient undergoing Chiari Type I Malformation surgery. These steps are standardized when performing the surgery of the posterior fossa, the pineal region and the occipital area. The different angles at which the surgical field has been observed is then achieved by manipulating the operative table. The first step in achieving an optimal prone position is to prepare the operating table (Fig. 9.1).

For the prone position, the patient is first anesthetized in the supine position on a bed or stretcher; the head is secured in a three-pronged head holder before the patient is turned prone [15] (Fig. 9.2).

A three-pronged head holder (e.g., the Mayfield head clamp) is often used to stabilize and maintain the head position of a patient during intracranial or posterior cervical spine surgeries. In adults, 60–80 pounds of force is applied across the three-point clamp to provide adequate fixation. In pediatric patients older than 3 years, a force of 30–40 pounds is applied, although for children ages 3–10 years, a horseshoe headrest can be used as an alternative. Complications associated with the use of the head clamp may include local puncture-site infection, scalp-vessel bleeding, air embolism, shunt-tube damage, epidural hematoma, chin and forehead pressure, skin necrosis, slippage of joints to the operating table, clamp breakage due to pressure of the transversal, and, rarely, depressed skull fracture. Twenty-six complications directly related to the use of head holders were identified through 19 papers published from 1981 to 2014: mainly skull fractures with or without a dural laceration (50%), epidural hematomas (23.8%), skull fractures with or without a dural laceration (50%), and air embolism (9.5%) [16]. To prevent these

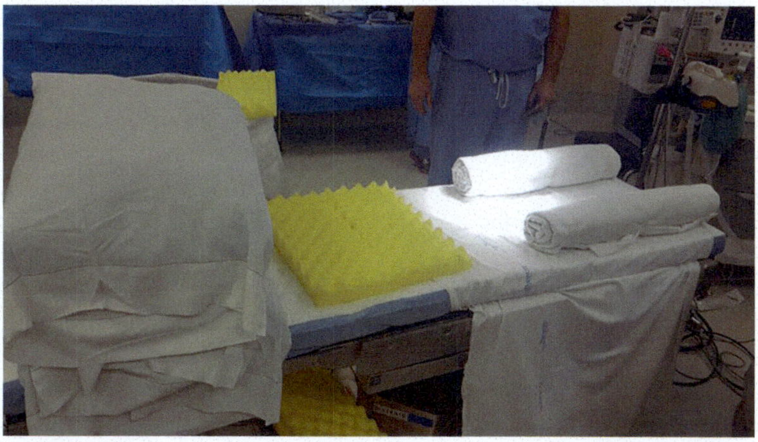

Fig. 9.1 Table setting for surgery in prone position. We use a standard sliding operating table. Note the previously prepared chest rolls, kneepads, padded footboard for the feet as well as pillows for elevation of the feet. Under the mattress is a towel which after the positioning is being performed is rolled around the positioned patient and secured with clamps

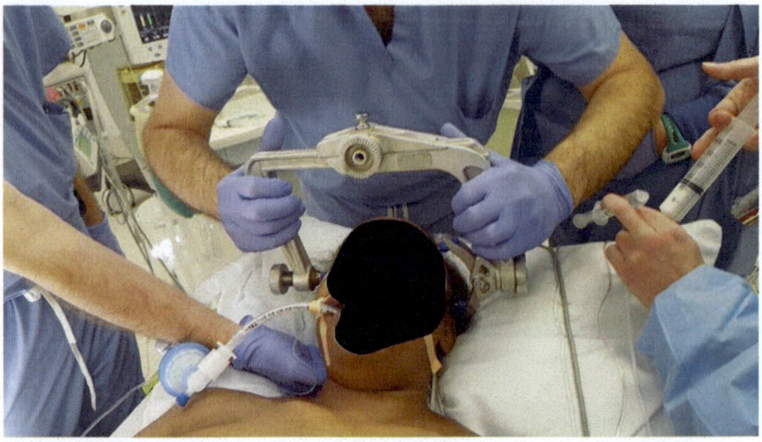

Fig. 9.2 First step in positioning the patient is to secure the head in a three-pronged head holder

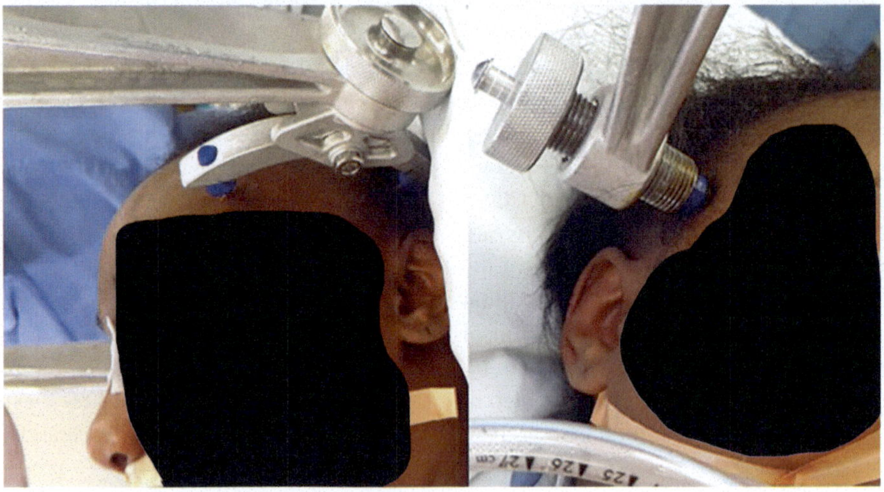

Fig. 9.3 Position of pins of three-pronged head holder (Mayfield)

complications, the surgeon must take special care when fixing the head; for the prone position, the pins should be positioned two fingerbreadths above the external meatus. The pins must be placed correctly to avoid the areas of the frontal sinus, temporal fossa, major blood vessels, nerves, previous bone flaps, bone defect, abnormally thin or disease involved bone. The skull clamp must be applied along the centerline of the patient's head with the pins entering the skull perpendicularly; the chin and forehead should not be in direct contact with the rocker arm because of the risk of pressure necrosis [16]. Pin positioning is also important to prevent pin sliding, skin laceration, and loosening of the head (Fig. 9.3).

It is often necessary to disconnect intravenous or arterial catheters and the tracheal tube (if in position) during body positioning and during rotation/movement of the operating table. These changes sometimes create a complete "blackout" state, when the patient may not be monitored or oxygenated. Therefore, pulse oximetry and blood pressure should be monitored throughout positioning whenever possible, and chest tubes should not be clamped. The head should be kept neutral. All catheters, invasive monitors, and the tracheal tube should be carefully secured before the patient is turned prone.

In order to move a patient from the supine position on a stretcher to the prone position on the procedure table, there are few standard steps

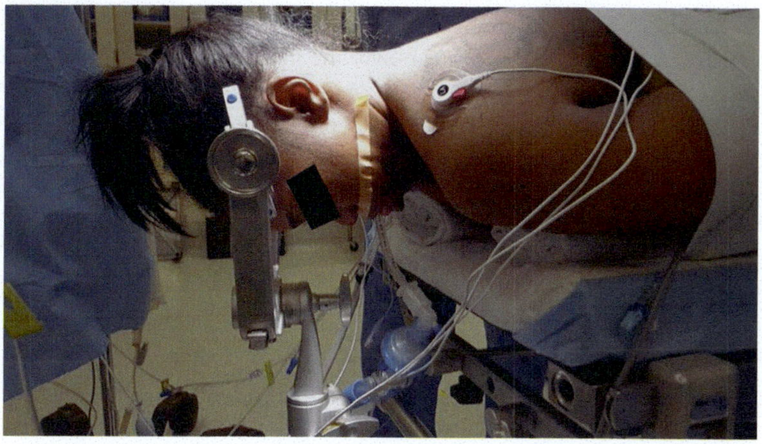

Fig. 9.4 Head positioning for the Chiari decompression. Note the slight anteroflexion. Special consideration is being taken in preserving the physiological cervical alignment as well as preventing the pressure sores of the chin and forehead

which need to be done [17]. First of all, make sure an adequate number of personnel are available to accomplish this maneuver safely (minimum of four). Anti-embolic or sequential compression stockings must be applied before. Ensure that the table and the stretcher are of equal heights and safely locked in position. Note the position of all lines and tubes and place the patient's arms at the sides. To avoid pinching the arm between the stretcher and the table or a possible shoulder dislocation, be sure that the arm that will be the down-side arm is secure [17].

To move the patient into the prone position, we use a log roll maneuver. The anesthesia provider coordinates the move and is responsible for the patient's head. Turners turn the patient from the stretcher side and receivers receive the patient on outstretched arms from the opposite side of the table. An additional assistant stands at the patient's feet. Remember to lift, not pull. Lifting will avoid shearing, which can result in tissue injury [17].

Once the patient has been successfully turned, the head will face down in a head support device. The core rule of positioning of the head is the preservation of the physiological cervical alignment. Therefore, hyperflexion or hyperextension should be avoided. For Chiari decompression, we would slightly perform a slight anteroflexion in order to expose the craniovertebral junction (Fig. 9.4), lesions of posterior fossa and pineal region require even more anteroflexion. Lesions of the occipital lobes could be positioned either in moderate flexion or extension. Changing the position of the table during the procedure (Trendelenburg and reverse-Trendelenburg) provides better view of the surgical field at the given moment of surgery.

It is essential to perform the preoperative neck evaluation in every patient. Between 17 and 86% of patients with rheumatoid arthritis will have evidence of cervical spine disease 5 years after diagnosis. The main concern is an iatrogenic spinal cord injury during the positioning of the head and neck during the intubation phase of the procedure, as well as when assessing the amount of flexion and extension in prone position. To overcome this, any patient with a spine classed as unstable the anesthetist may perform an awake fiber-optic intubation in place of the traditional intubation [18]. While there are no clinical guidelines regarding preoperative imaging of the cervical spine in patients with RA, clinicians must be aware of the risk of cervical instability, which may be asymptomatic. If performed, radiology imaging should include at least flexion-extension views of the cervical spine [19]. When placing patient prone special care needs to be taken when osteoporosis, instability in the cervical spine as well as metastatic spine disease are present.

Protecting the eyes is paramount, and appropriate lubrication and closure of the eyelids are necessary. The eyes are at particular risk for compression injuries. Direct pressure on the eyes should be avoided by not using a horseshoe-shaped headrest. The eyes should be gently taped shut. The patient's chin must be free of the table and frame.

Pressure sores (e.g., on eyes, breasts, the penis, soft tissue at the joints, ears) are the most frequent complications of prone positioning [15]. Prone position caries a high risk of eye compression, venous embolism, increased airway pressure, edema of face, tongue and neck, endotracheal tube migration as well as hypotension and dysrhythmias.

Special frames (e.g., Wilson, Relton-Hall, Andrews), which support the chest but leave the abdominal wall and pelvis free, may be used, as well as chest rolls. We prefer to use chest rolls in form of rolled sheets, as they are less traumatic to the breast, especially in female patient, furthermore chest rolls in contrast to frames do not press the diaphragm on its entire length and so enable the free motion of the abdomen (Fig. 9.5). Free movement of the abdominal wall is desirable for three reasons: improved excursion of the diaphragm and improved oxygenation ventilation, a decrease in intra-abdominal pressure and surgical bleeding, and improvement of venous return from the legs and pelvis [1]. Monitoring intra-abdominal pressure with an intravesicular transducer can be considered for high-risk patients or high-risk procedures.

The breasts, especially in women, must be medially displaced, with no pressure on the nipples. Large breasts are subject to greater direct pressure and these can be in exceptional cases moved laterally so that the patient's weight does not injure them. In addition, patients with breast implants have a theoretical risk of rupture and risk of breast necrosis with the direct pressure applied in prone position [20, 21]. The groin and knees should be appropriately padded, and the abdomen kept as free as possible. The femoral artery or peripheral leg pulses should be checked and recorded as they are an indicator that the abdominal aorta and femoral vessels are not unduly compressed. The presence of these pulses is evidence that the renal arteries are patent, with adequate perfusion to the kidneys. The male genitalia should be confirmed to be in a downward natural position to avoid compression or torsion injury. The electrocautery grounding plate must not be permitted to touch them.

The arms are positioned at the patient's side, with the palms facing the patient and the thumbs down. To prevent nerve compression, appropriate supportive padding should be used under bony surfaces where superficial nerves are known to travel. The axillas, elbows, and hands are padded. The shoulders may be taped so that they do not drift, and the arterial arm pulse should be checked after taping to detect any obstruction of blood flow [15]. If abduction is used, great care must be exercised to prevent hyperextension of the arms, thereby avoiding injury to the brachial plexus. Arm abduction, however, impedes the position of the surgeon [1] (Fig. 9.6).

Full neck flexion can be reduced with proper head and neck support. Body alignment is very important and should be confirmed by the surgical team. The cervical spine should be in alignment with the rest of the spine, with no torsion or

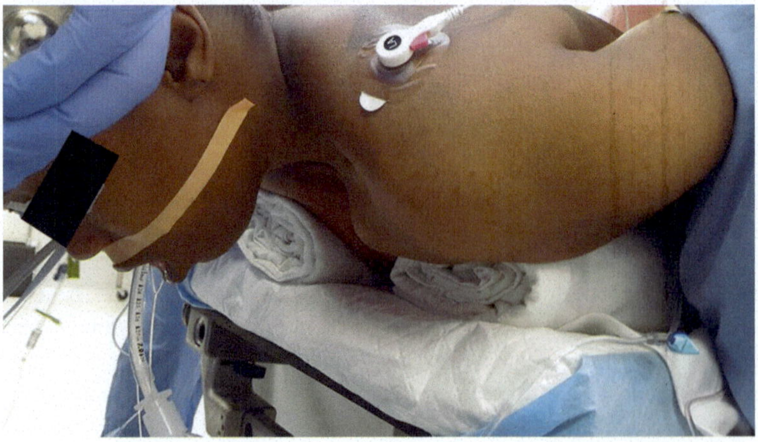

Fig. 9.5 Note the chest rolls with medially placed breasts. Chest rolls stretch from acromioclavicular joints to iliac crest, allowing chest movement and decreasing abdominal pressure. Be careful that the chest roll does not extend beyond the iliac crest, as this would compress the femoral nerve and artery [17]

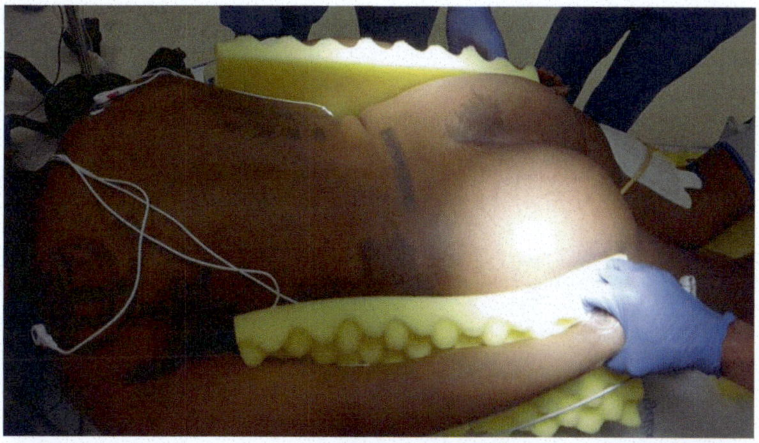

Fig. 9.6 Palms are turned inwards and padded with foam pads

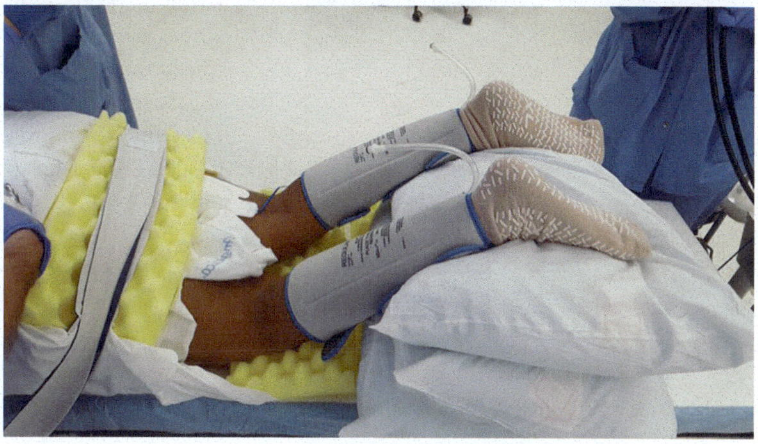

Fig. 9.7 Positioning of the legs. Sequential compression devices are applied to prevent blood clot formation in lower extremities

twisting, and the legs parallel to each other. A foot support or other method of stabilization, such as a belt apparatus placed strategically, may also be necessary to keep the patient from sliding down the table. The patient's feet should be kept off the bed surface to prevent pressure sores. Padding should be placed under each patella of the knee joints. A pillow should be placed under the ankle joints to elevate the foot to relieve tension on the sciatic nerve and prevent the toes from resting on the OR table mattress (Fig. 9.7).

The patient's face must be carefully checked when positioning is completed and the headrest and head should stay in the same relative positions. A chin bar can be used to reduce soft-tissue compression, and a bite block prevents tongue compression. In addition, oral airways can put increased pressure on the tongue, which should be taken into consideration. There should be no movement of the patient down the table, nor should the surgeon reposition the head during surgery without specifically checking for pressure on the patient's face. Obese patients may be at particular risk because of restricted diaphragmatic movement and high intrathoracic pressure [22] (Fig. 9.8).

The safety strap should not be placed until after the patient has been positioned. If the safety strap is placed prior to the positioning, such as during movement of the patient on the OR table, the safety strap could cause shearing and friction injuries.

After positioning of the arms and the legs as well as checking the potential pressure sites (acromion processes, breasts, iliac crest, male genitalia, patellae, and toes) the towel which lies underneath the chest rolls and the kneepads is being rolled around the patient and secured with clamps. Additional tape is stretched between shoulders and the foot pillows, retracting the shoulders posteriorly (Figs. 9.9 and 9.10).

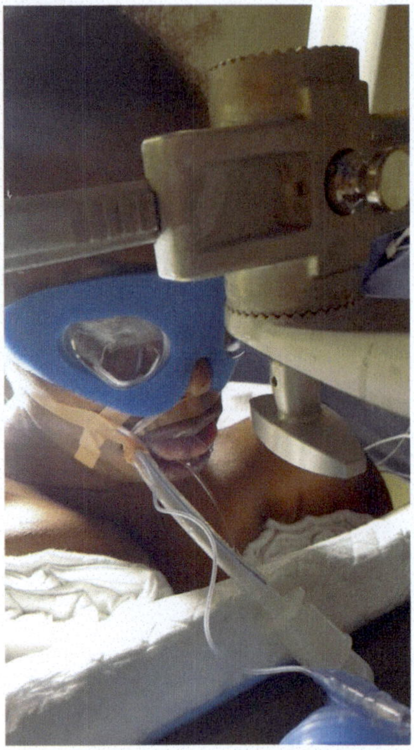

Fig. 9.8 Face position. Chin is not being compressed. Eyes are shut with tape with protective padded glasses. For procedures with motor evoked potential monitoring we include the bite block for the teeth which is not included in this slide

The Concorde Position: Technique and General Considerations

The Concorde position is a modification of the prone position and is used for occipital, transtentorial, and supracerebellar infratentorial surgical approaches. In this modification, the patient's head is typically skeletally flexed and fixed, but may be laterally flexed if needed. The body is placed in the reverse-Trendelenburg position and chest rolls are placed under the trunk. The patient's arms are tucked alongside the trunk, and the knees are flexed [1].

Positions used for pineal surgery include the sitting, prone, and semi-prone. In 1983, Kobayashi and associates [9] described a modified prone position, the Concorde position, for supracerebellar infratentorial approaches to this area. In this modification, the patient is placed prone as far to the surgeon's side of the operating table as possible, and the patient's head is fixed in the head frame with the head flexed and elevated higher than the heart. After craniectomy, the head is tilted to the right, away from the surgeon, and returned to the original position before wound closure. While operating from behind the patient's shoulder, the surgeon (right-handed) usually works on the left side of the patient (left Concorde position), or occasionally on the right side when a lesion is located on the left side (right Concorde position) [23]. The midline suboccipital craniotomy or craniectomy is made with the head in a neutral position. The surgeon is positioned to the left, right, or rostral side of

Fig. 9.9 Note the shoulder taping technique

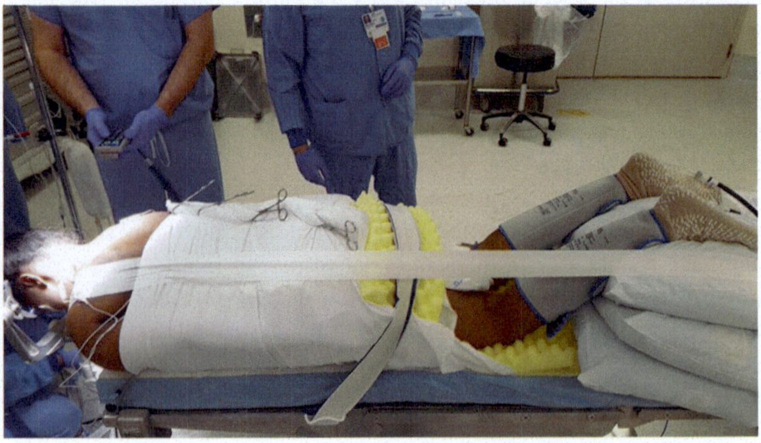

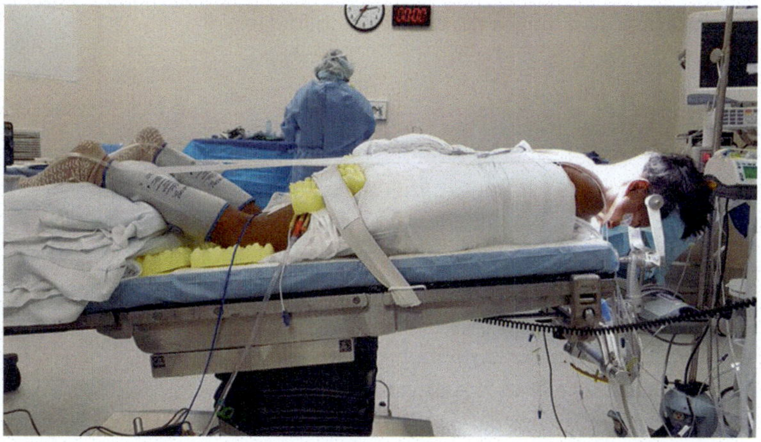

Fig. 9.10 Final preoperative position of the patient

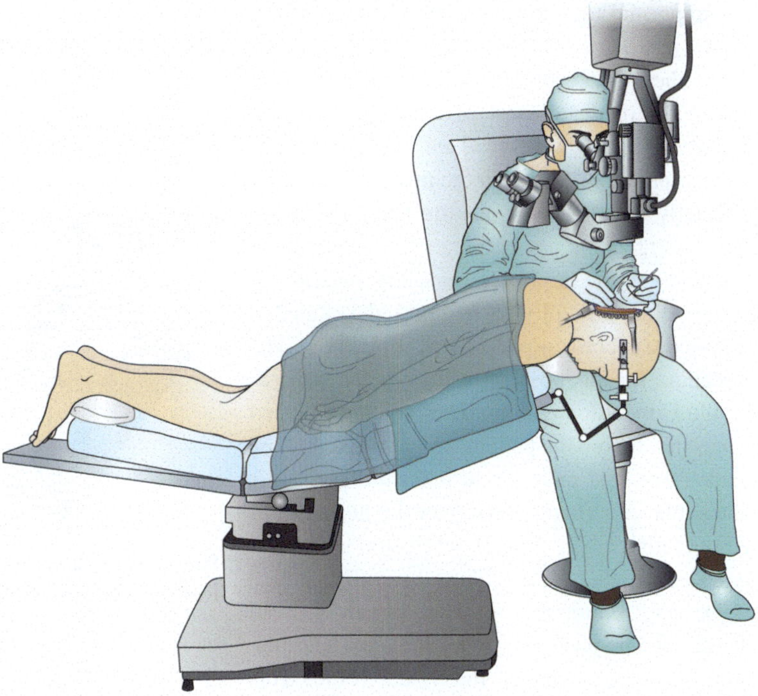

Fig. 9.11 Concorde position. The patient's head is positioned in flexion and is elevated above the level of the heart, while the surgeon sits on the left side of the patient and approaches from behind the patient's left shoulder

the patient, who is in the prone position for the craniotomy. The microscope is introduced at or after the opening of the dura mater, and the surgeon stands or sits to the left of the patient looking toward the cerebellum. The neutral head position is needed for the craniotomy to divide the occipital muscles symmetrically. Then, the patient's head is tilted to the right and the face is turned to the right before the microscope is introduced. The surgeon is able to keep the midline axis of the patient's head straight without discomfort and surgical manipulation is accurate and easy [24] (Fig. 9.11).

When the microscope is introduced after the craniotomy with the head neutral, there was formerly a need to release the holding arm of the head frame and adjust the position. It has also been necessary to reverse this adjustment during wound closure. To release the holding arm twice during the operation has proved troublesome, and Takasuna and Tanaka developed a modification to prevent this problem—the "skew head rotation"—in which the head can be tilted simultaneously only by rotating the head frame. In this maneuver, special care is required to prevent excessive rotation so as not to strain the patient's neck. The Sugita head holder, for example, offers a range of up to 36° of rotation to both the left and right. As the human cervical spine can rotate up to about 68°, this modified position is safer because the required head rotation is only about 30º. Nevertheless, there is individuality in the rotational range of the cervical spine, and the range of the patient's neck rotation should be verified before anesthesia is induced. In addition, it is important to confirm that the head is safely rotated just before draping [24].

In the Concorde position, however, the patient's shoulder closest to the surgeon occasionally interferes with the visual route and surgical manipulation. Although the involved shoulder is usually taped down from the neck and head, this arrangement is occasionally inadequate, especially in the case of a muscular patient. To prevent this difficulty, Kyoshima developed a modified Concorde position [25] (Fig. 9.12). The procedure for this position is almost the same as for the Concorde position. The patient is placed prone and, before the patient's head is fixed in the head frame, the patient's arm on the surgeon's side is placed to hang down over the head end of the operating table, with elbow flexion supported by an arm holder. The axilla is carefully padded to prevent compression. The patient's head should also be positioned with the chin—not the neck—down to enhance the visual route. This arm-down Concorde position allows good access to the pineal and supracerebellar regions and the pons in patients who are muscular, broad-shouldered, short-necked, or obese.

a

b

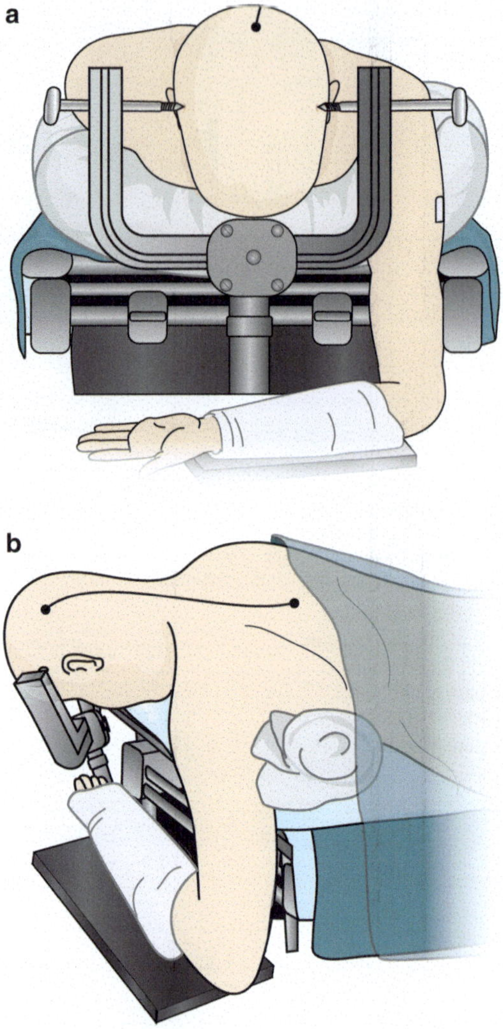

Fig. 9.12 Arm-down Concorde position. (**a**) The patient's left arm is placed hanging down over the head end of the operating table, with elbow flexion supported by an arm holder. (**b**) Note that the patient's left shoulder is lower than the right, and thus interferes less with the surgeon's view

Indications

The prone position can be used for both supra- and infratentorial surgery. Supratentorial lesions are those of the posterior parietal and occipital regions, and include intracerebral hematomas, metastases, gliomas, abscesses, meningiomas, cavernomas, arteriovenous malformations (AVMs), convexity meningiomas and meningiomas of the posterior third of the falx, falcotentorial meningiomas, and tumors of the pineal region. The full prone position is particularly useful in situations in which a bilateral craniotomy is needed (e.g., bilateral occipital falx meningiomas). Infratentorial lesions include inferior tentorial meningiomas, cerebellar primary tumors and metastases, brainstem tumors, posterior-inferior and anterior-inferior cerebellar artery aneurysms, Chiari malformations, fusion procedures in the craniocervical region, and intracerebellar hematomas [22, 26–28].

Supratentorial Lesions

The full prone position can be used for supratentorial approaches, particularly those utilizing the transcallosal route. This includes lesions of the posterior parietal and occipital regions, the posterior third of the falx, and the pineal region. The steep angle of the tentorium makes it difficult to use this approach for infratentorial lesions, and the Concorde position has been advocated for infratentorial lesions, particularly in the pediatric population (Fig. 9.13).

Infratentorial Lesions

There are four main positions to consider for surgery in the posterior fossa: the prone/Concorde position, the lateral decubitus/park-bench position, the supine position with rotation of the head, and the sitting position. The prone and Concorde positions are used when a midline approach is necessary, and the patient is lying prone with support for the thorax, pelvis, and legs. This support should leave the abdomen free. A U-cushion can be placed under the thorax, and the head is supported by a horseshoe cushion or fixed in the head clamp. The clamp allows more freedom to flex the head with concomitant better exposure of the lower occiput and neck. Such exposure can be exaggerated by lifting the upper thorax and shoulders and bending and lowering the head to the maximal flexion. In such a position, the surgeon may stand on one side

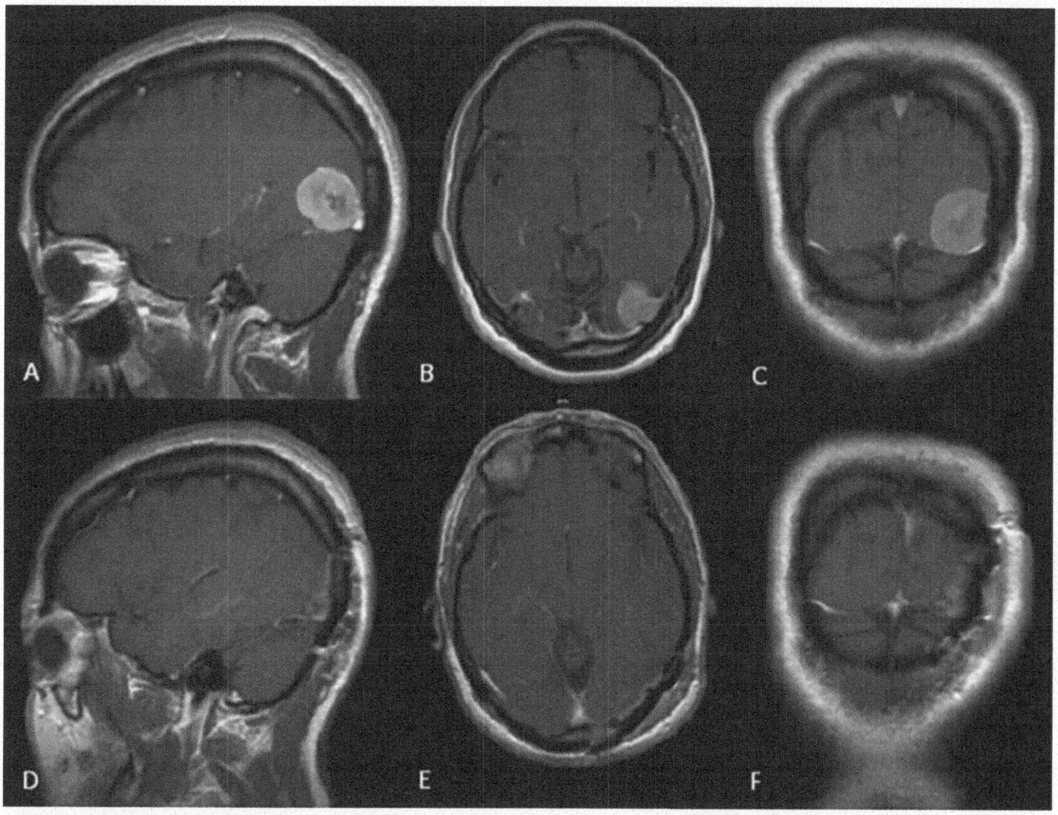

Fig. 9.13 A 38-year-old female patient with severe headaches and bilateral papilledema. Occipital meningioma with narrowing of the transversal sinus. (**a**) preoperative T1 post-contrast MRI of the brain, sagittal view. (**b**) axial view. (**c**) coronal view. (**d**) postoperative T1 post-contrast MRI of the brain, sagittal view. (**e**) axial view. (**f**) coronal view

of the body looking down toward the occipital region. Therefore, the head can even be angulated and tilted a little, according to the surgeon's preference. Especially in Concorde hyperflexion, the surgeon may work "upside down," standing and even sitting with the patient's head in his/her lap. The prone position can be also used for the far lateral approach. After full exposure, the table (with the patient well secured to it) may be turned and tilted as far as is necessary [29].

Lesions of the Cerebellum and Brainstem

A midline or a paramedian posterior approach is useful for cerebellar, fourth ventricular, and brainstem lesions. The most common lesions are metastatic brain tumors (Fig. 9.14), followed by cerebellar hemorrhages, cerebellar infarctions, and AVMs. A paramedian approach is also required for aneurysms of the distal posterior-inferior cerebellar artery.

A midline approach is used for suboccipital decompression of Chiari malformations (Fig. 9.15), as well as for dorsal foramen magnum meningiomas. Brainstem lesions that may be approached include cavernomas, small AVMs, exophytic brainstem gliomas, fourth ventricle cysts, choroid plexus granulomas, subependymal astrocytomas, and ependymomas (Fig. 9.16).

Vascular lesions, such as posterior-inferior cerebellar artery aneurysms and AVMs involving the cerebellar hemispheres and cerebellopontine angle, usually present with hemorrhage. Patients with increased intracranial pressure and hydrocephalus require initial placement of a ventriculostomy. The prone position is more suitable for

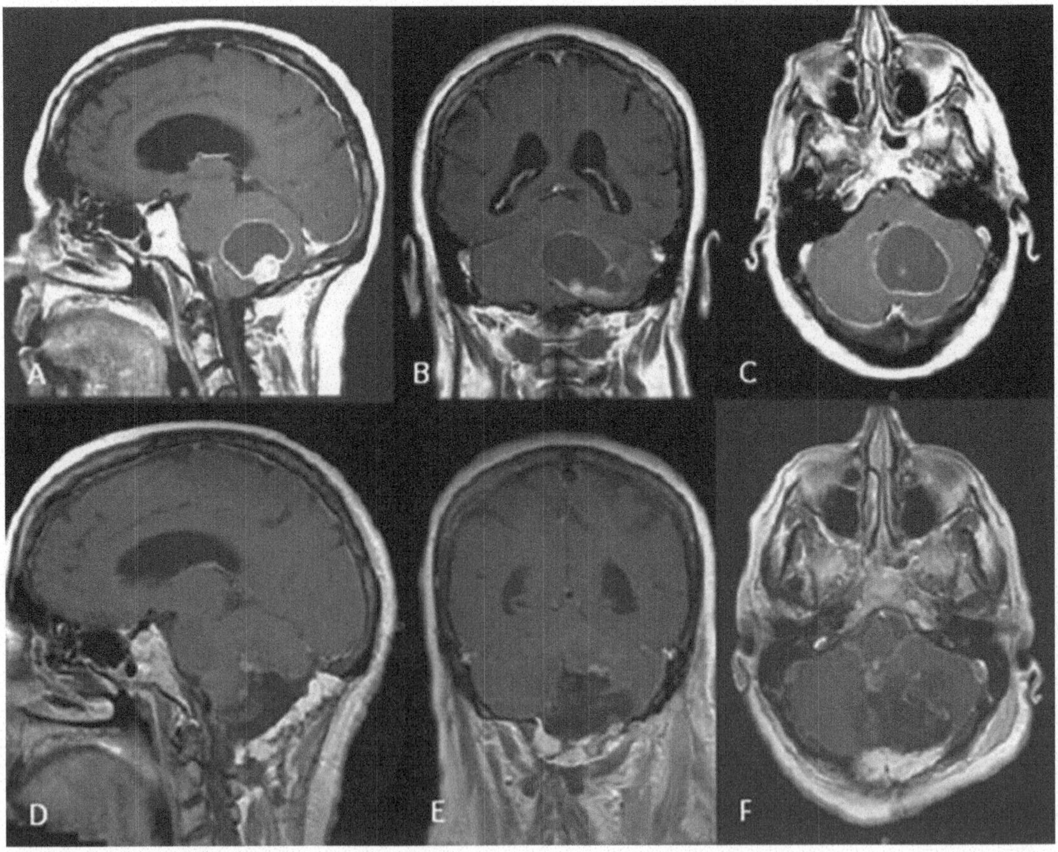

Fig. 9.14 A 62-year-old female patient with dizziness and balance problems. Metastatic lung adenocarcinoma. (**a**) preoperative T1-weighted post-contrast MRI of the brain, sagittal view. (**b**) coronal view. (**c**) axial view. (**d**) postoperative T1 post-contrast MRI of the brain, sagittal view. (**e**) axial view. (**f**) coronal view. Note the fat tissue graft placed along the dura for prevention of the CSF-related complications

midline lesions while the semi-prone position is better for paramedian lesions. These positions provide the same exposure as the semi-sitting position; in addition, the patient's table can be tilted up or down to decrease venous drainage in a controlled fashion. A vertical midline incision is made for midline lesions. For paramedian lesions, the incision starts in the midline and curves below the inion in an inverted U, toward the mastoid process [30].

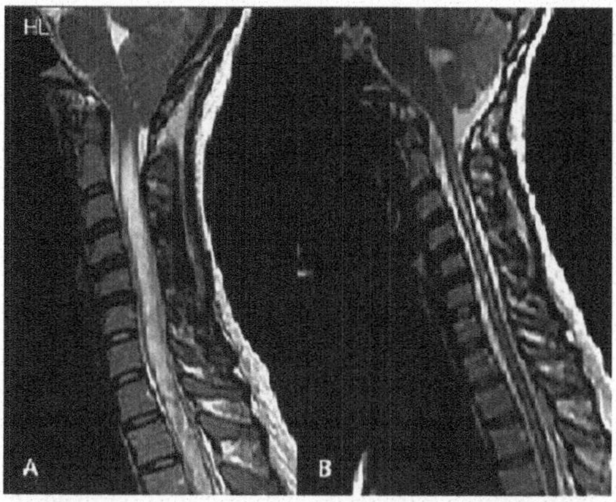

Fig. 9.15 A 32-year-old female patient with headaches. (**a**) preoperative T2-weighted MRI of the cervical spine depicting Chiari Malformation Type I with syringomyelia, sagittal view. (**b**) postoperative T2-weigted MRI of the cervical spine after the decompression of the posterior fossa with resection of the atlas arch, sagittal view. Note the resolution of the syrinx

AVMs of the vermis and cerebellar tonsils are best handled through a midline suboccipital exposure. For this, the patient is positioned prone on chest rolls with the back elevated. It is helpful to angle the head toward the opposite shoulder, allowing the surgeon better access to the midline without having to lean over the patient's back. A midline incision is made from above the inion to the level of the spinous processes of the fourth cervical vertebra [31].

Lesions of the Pineal Region

Although the sitting position is commonly used with approaches to the pineal region, several disadvantages may make the prone or semi-prone position, which provides identical exposure, a better choice. First, patients with pineal region lesions usually have to be placed in a more erect position than in the semi-sitting position, making the danger of air embolism considerable. The sitting position also makes the operation particularly difficult and tiring for the surgeon because it requires a long reach for the instruments and that the arms be held in an extended, elevated position for many hours [30]. Although this arrangement is generally comfortable for the surgeon, the operative field is considerably elevated, which can make it difficult for the surgeon to be seated. This position enables

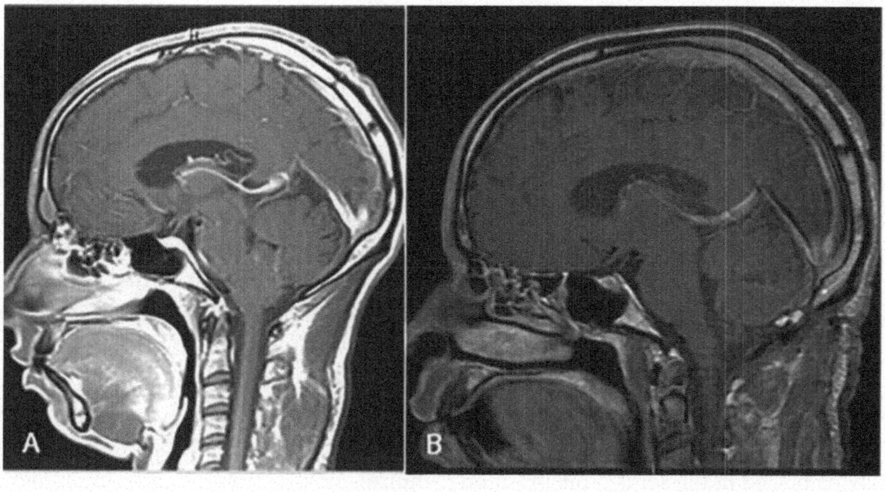

Fig. 9.16 A 39-year-old male patient with severe headaches and balance problems. (**a**) preoperative T1-weighted post-contrast MRI of the brain which shows the tumor on the floor of the fourth ventricle. (**b**) postoperative T1-weighted post-contrast MRI of the brain which shows the complete resection of the tumor (subependymoma)

the use of a bridge on the operating microscope, affording binocular vision for both the surgeon and the assistant. In the Concorde position, the patient's head may be rotated 15° away to facilitate occipital lobe retraction.

Posterior approaches to the pineal region may be divided into supra- and infratentorial. Supratentorial approaches include the occipital transtentorial, interhemispheric transcallosal, and interhemispheric retrocallosal. Infratentorial approaches include the median and paramedian supracerebellar infratentorial approaches. The occipital interhemispheric transtentorial approach and supracerebellar infratentorial approach are the ones most commonly used for the pineal region [32].

The posterior interhemispheric approach has traditionally been used for tumors located at the posterior third ventricle, pineal tumors growing superiorly or laterally to the trigone and lateral ventricle, tumors around the vein of Galen, and tumors of the median occipital lobe, as well as tumors of the splenium of the corpus callosum, brainstem tumors, vascular malformations, P2/3 segment aneurysms of the distal posterior-inferior cerebellar artery, cavernomas of the dorsal midbrain, and lesions of the superior vermian area. The advantage of this approach is that is allows early access to the superior cerebellar artery, a major artery feeding these tumors. It also affords better exposure of the veins in the quadrigeminal region and shortens the distance to the area because of the division of the tentorium [32]. Depending on the anatomy of the pineal region tumor (meningioma, pinealoblastoma, pineal cyst), additional resection of the splenium or tentorium is sometimes needed. Various positions have been described for this approach (semi-sitting, lateral, three-quarter prone, and semi-prone) [30].

The supracerebellar infratentorial approach is used for lesions in the pineal quadrigeminal area. For these, the patient may be placed prone with the surgeon seated near the patient's head, looking in the reverse direction. Alternatively, the patient may be placed in the semi-prone position with the surgeon looking at an angle from behind [30] (Fig. 9.17).

The combined occipital transtentorial supracerebellar trans-sinus approach is used for giant tumors of the pineal quadrigeminal area or meningiomas. It combines the advantages of the supracerebellar, infratentorial, and occipital transtentorial approaches [32] (Fig. 9.18).

Complications

Increased age, elevated body mass index, the presence of comorbidities, and long.

duration of surgery appear to be the most important risk factors for complications associated with prone positioning. The systematic use of checklists is recommended to guide operating room teams and to reduce prone position-related complications [33].

Complications associated with prone position include injury to the central and peripheral nervous system, ophthalmic injury, and pressure injuries [3]. Injury to the central nervous system occurs due to the rise of the intracranial pressure. There are few strategies which could be used in situation when intraoperative swelling occurs. These include releasing the cerebrospinal fluid from the cisterns, extending the decompression of the posterior fossa and placing a ventricular catheter at the Frazier point. Further maneuvers include tilting the table with head up, hyperventilation, hypertonic saline (especially in patients with renal failure), or mannitol. Injuries to central nervous system can occur when turning the patient from supine to prone or due to neck extension (occlusion of the carotid or vertebral arteries), as well as due to pneumorrhachis (air entrainment into the spinal canal) after posterior fossa exploration, which can result in quadriplegia [3, 34]. Quadriplegia can also occur due to excessive neck flexion in the "Concorde" position with the neck flexed and the chin approximately one fingerbreadth from the sternum in a patient with narrow spinal canal and herniated discs [35], which emphasizes the importance of the preoperative neck evaluation. Pressure injuries can be divided into direct and indirect [3]. Direct pressure injuries include pressure necrosis of the skin, contact dermatitis, tracheal

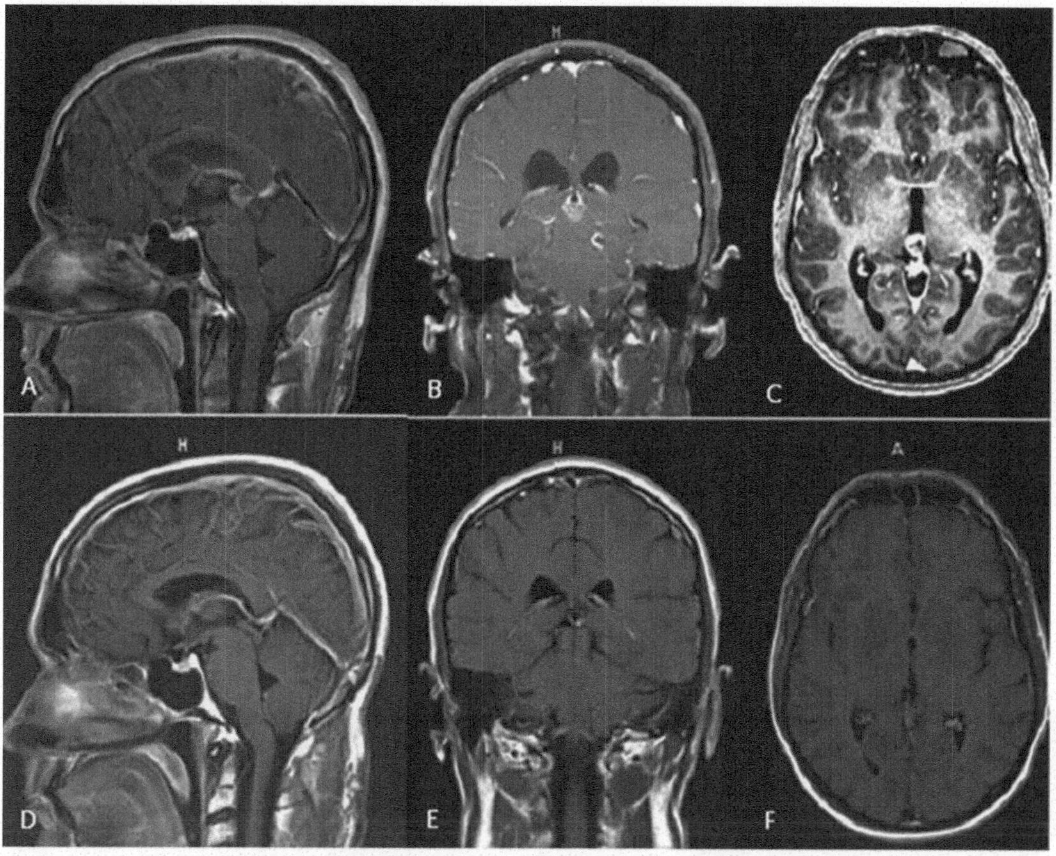

Fig. 9.17 A 31-year-old patient with diplopia and Parinaud syndrome. (**a**) preoperative T1-weighted post-contrast MRI of the brain, sagittal view, which shows lesion in the pineal region (germinoma), (**b**) coronal view; note the enlarged ventricles due to occlusive hydrocephalus; (**c**) axial view. (**d**) postoperative T1-weighted post-contrast MRI of the brain, sagittal view, which shows the complete resection of the tumor. The procedure was performed in the prone position with supracerebellar infratentorial approach performing the resection of the tentorium. (**e**) coronal view; note the fat patch used to prevent complications due to leak of the cerebrospinal fluid; (**f**) axial view, note that the ventricles returned to normal size

compression, salivary gland swelling, and shoulder dislocation. Indirect pressure injuries involve macroglossia and oropharyngeal swelling, mediastinal compression, visceral ischemia, avascular necrosis of the femoral head, peripheral vessel occlusion, and limb compartment syndromes and rhabdomyolysis.

Three types of complications have been associated with the prone position in cranial and spine surgery: those arising as a direct result of the positioning method, those due to venous air embolism, and those resulting from anesthesia [15].

Complications that arise as a direct result of the method of positioning include postoperative vision loss, myocardial ischemia, increased abdominal pressure and bleeding, abdominal compartment syndrome, limb compartment syndrome, shoulder dislocation, nerve palsies, pressure sores, hepatic dysfunction, and cardiovascular compromise. Rates of pressure sores as an intraoperative complication have been reported to range from 5 to 66%. As such, pressure sores lead to longer hospital stays and higher healthcare costs [20]. Retinal artery occlusion as a result of direct pressure on the eye lobe can lead to postoperative blindness. The rate at which this complication occurs increases relative to risk factors such as diabetes, obesity, smoking, and

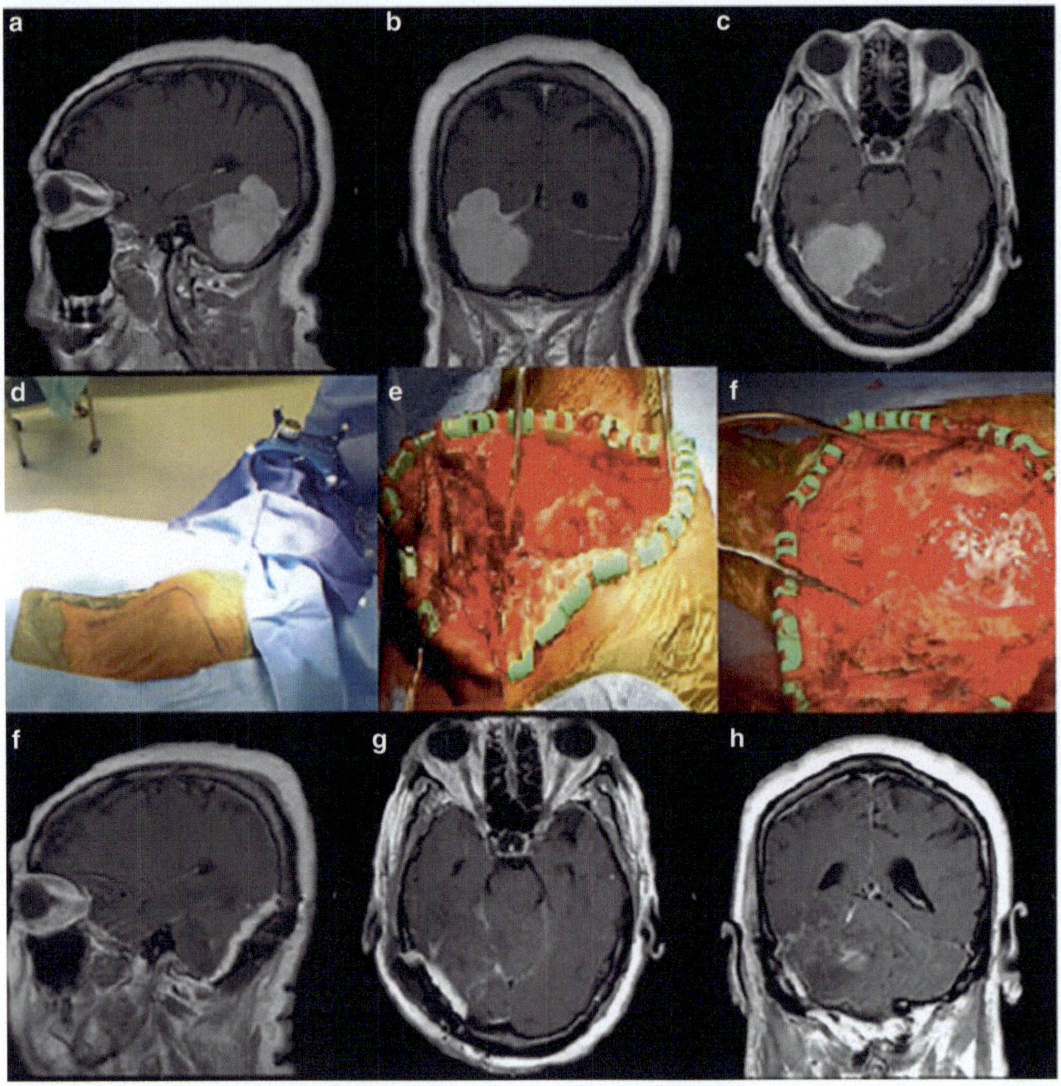

Fig. 9.18 A 74-year-old female patient with headaches, dizziness, and balance problems. (**a**) preoperative T1-weighted post-contrast MRI of the brain, sagittal view, which shows supra- and intratentorial meningioma. (**b**) coronal view; (**c**) axial view. (**d**) Note the midline incision which is curved to the right above the inion; (**e**) intraoperative photo, exposing the bone; (**f**) supra- and infratentorial craniotomy. (**g**) postoperative T1-weighted post-contrast MRI of the brain, sagittal view, which shows the complete resection of the tumor. (**h**) axial view; note the fat patch used to prevent CSF complications; (**i**) coronal view

hypertension, and risk factors related to the surgical procedure such as anemia, decreased venous return, and prolonged hypotension. Corneal abrasion is also very often complication of Trendelenburg position [34]. Anemia, hemodilution, blood loss (>1000 mL), and hypotension, in combination with the increased ocular pressure in the prone position, can reduce perfusion pressure to the optic nerve and cause ischemic optic neuropathy [20].

Skin excoriations can occur on shoulders associated with taping. Wrist drop can be associated with pressure on the radial nerve above the elbow associated with securing straps or equipment compression. Brachial plexus injuries or lesions can occur as a result of excessive stretching and incorrect shoulder positioning that may cause transitory or permanent sensory and/or motor deficit. Another complication reported is ulnar neuropathy, which may be caused by entrapment of the ulnar nerve at the elbow or wrist with resultant numbness and tingling in the fourth and fifth fingers. This complication may be caused by mal-positioning or the lack of adequate padding during surgical positioning. There have also been a few cases of reported in association with prone positioning during surgery, with visceral hypo-perfusion implicated in those cases4. When a surgical patient is in the prone position (Jackson table), increased pressure on muscles can lead to muscle hypo-perfusion and ischemia as well as subsequent reperfusion injury with release of myoglobin. This could lead to rhabdomyolysis and acute renal failure [36]. Pressure to penis and scrotum can lead to scrotal edema.

Luostarinen and associates showed that, compared with the prone position, surgery with the patient in the sitting position does not require excessive fluid administration to achieve stable hemodynamics [37]. Risk factors for reduced stroke volume, cardiac index, raised central venous pressure, and low blood pressure include massive blood loss, hypothermia, fluid shifts, cardiac comorbidities, venous air embolism, and anatomic deformities such as thoracic lordosis or pectus excavatum, which can aggravate hypotension. Also, an increase of intra-abdominal pressure in the prone position of more than 12 mmHg increases the risk for abdominal compartment syndrome, as visceral compression and intra-abdominal hypertension caused by decreased perfusion pressure lead to multi-organ failure. Patients with previous abdominal surgeries are at particularly high risk as tight abdominal closures can reduce abdominal compliance, increasing abdominal pressure. Lower limb compartment syndrome and rhabdomyolysis are common complications associated with placement in non-supine positions.

The risk of venous air embolism (VAE) is not confined to neurosurgical procedures done with the patient in the sitting position, nor is it eliminated by placing the patient horizontally. Avoiding techniques that enhance air entrainment or increase bubble size is imperative, as is identifying the population at risk of its devastating sequela, paradoxical air embolism. Children are at increased risk of VAE, as their reported rate of VAE (73%) is significantly higher compared with that of adults (37%) [38]. Surgery with the patient in the sitting position has the highest rate of VAE. It may also occur in patients in the prone position during intracranial procedures; the reported rate ranges from 10 to 25% [38]. The diagnosis of VAE can be made with capnography (a sudden drop in end-tidal CO_2), precordial Doppler (with the transducer placed in the area of right atrium), and transesophageal echocardiography (the most sensitive invasive method, essential in patients with a patent foramen ovale). Supplementary monitoring is directed toward prompt detection and early treatment of VAE. Transesophageal echocardiography and Doppler were found to be equally sensitive with respect to air detection, and transesophageal echocardiography provided the added benefit of localizing intracardiac air within a specific cardiac chamber. Cardiovascular changes occur late and include hypotension, elevation of central venous pressure, and electrocardiogram changes. TEE is not routinely used in prone position for monitoring due to the risk of compression of the base of the tongue with postoperative edema.

VAE may increase airway pressure during mechanical ventilation as a result of bronchoconstriction and reduced pulmonary compliance. Intermittent positive-pressure ventilation has been advocated to prevent the reflex gasp that occurs with an air embolus and may cause a bolus of air to be sucked into an open vein. Initial exposure of the posterior fossa, when air may enter the diploic and emissary veins or the dural sinuses, is the time of greatest concern for the development of VAE. Sources of VAE are often not identified, but careful surgical technique is paramount. Bone was identified as a source of VAE in 16% of cases in one study; hence, the recommendation that all bone edges be waxed. Pin-type head holders have also been implicated, and it has been suggested that these pins be wrapped with gauze impregnated with petrolatum or bismuth tribromophenate [38, 39] Alternatively, bleeding from pinholes can be stopped with stitching or gel foam powder. When performing posterior fossa surgery, special care needs to be done when opening above or in the region of sinus transversus, sinus sigmoideus, and torcula. Communication with the anesthesiologist which monitors the TEE is essential, as well as preparation for hemostasis in possible sinus bleeding.

One potential source of venous air embolism during surgery in the posterior fossa is the suboccipital cavernous sinus, specifically the area of the third segment of the vertebral artery, which extends from the transverse foramen of the axis to the dural penetration of the vertebral artery, its loops, branches, supporting fibrous rings, adjacent nerves, and surrounding venous structures [40]. If venous embolism is suspected, the anesthesiologist must immediately inform the neurosurgeon to begin irrigating the surgical field and cover any exposed blood vessels. Oxygen (100%) should be used, and air lodged between the superior vena cava and the right atrium should be aspirated through the central venous catheter. In the case of a massive embolism, advanced resuscitation maneuvers should be quickly initiated and a pneumatic counter-pressure device may be used. An example of this device is MAST, military anti-shock trousers, which extend from the hip to the ankles and are inflated if the patient's condition becomes hypotensive.

Complications due to anesthetic technique include dislodgement of the endotracheal tube. This could be a major complication when oropharyngeal and facial swelling are present (Fig. 9.12). The critical preventive factor is the correct placement and securing of a non-kinking endotracheal tube to prevent an unrecognized disconnection or occlusion. Oral secretions draining from the mouth may loosen the retaining straps, and inadvertent endobronchial intubation may be produced by changes in the head position associated with the turning procedure. The endotracheal tube (ETT) kink during posterior fossa surgery might result from overbending of the softening tube due to oral temperature and neck flexion [41]. The smaller size tubes may be more prone for airway obstruction. It could be difficult to carry out reintubation in such an awful situation when the patient was prone and in pins with surgery in process. Manual straightening of the tube may be helpful to relive kinking of ETT. Emphasis should also be laid on the proper positioning of the head and neck prior to surgery. The use of reinforced, non-kinking ETT may be considered in high-risk patients [42] (Fig. 9.19).

Particular attention should be exercised to prevent a tongue-biting injury by applying one of the forms of protection. The use of the plastic oral airways that place pressure on the posterior

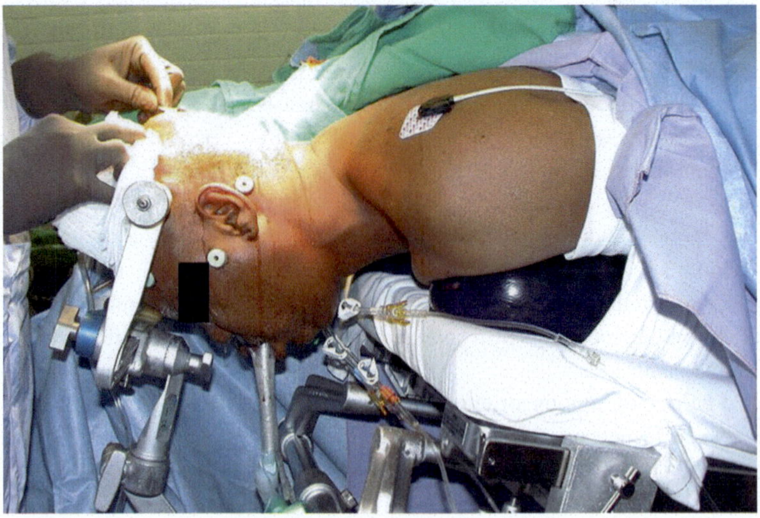

Fig. 9.19 Patient positioned prone with reinforced, non-kinking endotracheal tube

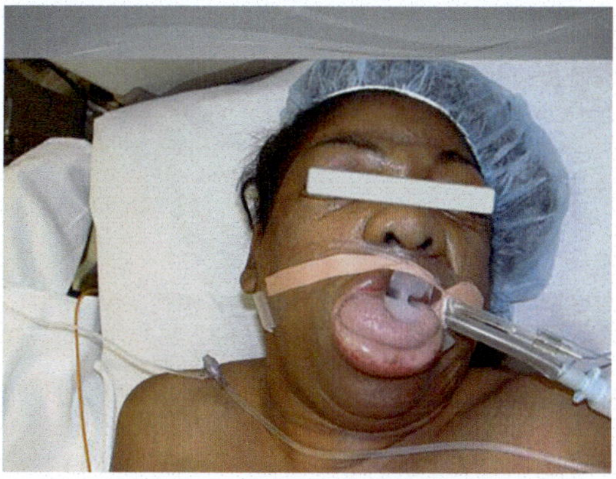

Fig. 9.20 Orofacial swelling following the surgery in prone position

aspect of the tongue results in the edema. Bite blockers that do not extend into the posterior pharynx are recommended. Problems with extubation may occur due to facial edema, swelling of the soft palate, swelling of the tongue causing macroglossia, upper airway edema (because of head flexion and compression of lingual and pharyngeal venous drainage), and swelling of submandibular glands (from compression of the salivary duct) [43]. Proposed mechanism of macroglossia and oropharyngeal swelling suggests that excessive flexion of the head and the presence of a tracheal tube cause kinking and obstruction of the internal jugular vein in the neck, which in turn obstructs venous drainage from the lingual and pharyngeal veins (Fig. 9.20). There were two described reports on postoperative macroglossia with swelling in patients with Chiari malformation, one of them being extubated after 3 days on the respirator and the other one requiring emergency tracheotomy to relieve the obstruction, both without long-term sequelae [3, 44–46].

Neuronavigation in the Prone Position

Navigation systems have become essential tools in neurosurgery, and precise registration is indispensable for its accuracy. Rapid and precise registration by surface matching on the facial skin is possible by using the landmarks of the face with the patient supine. On the other hand, incomplete registration may occur in the prone position because of the ventral direction of the face, displacement of the skin by headpins, and obscuring of the skin by the bispectral index monitor, the many electrodes on the forehead, and the eye patch. Surface matching on the occipital scalp may not be suitable for registration because the occipital scalp is flat and is compressed in the supine position during preoperative neuroimaging. To improve accuracy, fiducial markers can be placed prior to magnetic resonance imaging and left in place for neuronavigation registration after positioning.

To overcome the problem of failed registration, Ogiwara and colleagues have developed a method of registration designated as bony surface registration, in which surface matching is achieved by using the bony surface of the skull after exposure. After the skin flap is created and before the craniotomy, bony surface registration is carried out by exposing the skull surface in a sterile environment [47].

In tumor surgery, updated image data allow a reliable identification of a tumor remnant or correction of a catheter position. With the help of intraoperative imaging (intraoperative MRI) navigation data can be updated, so that brain shift can be compensated for and initially missed tumor remnants can be localized reliably [48]. Electromagnetic guided neuronavigation is a recently developed technique which enabled fast and accurate referencing without loss of navigation accuracy despite repositioning of the patient in the semi-sitting position [49]. In the surgery of the posterior fossa, neuronavigation is important tool in localizing the venous sinuses.

Neuromonitoring in the Prone Position

Positioning maneuvers during surgical cases can place the patient at risk for spinal cord and/or peripheral nerve injury. The initial transition of the patient from supine to prone, as well as passive neck flexion or extension, are potentially high-risk portions of the procedure, especially during spine surgery. Intraoperative neurophysiologic monitoring, including transcranial motor evoked potentials (MEPs), somatosensory evoked potentials (SEPs), and electromyography (EMG) can be of use before the initial patient positioning. Their use can facilitate prompt identification of potentially reversible changes that may indicate impending positioning-related injuries [50]. Appropriate mouth gag or bite blocker should be applied when performing MEPs. The use of somatosensory evoked potentials (SSEP) as an indirect indicator of potential injury has been proposed as a useful detector of positioning-related peripheral nerve injury [3]. When performing SSEPs and MEPs, we recommend first to position the patient and then to place the electrodes and afterwards to perform the padding of the hands and feet. The hands and feet should be properly padded while undergoing electrical stimulation in an unparalysed patient.

References

1. Rozet I, Vavilala MS. Risks and benefits of patient positioning during neurosurgical care. Anesthesiol Clin. 2007;25(3):631–53. x.
2. Backofen JE, Schauble JF. Hemodynamic changes with prone position during general anaesthesia. Anesth Analg. 1985;64:194.
3. Edgcombe H, Carter K, Yarrow S. Anaesthesia in the prone position. Br J Anaesth. 2008;100(2):165–83.
4. Sudheer PS, Logan SW, Ateleanu B, Hall JE. Haemodynamic effects of the prone position: a comparison of propofol total intravenous and inhalation anaesthesia. Anaesthesia. 2006;61(2):138–41.
5. Rolighed Larsen JK, Haure P, Cold GE. Reverse Trendelenburg position reduces intracranial pressure during craniotomy. J Neurosurg Anesthesiol. 2002;14(1):16–21.
6. Reinprecht A, Greher M, Wolfsberger S, Dietrich W, Illievich UM, Gruber A. Prone position in subarachnoid hemorrhage patients with acute respiratory distress syndrome: effects on cerebral tissue oxygenation and intracranial pressure. Crit Care Med. 2003;31(6):1831–8.
7. Rasmussen M, Cold GE. Subdural intracranial pressure, cerebral haemodynamics, dural tension and degree of swelling after opening of dura in patients with infratentorial tumors. In: Cold GE, Juul N, editors. Monitoring of cerebral and spinal haemodynamics during neurosurgery. Berlin: Springer; 2008.
8. Rosin D, Rosenthal RJ. Adverse hemodynamic effects of intraabdominal pressure—is it all in the head? Int J Surg Investig. 2001;2(5):335–45.
9. Kamine TH, Papavassiliou E, Schneider BE. Effect of abdominal insufflation for laparoscopy on intracranial pressure. JAMA Surg. 2014;149(4):380–2.
10. Artigas A, Bernard GR, Carlet J, Dreyfuss D, Gattinoni L, Hudson L, et al. The American-European Consensus Conference on ARDS, part 2. Ventilatory, pharmacologic, supportive therapy, study design strategies and issues related to recovery and remodeling. Intensive Care Med. 1998;24(4):378–98.
11. Beuret P, Carton MJ, Nourdine K, Kaaki M, Tramoni G, Ducreux JC. Prone position as prevention of lung injury in comatose patients: a prospective, randomized, controlled study. Intensive Care Med. 2002;28(5):564–9.
12. Georgiadis D, Schwarz S, Kollmar R, Baumgartner RW, Schwab S. Influence of inspiration:expiration ratio on intracranial and cerebral perfusion pressure in acute stroke patients. Intensive Care Med. 2002;28(8):1089–93.
13. Robba C, Bragazzi NL, Bertuccio A, Cardim D, Donnelly J, Sekhon M, et al. Effects of prone position and positive end-expiratory pressure on noninvasive estimators of ICP: a pilot study. J Neurosurg Anesthesiol. 2017;29(3):243–50.
14. Young N, Rhodes JK, Mascia L, Andrews PJ. Ventilatory strategies for patients with acute brain injury. Curr Opin Crit Care. 2010;16(1):45–52.
15. Winn HR. Positioning for cranial surgery. In: Webster Crowley R, Dumont AS, Sean McKisic M, Jane Sr JA, editors. Youmans neurological surgery, 4-Volume Set: Expert Consult - Online and Print, (Winn, Neurological Surgery). 6th ed. Philadelphia: Saunders; 2011.
16. Beuriat PA, Jacquesson T, Jouanneau E, Berhouma M. Headholders'—complications in neurosurgery: a review of the literature and recommendations for its use. Neurochirurgie. 2016;62(6):289–94.
17. Dybec RB, Kneedler JA, Pfiester JI. Basic principles of patient positioning (Online Continuing Education Activity) Pfiedler Enterprises; 2013. www.pfiedler.com/1079/.
18. Lopez-Olivo MA, Andrabi TR, Palla SL, Suarez-Almazor ME. Cervical spine radiographs in patients with rheumatoid arthritis undergoing anesthesia. J Clin Rheumatol. 2012;18(2):61–6.
19. Krause ML, Matteson EL. Perioperative management of the patient with rheumatoid arthritis. World J Orthop. 2014;5(3):283–91.
20. Kwee MM, Ho YH, Rozen WM. The prone position during surgery and its complications: a systematic review and evidence-based guidelines. Int Surg. 2015;100(2):292–303.
21. Mobley SR, Miller BT, Astor FC, Fine B, Halliday NJ. Prone positioning for head and neck reconstructive surgery. Head Neck. 2007;29(11):1041–5.
22. Arnautovic KI, Muzevic D, Splavski B, Boop FA. Association of increased body mass index with

Chiari malformation Type I and syrinx formation in adults. J Neurosurg. 2013;119(4):1058–67.
23. Kobayashi S, Sugita K, Tanaka Y, Kyoshima K. Infratentorial approach to the pineal region in the prone position: concorde position. Technical note. J Neurosurg. 1983;58(1):141–3.
24. Takasuna H, Tanaka Y. The modified concorde position with an intraoperative skew head rotation: technical note. Neurol Med Chir (Tokyo). 2015;55(8):680–2.
25. Kyoshima K. Arm-down concorde position: a technical note. Surg Neurol. 2002;57(6):443–5. discussion 5–6.
26. Broadway SJ, Arnautovic KI, Zhang Y. Xanthoma of the occipital bone and with preserved inner and outer bone cortex: case report. J Neurol Surg Rep. 2013;74(1):29–32.
27. Lakičević G, Arnautović K, Muževič D, Chesney T. Cerebellar glioblastoma multiforme presenting as hypertensive cerebellar hemorrhage: case report. J Neurol Surg Rep. 2014;75(1):e117–21.
28. Pait TG, Al-Mefty O, Boop FA, Arnautovic KI, Rahman S, Ceola W. Inside-outside technique for posterior occipitocervical spine instrumentation and stabilization: preliminary results. J Neurosurg. 1999;90(1 Suppl):1–7.
29. Mooij JJA. How to perform posterior fossa approaches. In: Sindou M, editor. Practical handbook of neurosurgery from leading neurosurgeons. New York: Springer; 2009.
30. Sekhar L, Oliveira E. Cranial microsurgery: approaches and techniques. Stuttgart: Thieme; 1998.
31. Samson D, White JA, Welch BG. Posterior fossa Arteriovenous malformations. In: Macdonald RL, editor. Neurosurgical operative atlas vascular neurosurgery. Stuttgart: Thieme; 2008.
32. Vannemreddy P, Ezer H, Nanda A. Posterior Interhemispheric approach to pineal region and brainstem. In: Nanda A, editor. Principles of posterior fossa surgery. Stuttgart: Thieme; 2012.
33. Chui J, Craen RA. An update on the prone position: continuing professional development. Can J Anaesth. 2016;63(6):737–67.
34. Prabhakar H, Bithal PK, Ghosh I, Dash HH. Pneumorrhachis presenting as quadriplegia following surgery in the prone position. Br J Anaesth. 2006; 97(6):901–3.
35. Rau CS, Liang CL, Lui CC, Lee TC, Lu K. Quadriplegia in a patient who underwent posterior fossa surgery in the prone position. Case report. J Neurosurg. 2002;96(1 Suppl):101–3.
36. Ziser A, Friedhoff RJ, Rose SH. Prone position: visceral hypoperfusion and rhabdomyolysis. Anesth Analg. 1996;82(2):412–5.
37. Luostarinen T, Lindroos AC, Niiya T, Silvasti-Lundell M, Schramko A, Hernesniemi J, et al. Prone versus sitting position in neurosurgery—differences in patients' hemodynamic management. World Neurosurg. 2016; 97:261–6.
38. Matjasko J, Petrozza P, Cohen M, Steinberg P. Anesthesia and surgery in the seated position: analysis of 554 cases. Neurosurgery. 1985;17(5):695–702.
39. Domaingue CM. Anaesthesia for neurosurgery in the sitting position: a practical approach. Anaesth Intensive Care. 2005;33(3):323–31.
40. Arnautović KI, al-Mefty O, Pait TG, Krisht AF, Husain MM. The suboccipital cavernous sinus. J Neurosurg. 1997;86(2):252–62.
41. Hübler M, Petrasch F. Intraoperative kinking of polyvinyl endotracheal tubes. Anesth Analg. 2006; 103(6):1601–2.
42. Bharti N, Bala I. Kinking of endotracheal tube during posterior fossa surgery. Indian J Anaesth. 2010;54(2):172–3.
43. Hans P, Demoitié J, Collignon L, Bex V, Bonhomme V. Acute bilateral submandibular swelling following surgery in prone position. Eur J Anaesthesiol. 2006;23(1):83–4.
44. Tsung YC, Wu CT, Hsu CH, Yeh CC, Lin SL, Wong CS. Macroglossia after posterior fossa surgery in the prone position--a case report. Acta Anaesthesiol Taiwanica. 2006;44(1):43–6.
45. Sinha A, Agarwal A, Gaur A, Pandey CK. Oropharyngeal swelling and macroglossia after cervical spine surgery in the prone position. J Neurosurg Anesthesiol. 2001;13(3):237–9.
46. Pivalizza EG, Katz J, Singh S, Liu W, McGraw-Wall BL. Massive macroglossia after posterior fossa surgery in the prone position. J Neurosurg Anesthesiol. 1998;10(1):34–6.
47. Ogiwara T, Goto T, Aoyama T, Nagm A, Yamamoto Y, Hongo K. Bony surface registration of navigation system in the lateral or prone position: technical note. Acta Neurochir. 2015;157(11):2017–22.
48. Nimsky C, Kuhnt D, Ganslandt O, Buchfelder M. Multimodal navigation integrated with imaging. Acta Neurochir Suppl. 2011;109:207–14.
49. Hermann EJ, Petrakakis I, Polemikos M, Raab P, Cinibulak Z, Nakamura M, et al. Electromagnetic navigation-guided surgery in the semi-sitting position for posterior fossa tumours: a safety and feasibility study. Acta Neurochir. 2015;157(7):1229–37.
50. Lee L, Cho S, Nguyen V, Rattlif J, Park J, Lopez J. Critical intraoperative neurophysiologic monitoring (IONM) changes associated with patients positioning maneuvrs. Neurology. 2014;82(10 Supplement):P6.336.

10 Spinal Surgery Positioning Overview

Kevin Foley

Introduction

Patient positioning is often underappreciated, but it is critical to the success of spinal surgical procedures. When optimized, it maximizes the likelihood of accomplishing the surgical goals in a timely manner and decreases the risk for complications. The three positions that are most commonly utilized in spinal surgery are the supine, prone, and lateral positions. These positions are discussed in detail in the following chapters. Less common positions such as the sitting position are also described. In this chapter, we present an overview of positioning for spinal surgery and discuss some positioning pearls that we have found to be quite useful. The goals of successful positioning are to provide optimal exposure to the pathology while ensuring the overall safety of the patient. In this regard, three principles must be taken into consideration.

Optimal Surgical Exposure

The ideal surgical position is one that provides the best visualization of and access to the surgical pathology while minimizing positioning-related morbidity. The selection of the surgical position is at the discretion of the surgeon, but patient factors, surgical anatomy, and operating room resources must also be taken into consideration. Patient factors include the nature of the surgical pathology as well as the intended surgical goals. Other patient-specific positioning limitations can be determined from the physical examination and/or the past medical/surgical history that might preclude certain positions or limit operative approaches due to such things as limited patient mobility. For example, the inability to fully abduct or rotate the patient's shoulder (due to prior injury, prior shoulder surgery, etc.) may limit one's ability to position the patient prone while providing optimal access to or fluoroscopic visualization of the thoracolumbar spine. The patient's body habitus is also very important to appreciate as it relates to the surgical approach and in determining the equipment necessary to safely support the patient on the operating room table.

Any concerns from the surgeon's preoperative evaluation should be communicated to the operating room support staff, including the anesthesia team, nurses, and surgical technologists involved with the procedure. This team-based approach is critical to optimizing the operative environment to maximize the probability of surgical success. Some important considerations with regard to ideal positioning that should be communicated to the surgical team preoperatively and addressed in

K. Foley (✉)
Semmes-Murphey Clinic, University of Tennessee Health Science Center, Memphis, TN, USA
e-mail: kfoley@semmes-murphey.com

A. Arthur et al. (eds.), *Perioperative Considerations and Positioning for Neurosurgical Procedures*,
https://doi.org/10.1007/978-3-319-72679-3_10

the operating room while positioning the patient include the type of surgical table, the position of the arms, pressure point support, and padding for any vulnerable areas (see "Patient Safety" below). Depending upon the specific spinal surgical procedure, the position of essential equipment such as the c-arm fluoroscope, the operative microscope, intraoperative navigation system, and electrophysiologic monitoring equipment should also be discussed with the operative staff to minimize surgical inefficiency and any impact upon patient positioning. Although such technological advances have contributed greatly to decreasing surgical morbidity, they also necessitate a greater degree of preparation preoperatively.

An additional consideration when positioning a spinal surgery patient is to optimize the spinal alignment for the surgery as well as diminish the probability of epidural venous bleeding. For decompression of the lumbar spine, flexion is ideal to open the interlaminar spaces for improved access to the spinal canal and disc spaces. Placement of the patient on a kyphosis positioning device (such as a Wilson frame) can provide for flexion of the lumbar spine to open the interlaminar spaces as well as lift the patient's abdominal wall off the operating room table to diminish intra-abdominal pressure/epidural venous distention. For posterior cervical surgery, placing the patient in the reverse Trendelenburg position can raise the patient's head above the heart and diminish intraoperative venous bleeding. In fusion procedures, the spinal alignment achieved through optimal positioning should reflect the natural spinal curvature (lordosis for the cervical and lumbar regions, kyphosis for the thoracic spine). This goal can be verified with a c-arm fluoroscope. The operating room table and various accessories (chest rolls, Wilson frame, etc.) can be utilized to optimally produce the desired spinal curvature, as will be discussed in the following chapters.

Patient Safety

A paramount goal of proper operative positioning is to minimize complications. With regard to spinal surgical positioning, the most common concerns are the development of neuropathies. An ulnar neuropathy is the most common neuropathy related to positioning and can be caused by compression or ischemia. The ulnar nerve is most susceptible at the superficial condylar groove at the medial aspect of the elbow, and thus excessive flexion or compression in this region should be avoided. In the supine position, this risk can be minimized by ensuring the medial elbow is properly padded, and the arm is in a "natural" position with the palms facing medially. In the prone position, the upper extremity should be abducted no more than 90° at the shoulder and the elbow should be flexed, with the axilla padded to prevent brachial plexus compression. Lower extremity neuropathies can also occur although they are infrequent with spine surgery. The knees and ankles should be properly padded. The anterior superior iliac spine and surrounding area should be padded as well to minimize the risk of meralgia paresthetica when patients are positioned prone. The lateral femoral cutaneous nerve exits the abdominal fascia near the anterior superior iliac spine and is vulnerable to compression in this region.

An additional consideration when positioning a spinal surgical patient is to provide proper support to pressure points to prevent soft tissue injury. The points of greatest susceptibility are the dependent areas, especially those adjacent to bony prominences (e.g., the heels in the supine position and the knees in the prone position). The best method of minimizing the risk of skin breakdown is to decrease the operative time. As this is not always possible, other means to decrease the pressure on vulnerable areas include allowing them to be free from compression and/or padding them.

Operative Ergonomics

The ideal ergonomic position for the surgeon is one that maintains cervical and lumbar lordosis such that the surgeon's head remains above his or her shoulders and hips in relative spinal balance. Unfortunately, the importance of proper surgeon positioning, especially over a long career, is underappreciated, and it is seldom achieved. The use of the operating microscope or surgical endoscope can improve surgeon ergonomics, as they allow the surgeon to view operative anatomy by moving the means of visualization, rather than the surgeon's neck or back. Still, spinal surgeons may find that they have to contort themselves to adequately view the surgical anatomy in certain situations (e.g., spondylolisthesis at L5-S1 in patients with a high slip angle). Adjusting the operating room table can help the surgeon to compensate for less than ideal ergonomic situations (e.g., placing patients with L5-S1 spondylolisthesis in the reverse Trendelenburg position). Ongoing developments in surgical technology, such as "head's up" display technologies, may help improve operative ergonomics.

Conclusion

Proper patient positioning is absolutely critical to the success of spinal surgical procedures. A multitude of factors must be considered to adequately position the spinal surgical patient, including optimal surgical exposure, patient safety, and ergonomics for the surgeon. By addressing these factors, spinal surgeons can minimize complications and improve outcomes.

The Supine, Sitting, and Lithotomy Positions

11

Shaheryar F. Ansari and Jean-Pierre Mobasser

Introduction

Positioning is a critical component of the operation in any neurosurgical case. Inadequate positioning can impede access to the site of interest, limit the surgeons view, or injure the patient. On the other hand, appropriate positioning can facilitate the efficient completion of an operation, divert blood to optimize visualization, and protect the patient from injuries such as pressure ulcers or neuropathies. In this chapter, the authors discuss sitting, supine, and lithotomy positions. Indications for each position will be discussed, along with advantages and drawbacks of each position.

The Sitting Position

The sitting position for neurosurgical procedures was first described by De Martel in 1931 [1]. It has seen variable popularity over the intervening years, and controversy continues in the literature to this day. While it certainly has its advantages, it presents many challenges to the operative team and has the potential for significant complications for the patient. While commonly used for posterior fossa cranial surgery, it is also useful in certain spinal operations. On the whole, though, its use has been in decline [2].

Positioning the Patient

After induction of general anesthesia and placement of appropriate lines, monitors, and catheters, the patient is positioned in a Mayfield head holder. The AORN recommends use of a lateral transfer device and for multiple caregivers to work together to place the patient into position [3]. The table is then raised slowly to bring the patient into a sitting position. It is recommended to perform this change in position over several minutes to avoid major hemodynamic shifts, as patients have depressed cardiovascular reflexes under general anesthesia [4, 5]. The neck is then secured in a neutral and slightly flexed position [6]. The severe flexion needed for posterior fossa cranial surgery is not necessary in the case of sitting posterior cervical surgery. The Mayfield clamp is secured to a cross bar which is anchored to the operative table. Care is taken to ensure that the patient's hip and knees are not excessively flexed and that prominences are carefully padded. The arms are

S. F. Ansari J. -P. Mobasser (✉)
Goodman Campbell Brain and Spine,
Indianapolis, IN, USA

Department of Neurological Surgery,
Indiana University School of Medicine,
Indianapolis, IN, USA
e-mail: sfansari@iu.edu;
jmobasser@goodmancampbell.com

A. Arthur et al. (eds.), *Perioperative Considerations and Positioning for Neurosurgical Procedures*,
https://doi.org/10.1007/978-3-319-72679-3_11

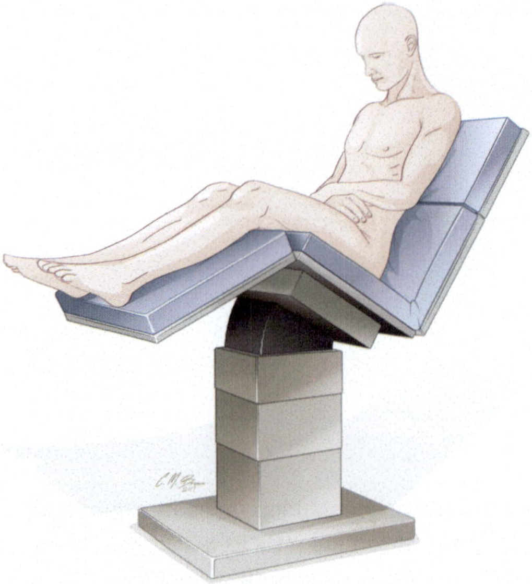

Fig. 11.1 The sitting position (illustration credit: Christopher Brown)

secured on arm boards and accessible to the anesthetist. The fluoroscope is then positioned with the base at the foot of the bed. Figure 11.1 illustrates the patient in the sitting position.

Procedures Performed

The most common spinal procedure performed in the sitting position is the cervical laminotomy or laminectomy, though some groups have reported performing thoracic laminectomies, as well [4–12]. Decompressive surgery for radiculopathy has been widely reported with a large number of patients [6, 11], and tumors can also be resected in the sitting position [13]. There is a single case report about a combined anterior and posterior reconstruction in the sitting position [5].

Anesthesia and Monitoring

Induction of anesthesia for surgery in the sitting position should follow the anesthesiologist's routine, with the same attention to neck positioning as other cervical operations. If intraoperative neuromonitoring is to be used, then total intravenous anesthesia will be necessary. Careful attention should be paid to hemodynamic status during positioning. Patients with poor autoregulation may be especially susceptible to drops in blood pressure during this phase [10]. Venous pooling in the lower extremities also limits venous return and may lower cardiac output [3, 10, 14].

Standard hemodynamic monitoring, electrocardiogram, noninvasive and invasive blood pressure, capnography, and oximetry are employed in all cases. Monitoring for air embolus is mandatory during sitting position surgery, given the catastrophic nature of this complication [2, 7, 11, 14–16]. The ASA does not provide a specific guideline for what kind of monitoring to use, but the literature contains considerable information to help practitioners make this decision. The use of precordial Doppler was first described by Michenfelder et al. in 1972 [16]. This provides a characteristic auditory signal to the entry of air into the heart. Recent analyses have indicated this to be a highly sensitive way to detect air emboli—Standefer et al. indicate that it detected 91% of air emboli in their population [12], though others place the detection rate closer to 50% [4]. Even more sensitive than Doppler is intraoperative transesophageal echocardiography (TEE). This technique was first described by Cucchiara et al. in 1984, and they described the ability of TEE to detect as little as one air bubble in the cardiac chambers, and point out that TEE provides excellent spatial localization of the air, which Doppler is unable to provide [15]. Ganslandt et al. found that a much higher incidence of air embolism in a group monitored with TEE than they did with the Doppler [4]. Many groups also recommend preoperative evaluation for a patent foramen ovale to avoid paradoxical air emboli [8, 15, 17].

Advantages

The sitting position does create certain advantages for the surgeon—it places the head above the heart and can enhance venous drainage, leading to lower intracranial pressure, which is particularly important for posterior fossa tumor operations [7, 12]. This also decompresses the epidural venous plexus, which may decrease epidural bleeding. For cervical spine surgery, allowing the shoulders to drop out of the way affords better visualization on fluoroscopy, and upright alignment is very evident [18]. It also allows drainage of blood and CSF out of the field by way of gravity, thus providing superior visualization of the operative field [7, 12, 18]. Furthermore, this position is much better tolerated by obese patients with regard to ventilation than is the prone position. The anesthesiologist also has easy access to both arms in case of problems with intravenous access or need for more lines.

Complications and Disadvantages

Air Embolism

Perhaps the most feared complication of sitting position surgery, air embolism carries with it the potential for catastrophic injury to the patient. Much has been written about this complication and how to manage it. There is variability in reporting, and the incidence may vary from as little as 1.6% to as high as 76% [4, 6, 12, 13, 15, 17, 19]. Part of the variability is due to differences in monitoring technique, but there is also variability in reporting. Some publications report all air emboli whereas others report only those that are "clinically significant"—the definition of which varies. The Tübingen group has published a grading scale in the hopes of standardizing the way that air emboli are reported and discussed in the literature with an emphasis on the patient's clinical status [7].

There does seem to be a difference between posterior fossa cranial operations and cervical spine operations with regard to the incidence of air embolism, with much less frequent air embolism in cervical operations—as low as 0.7% in the population of Himes et al. [8], 2.3% in the study by Zeidman and Ducker [11], and Standefer et al. found that there were a very small number of patients who had cervical laminectomies among their population of patients with significant embolic events [12]. Likely, this difference is accounted for by the fact that no large venous sinus is encountered in cervical surgery as opposed to posterior fossa operations. No group reported ischemic sequalae following air embolus detection intraoperatively, and it may be that small amounts of air pass frequently into the circulation but clinically have no effect [8].

Quadriplegia

Midcervical quadriplegia is an exceedingly rare but reported complication after sitting position surgery. It was first reported by Hitselberger and House in 1980 in the setting of acoustic neuroma surgery [14] but has since been reported again [20, 21]. The theorized mechanism is stretched on the cervical spinal cord when the neck is flexed may cause impaired autoregulation of spinal cord blood flow. Combined with the already reduced cardiac output in the setting of general anesthesia and the hemodynamics of the sitting position, the spinal cord may see significant ischemia, especially during prolonged surgery [22]. The spinal cord may elongate up to 2.8 cm from full extension to full flexion [21], and overlying cervical stenosis may contribute to constriction of the arteries.

Peripheral Neuropathies

Sciatic and peroneal neuropathies have been reported after surgery in the sitting position. Bilateral sciatic neuropathy in a patient who underwent surgery in the sitting position was described by Wang et al. and is only the fourth reported case of sciatic neuropathy causing weakness of plantarflexion, all of which occurred after prolonger operations [23]. Peroneal neuropathy causing a foot drop is more common, though still occurs less than 1% of the time after sitting position surgery, and patients are able to recover function with time and therapy [10, 23, 24]. Patient factors that may increase the risk of peripheral nerve injury include a low BMI, old age, smoking, and pre-existing peripheral neuropathies [23]. Careful padding and patient selection can aid in minimizing this complication.

Face and Tongue Swelling

Tattersall reports a case of massive facial and tongue swelling that necessitated reintubation and a prolonged stay in the ICU, culminating in

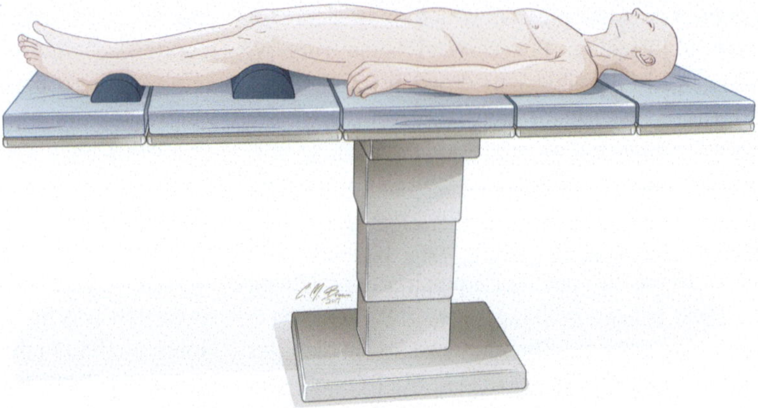

Fig. 11.2 The supine position (illustration credit: Christopher Brown)

patient death [25]. This was suspected to be due to excessive flexion of the neck which caused venous hypertension and ultimately thrombosis with no drainage of the head. Porter et al. recommend use of a small diameter echo probe and the avoidance of a rigid oral airway to minimize the risk of this complication [10].

Ergonomics and Learning Curve

The sitting position places a great deal of strain on the surgeon, who must keep his arms elevated for the duration of the surgery. This necessitates the surgeon to either work quickly or formulate a sterile solution upon which to rest his arms. Surgeon fatigue can lead to errors and potential complications. The learning curve for sitting position surgery can be significant for the operative team. Because this position is not commonly used, the first few cases will require extra time to get the patient safely into position. Repetition, however, will build competence and comfort for the team with the sitting position. Similarly, the anesthesiologist must be comfortable with the patient in this position and the accompanying changes as outlined above.

The Supine Position

The supine position is one of the most commonly used positions in neurosurgery and many other surgical subspecialties. Its ubiquity makes it straightforward for the operative team, but there are precautions that must be taken to prevent injury to the patient.

How to Position the Patient

The supine position is illustrated in Fig. 11.2. The patient may move onto the operating table under his or her own power if able, or he or she may be moved by the operative team. The AORN recommends the use of a lateral transfer device in the latter case, with at least four people (including the anesthesiologist) to assist with the transfer [3]. A pillow should be placed under the patient's knees to avoid any strain on the hamstrings and back muscles. The head should be on a headrest. The heels should be elevated or sufficiently padded with foam to avoid pressure ulcers. Some institutions may also pad the sacrum. A safety belt should be placed approximately two inches above the knees to protect the patient from falling off of the table [26]. If the arms are to be abducted on arm boards, care should be taken to avoid abducting the arms more than 90° to lower the risk of brachial plexus injury [3, 27]. If arms are to be tucked at the sides, the AORN recommends against "tucking" by wrapping the sheet around the patient's arm and securing it under the table, but rather supports "papoosing" the patient by wrapping the sheet around the patient to secure the arms [3]. If securing the patient's arms at the sides, care should be taken to pad all prominences at the elbow and wrist and pad the intravenous lines against the skin. The draw sheet should extend above the elbows [3, 26]. The IV lines should be carefully checked to ensure they are still running, as tubes can get kinked during arm positioning.

Depending on the patient's size and spinal levels of interest, there may be a need to push the shoulders down with a brace or with tape to obtain better exposure of the lower cervical spine for fluoroscopy. In myelopathic patients, care should be taken with neck position and neck manipulation during anesthetic induction. The need for cervical traction is determined by the surgeon on a case-by-case basis. The neck should be placed in slight lordosis to maintain the anatomic alignment after fusion.

Procedures Performed in the Supine Position

The supine position is ideal for anterior cervical exposure for discectomy or corpectomy. The surgeon can access almost the entire cervical spine from the anterior exposure. Access to the C2-C3 level may be somewhat limited by the mandible. One group from Japan places the patient in extension and rightward rotation to move the mandible out of the way, but has found that this can affect the extent of decompression and place the vertebral artery at risk of injury [28]. Anterior odontoid screw fixation is also best accomplished in this position. The supine position also allows for anterior lumbar spine exposure. This often requires the spine surgeon to work with a general or vascular surgeon for access to the surgical site.

Anesthesia and Monitoring

Induction of anesthesia is relatively straightforward and can follow the attending anesthesiologist's routine. Total intravenous anesthesia is used if intraoperative neuromonitoring is to be utilized. Great care should be utilized in myelopathic patients or patients with unstable cervical spine injuries, in whom intubation should be carried out either while the patient is awake and/or with minimal neck manipulation. Light wand and GlideScope™ are optimal tools to use for intubation in the setting of myelopathy. Standard monitoring should include EKG, pulse oximetry, capnography, noninvasive blood pressure, and invasive blood pressure at the discretion of the anesthesiologist. Monitoring of motor and somatosensory evoked potentials and electromyography should be used at the discretion of the surgeon. For anterior lumbar operations, in which the iliac arteries and veins are retracted, use of lower extremity oximetry may be used at the discretion of the surgical team [29–31].

Advantages

The supine position is common and thus easy for the surgical team. This also allows for the patient to be positioned relatively quickly (in contrast to the sitting position, which can add considerable time to the positioning portion of a case). The anesthetic is also usually straightforward in the supine position though very obese patients or patients with significant pulmonary disease can have some difficulty with ventilation in this position [3]. The supine position is also ergonomically familiar and comfortable for the surgeon and surgical technician.

Disadvantages and Complications

Visualization

Adequate visualization can be difficult in the supine position, especially in large patients. The fluoroscopic image is significantly limited by the patient's shoulders in the lower cervical spine. This creates a hazard when localizing and requires the surgeon take extra steps to ensure that the correct level is exposed. Seeing into the operative field is also difficult in large patients, especially if the chest is prominent, creating limited working space between the chest and the chin. Limited light and a long reach for instruments can make the surgery both more technically challenging and raise the risk of complications for the patient.

Working angles can be a challenge for hardware placement at the extremes of the cervical spine. At C3-4 (and indeed at C2-3), the chin and mandible can create difficulty with appropriately angling fixation screws for the anterior plate. Similarly, at C7-T1, the manubrium can create difficulty with placing hardware. In a patient with a large chest, obtaining the correct angle for an odontoid screw can be particularly challenging.

Venous Congestion

Lying flat allows redistribution of venous blood to the head and neck and can engorge the epidural venous plexus. In contrast to the sitting position, where there may be little to no epidural bleeding, this can be much more significant in the supine position. Furthermore, if a chin strap is used for cervical traction, this can further worsen venous congestion by compressing the jugular vein. Congestion can be somewhat mitigated by placing the patient in a slight reverse Trendelenburg position.

Patient Anatomy

In the setting of a patient with a very steep sacral slope, it may be difficult or impossible to access the L5-S1 disc space to perform an anterior discectomy and fusion. In such cases, it may become necessary to use the lithotomy position (to retrovert the pelvis) or use an alternative procedure. Patients with previous shoulder operations or pre-existing shoulder conditions may suffer from worsened shoulder discomfort or stiffness after prolonged taping of the shoulders.

Neck Positioning

In anterior cervical operations with significant stenosis, the patient may develop monitoring changes if the neck is extended to create lordosis. In such a case, the neck should be kept neutral or moved back into the last position with intact evoked potentials until the spinal cord is adequately decompressed, then lordosis can be created intraoperatively by removing bolsters under the head.

Peripheral Nerve Injuries

The brachial plexus is particularly vulnerable in any surgery where the arm may be abducted or the shoulder manipulated. This is because of its long course, relatively superficial position, and the fact that it is anchored at two fixed points—the spine and the axillary fascia as it passes into the arm [32]. The plexus also contacts the clavicle, first rib, and the head of the humerus along its course, all of which can cause stretch or compression on the plexus [32]. Uribe et al. describe brachial plexus injury after spine surgery in their population, with 44 of 514 patients suffering from brachial plexus injuries after being in the supine or lateral position. Fortunately, most patients recover completely and only a very small fraction have deficits persisting beyond 3 months [32]. Ben-David and Stahl similarly found in their population of patient with postoperative brachial plexus injuries that most patients recover full within 3 months and that a small proportion have a persistent deficit beyond that time period, but they noted that even patients with a persistent deficit tend to show continued functional improvement [33]. The mechanism of injury is likely prolonged stretch and/or compression along the course of the brachial plexus, especially in cases where the shoulders are taped down aggressively for visualization or if the arms are abducted beyond 90 degrees [3, 27]. Under general anesthesia, the normal defensive muscle reflexes and the ability to move the arm into a more comfortable position are absent, creating a situation in which nerve injuries are more likely [32].

The ulnar nerve, with its relatively superficial course, is also susceptible to injury due to malposition of the arm. The ASA recommends taking care to pad the elbow and keep the arm in a neutral position if tucked/wrapped or to keep the arm in a supinated or neutral position if placed on an arm board [27]. There is less concern regarding the radial and median nerves, as these are relatively protected by muscle along their respective courses, though the ASA does recommend taking care to avoid putting pressure on the spiral groove of the humerus [27].

The Lithotomy Position

Though the lithotomy position is uncommonly used in the neurosurgical world, it is useful to access the pelvis and perineal region and thus often used in urology, gynecology, and colon and rectal surgery. The lack of familiarity with this position can be a major challenge for operative teams, but it can be highly useful for select indications.

How to Position the Patient

The process of placing the patient in the lithotomy position begins with the patient supine on the operating table for induction. The legs are then elevated, abducted, and placed in stirrups for support [34]. The patient is moved so that the buttocks are on the end of the table. The legs are elevated such that the pelvis can be retroverted. It is recommended to position the legs slowly and simultaneously, with support on both the foot and the lower leg [34]. The bottom section of the table should only be lowered after the legs are secured. Padding should be placed under the sacrum to prevent lumbosacral strain. Care should be taken to avoid excess pressure on the popliteal region and the heels should be padded to prevent pressure ulcers [3]. The arms are placed on arm boards and abducted less than 90 degrees. The patient should be secured to the table with a safety strap and/or tape. If any Trendelenburg posture is used, some authors recommend the use of a soft shoulder brace to prevent the patient from sliding cranially [35]. When taking the patient out of lithotomy position, the lower section of the table should be raised before the legs are removed from the stirrups, and they should be removed simultaneously and extended fully before lowering onto the table [34]. Figures 11.3 and 11.4 illustrate this position.

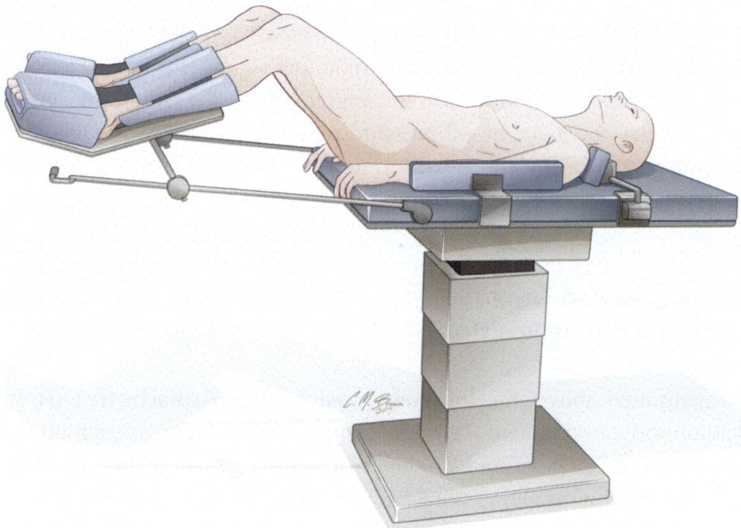

Fig. 11.3 The lithotomy position with Trendelenburg (illustration credit: Christopher Brown)

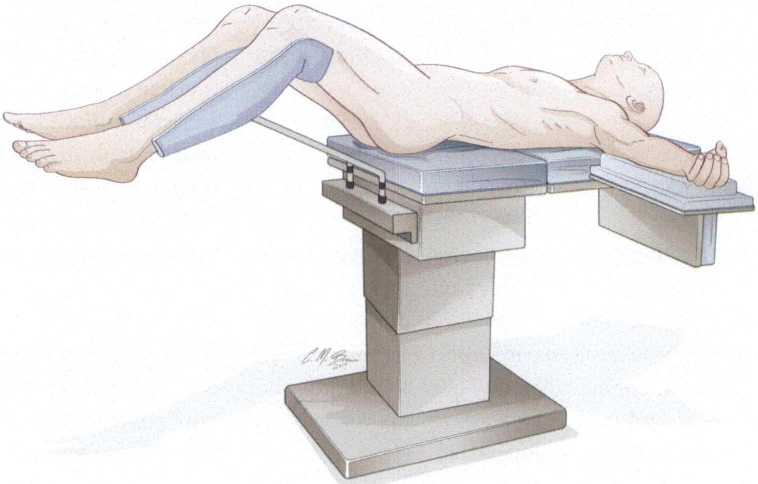

Fig. 11.4 The lithotomy position with less elevation of the legs (illustration credit: Christopher Brown)

Anesthesia and Monitoring

Anesthesia induction and maintenance should follow the anesthesiologist's routine for intra-abdominal surgery. It has been reported that physiological dead space is increased in lower abdominal surgery performed in the lithotomy and Trendelenburg position, and that respiratory compliance is decreased as a result of pressure on the lungs from the intra-abdominal contents [36]. The oxygen tension in the blood has been shown to be lower in patients in the lithotomy position after about 10 min, relative to the supine position [36]. This effect may be augmented in obese patients, requiring increased ventilator support while in this position. Monitoring should consist of standard intraoperative anesthetic monitors—EKG, noninvasive blood pressure, capnography, and oximetry. Invasive blood pressure monitoring can be performed at the discretion of the anesthesiologist.

Procedures Performed in the Lithotomy Position

As mentioned above, the lithotomy position is uncommonly used in neurosurgery. The primary indication for this position is for anterior lumbar interbody fusion involving the L5/S1 interspace in which there is a very steep sacral inclination which is difficult to access in the supine position. The lithotomy position allows for retroversion of the pelvis and brings the interspace more perpendicular to the floor and thus more accessible.

Advantages

By allowing the surgeon access to a steep L5/S1 disc or patients with a very high grade spondylolisthesis, the lithotomy position allows for solid interbody arthrodesis in group of patients with very challenging anatomy in whom traditional anterior and posterior interbody approaches are very difficult, if not impossible.

Disadvantages and Complications

Lack of Familiarity

The lack of experience among neurosurgical teams with this position is a major challenge and arises from the infrequency with which this position is used. As such, the risk of complications is higher if careful attention is not paid to each individual detail of positioning. Similarly, the surgeon's own comfort level with the lithotomy position and the anatomy when in this position may increase the risk of complications until sufficient experience is gained [37]. The perioperative team should consider utilizing the experience from other surgical departments for optimal patient safety.

From the perspective of surgical education, the lithotomy position is somewhat suboptimal. Because the lithotomy position places the surgeon between the patient's legs, there is limited room for others to view the operative field. This creates difficulty for trainees and academic surgeons who wish to teach the procedure, whereas in prone and supine positions, the surgeon and assistant are able to stand across from each other.

Anesthetic Difficulties

As mentioned above, there are significant pulmonary changes while in the lithotomy position, especially if this is combined with Trendelenburg. The abdominal contents compress the diaphragm, raising pressure in the chest. In a high lithotomy position, especially in an obese patient, the thighs place pressure on the abdomen and further increase pressure on the lungs [36, 38, 39]. Fahy et al. mention that there is an expected reduction in PaO_2 and increase in $PaCO_2$, and while these shifts are not unacceptable in healthy patients, patients with preexisting cardiopulmonary comorbidity may not tolerate them as well [38]. Ryniak et al. mention that lung elasticity and compliance increase when in the Trendelenburg position, and elasticity increase further with lithotomy positioning [39]. This knowledge necessitates careful monitoring of the respiratory status of patients while in the lithotomy position and implies that certain patients may be unable to tolerate being in this position.

Peripheral Neuropathies

Because of the unique positioning of the legs in lithotomy, multiple peripheral nerves are at risk for injury. The ASA recommends limiting hip flexion to 90 degrees, as this minimizes stretch on the sciatic nerve [27]. Gumus et al. found a postoperative neurapraxia in 12 of 1170 patients undergoing surgery in the lithotomy position. They, too, comment that excess hip flexion places the sciatic nerve under stretch which over time can result in injury. In their series, only two patients had a deficit persist beyond 1 month. They concluded that age over 70 and operative time longer than 3 h contributed to an increased risk of postop neurapraxia [37]. The ASA indicates that the femoral nerve may also be at risk with excessive abduction and external rotation of the hips [27]. Finally, both the ASA and the AORN recommend careful padding of the fibular head, as prolonged pressure on this region can lead to peroneal neuropathy and foot drop [3, 27].

Compartment Syndrome

This is a dreaded, though rare, complication of lithotomy positioning. Zappa et al. describe in their series of 473 patients undergoing gynecologic surgery in the lithotomy position, 8 patients developed compartment syndrome requiring fasciotomy [35]. Sajid et al. mention that the incidence of compartment syndrome requiring fasciotomy in colorectal patients is about 1/3500 [40]. The pathophysiology of compartment syndrome is prolonged ischemia followed by reperfusion and edema [35, 40–43]. It is suspected that raising the legs above heart level, combined with pressure on the leg musculature and vasculature while in stirrups, impedes blood flow to the calf musculature. The prolonged ischemia results in breakdown of the basement membranes around the blood vessels and leads to the leakage of fluid into the interstitial space, resulting in swelling of the muscle [41–43]. Consensus in the literature suggests that 3–4 h of operative time is the point at which the risk of compartment syndrome rises [40, 41]. Rapid diagnosis and treatment with fasciotomy is then necessary to prevent permanent neurologic damage or loss of limb [35, 40]. Recommended preventive measures include careful padding of the calf and heel, minimizing Trendelenburg positioning, and minimizing hypovolemia [40].

Realistically speaking, the lithotomy position is rarely used in spine surgery and is somewhat limited to centers where it is used in conjunction with vascular and general surgeons who are comfortable with set up and patient positioning. While it is not a necessary tool for the spine surgeon's armamentarium, it could be a useful adjunct from time to time, when a patient has a steep sacral inclination, and an anteriorly placed graft is required.

Conclusion

This chapter discussed the sitting, supine, and lithotomy positions in spine surgery. Methods of positioning were explained and nuances described. Advantages and disadvantages to each position were explored. Each position has specific indications. Surgeons must choose the position best suited for the individual operation and patient in order to optimize surgical access and minimize position-related injury.

Acknowledgment The authors thank Christopher Brown for assistance with illustrations.

References

1. De Martel T. Surgical treatment of cerebral tumours. Technical considerations. Surg Gynecol Obstet. 1931;52:381–5.
2. Elton RJ, Howell RS. The sitting position in neurosurgical anaesthesia: a survey of British practice in 1991. Br J Anaesth. 1994;73(2):247–8.
3. Recommended Practices for Positioning the Patient in the Perioperative Practice Setting. In: Nurses AoOR, editor. 2009 Perioperative Standards and Recommended Practices. 2009.
4. Ganslandt O, Merkel A, Schmitt H, Tzabazis A, Buchfelder M, Eyupoglu I, et al. The sitting position in neurosurgery: indications, complications and results. A single institution experience of 600 cases. Acta Neurochir. 2013;155(10):1887–93.
5. Han Y, Xia Q, Hu YC, Zhang JD, Lan J, Ma XL. Simultaneously combined anterior-posterior approaches for subaxial cervical circumferential reconstruction in a sitting position. Orthop Surg. 2015;7(4):371–4.

6. Adamson TE. Microendoscopic posterior cervical laminoforaminotomy for unilateral radiculopathy: results of a new technique in 100 cases. J Neurosurg. 2001;95(1 Suppl):51–7.
7. Feigl GC, Decker K, Wurms M, Krischek B, Ritz R, Unertl K, et al. Neurosurgical procedures in the semi-sitting position: evaluation of the risk of paradoxical venous air embolism in patients with a patent foramen ovale. World Neurosurg. 2014;81(1):159–64.
8. Himes BT, Mallory GW, Abcejo AS, Pasternak J, Atkinson JL, Meyer FB, et al. Contemporary analysis of the intraoperative and perioperative complications of neurosurgical procedures performed in the sitting position. J Neurosurg. 2016;127(1):1–7.
9. Leslie K, Hui R, Kaye AH. Venous air embolism and the sitting position: a case series. J Clin Neurosci. 2006;13(4):419–22.
10. Porter JM, Pidgeon C, Cunningham AJ. The sitting position in neurosurgery: a critical appraisal. Br J Anaesth. 1999;82(1):117–28.
11. Zeidman SM, Ducker TB. Posterior cervical laminoforaminotomy for radiculopathy: review of 172 cases. Neurosurgery. 1993;33(3):356–62.
12. Standefer M, Bay JW, Trusso R. The sitting position in neurosurgery: a retrospective analysis of 488 cases. Neurosurgery. 1984;14(6):649–58.
13. Basaldella L, Ortolani V, Corbanese U, Sorbara C, Longatti P. Massive venous air embolism in the semi-sitting position during surgery for a cervical spinal cord tumor: anatomic and surgical pitfalls. J Clin Neurosci. 2009;16(7):972–5.
14. Hitselberger WE, House WF. A warning regarding the sitting position for acoustic tumor surgery. Arch Otolaryngol. 1980;106(2):69.
15. Cucchiara RF, Nugent M, Seward JB, Messick JM. Air embolism in upright neurosurgical patients: detection and localization by two-dimensional transesophageal echocardiography. Anesthesiology. 1984;60(4):353–5.
16. Michenfelder JD, Miller RH, Gronert GA. Evaluation of an ultrasonic device (Doppler) for the diagnosis of venous air embolism. Anesthesiology. 1972; 36(2):164–7.
17. Fathi AR, Eshtehardi P, Meier B. Patent foramen ovale and neurosurgery in sitting position: a systematic review. Br J Anaesth. 2009;102(5):588–96.
18. Sandwell S, Kimmell KT, Silberstein HJ, Rodenhouse TG, Maurer PK, Pilcher WH, et al. 349 safety of the sitting cervical position for elective spine surgery. Neurosurgery. 2016;63(Suppl 1):203.
19. Papadopoulos G, Kuhly P, Brock M, Rudolph KH, Link J, Eyrich K. Venous and paradoxical air embolism in the sitting position. A prospective study with transoesophageal echocardiography. Acta Neurochir. 1994;126(2–4):140–3.
20. Mostafa RM, Mejadi A. Quadriplegia after interscalene block for shoulder surgery in sitting position. Br J Anaesth. 2013;111(5):846–7.
21. Morandi X, Riffaud L, Amlashi SF, Brassier G. Extensive spinal cord infarction after posterior fossa surgery in the sitting position: case report. Neurosurgery. 2004;54(6):1512–5. discussion 5–6.
22. Wilder BL. Hypothesis: the etiology of midcervical quadriplegia after operation with the patient in the sitting position. Neurosurgery. 1982;11(4):530–1.
23. Wang JC, Wong TT, Chen HH, Chang PY, Yang TF. Bilateral sciatic neuropathy as a complication of craniotomy performed in the sitting position: localization of nerve injury by using magnetic resonance imaging. Childs Nerv Syst. 2012;28(1):159–63.
24. Keykhah MM, Rosenberg H. Bilateral footdrop after craniotomy in the sitting position. Anesthesiology. 1979;51(2):163–4.
25. Tattersall MP. Massive swelling of the face and tongue. A complication of posterior cranial fossa surgery in the sitting position. Anaesthesia. 1984;39(10): 1015–7.
26. St-Arnaud D, Paquin MJ. Safe positioning for neurosurgical patients. Can Oper Room Nurs J. 2009;27(4):7–11. 16, 18–19 passim.
27. Apfelbaum JLCR, Caplan RA, Nickinovich DG. Practice advisory for the prevention of perioperative peripheral neuropathies. Anesthesiology. 2011;114(4):741–54.
28. Tanahashi H, Miyamoto K, Hioki A, Iinuma N, Ohno T, Shimizu K. Alterations in axial curvature of the cervical spine with a combination of rotation and extension in the conventional anterior cervical approach. Eur Spine J. 2013;22(12):2850–6.
29. Crofts KM, Wong DA, Murr PC. Anterior paramedian retroperitoneal surgical approach to the lumbar spine. Orthopedics. 1994;17(8):699–702.
30. Czerwein JK Jr, Thakur N, Migliori SJ, Lucas P, Palumbo M. Complications of anterior lumbar surgery. J Am Acad Orthop Surg. 2011;19(5):251–8.
31. Edgard-Rosa G, Geneste G, Negre G, Marnay T. Midline anterior approach from the right side to the lumbar spine for interbody fusion and total disc replacement: a new mobilization technique of the vena cava. Spine. 2012;37(9):E562–9.
32. Uribe JS, Kolla J, Omar H, Dakwar E, Abel N, Mangar D, et al. Brachial plexus injury following spinal surgery. J Neurosurg Spine. 2010;13(4):552–8.
33. Ben-David B, Stahl S. Prognosis of intraoperative brachial plexus injury: a review of 22 cases. Br J Anaesth. 1997;79(4):440–5.
34. Positioning the patient for surgery. In: Goodman T, Cynthia Spry, editor. Essentials of perioperative nursing. 7th ed. Burlington, MA: Jones & Bartlett Learning; 2017. p. 141–65.
35. Zappa L, Sugarbaker PH. Compartment syndrome of the leg associated with lithotomy position for cytoreductive surgery. J Surg Oncol. 2007;96(7):619–23.
36. Unoki T, Mizutani T, Toyooka H. Changes in respiratory physiological dead space and compliance during non-abdominal, upper abdominal and lower abdominal surgery under general anaesthesia. Eur J Anaesthesiol. 2004;21(4):302–8.
37. Gumus E, Kendirci M, Horasanli K, Tanriverdi O, Gidemez G, Miroglu C. Neurapraxic complications

in operations performed in the lithotomy position. World J Urol. 2002;20(1):68–71.
38. Fahy BG, Barnas GM, Nagle SE, Flowers JL, Njoku MJ, Agarwal M. Effects of Trendelenburg and reverse Trendelenburg postures on lung and chest wall mechanics. J Clin Anesth. 1996;8(3):236–44.
39. Ryniak S, Brannstedt S, Blomqvist H. Effects of exaggerated lithotomy position on ventilation and hemodynamics during radical perineal prostatectomy. Scand J Urol Nephrol. 1998;32(3):200–3.
40. Sajid MS, Shakir AJ, Khatri K, Baig MK. Lithotomy-related neurovascular complications in the lower limbs after colorectal surgery. Color Dis. 2011;13(11):1203–13.
41. Chow CE, Friedell ML, Freeland MB, Dejesus S. A pitfall of protracted surgery in the lithotomy Position: lower extremity compartment syndrome. Am Surg. 2007;73(1):19–21.
42. Stornelli N, Wydra FB, Mitchell JJ, Stahel PF, Fabbri S. The dangers of lithotomy positioning in the operating room: case report of bilateral lower extremity compartment syndrome after a 90-minutes surgical procedure. Patient Saf Surg. 2016;10:18.
43. Wassenaar EB, van den Brand JG, van der Werken C. Compartment syndrome of the lower leg after surgery in the modified lithotomy position: report of seven cases. Dis Colon Rectum. 2006;49(9):1449–53.

12 Spinal Procedures in the Lateral Position

Matthew T. Brown, Raul Cardenas, and Julius Fernandez

Introduction

Lateral approaches to the thoracolumbar spine were initially described by Mayer and McAfee in 1997 and 1998. These approaches have become a more frequently used technique following the series published by Pimenta in 2006 and the implementation of minimally invasive techniques [1–3]. Most commonly touted as an alternative to the muscle-disruptive posterior approaches while avoiding the vascular and abdominal complications of anterior approaches, the lateral approach presents a unique set of risks to the patient while offering an alternative for decompression and stabilization of the thoracolumbar spine [4].

The two most common indications for utilization of the lateral approach include both trauma of the thoracolumbar junction and degenerative disease of the lumbar spine. Additionally, the lateral position can be utilized when other lesions or pathology preclude safe prone positioning with compression of a large vessel or airway. Although a lateral approach can be utilized for thoracic disc disease, our institution feels a posterior approach provides both adequate exposure and a more familiar approach for these rare lesions when able.

Positioning for the Elective Spine

Once the patient has been identified for the procedure, the first critical step in positioning is the choice of operating tables. For the minimally invasive lateral, trans-psoas approach used by our group for lateral lumbar interbody fusion (MIS-LLIF) the Skytron operating bed is utilized. This bed allows for both an appropriate break, when necessary, as well as the option for the bed to be translated cranially or caudally. The translation allows for the primary operative site to be moved away from the base of the table, allowing for sufficient under-bed clearance for the C-arm fluoroscopy unit. Tables that are unable to translate will often limit C-arm positioning over the break, and/or the lumbar spine, significantly reducing the adequate visualization of the spine throughout the procedure; without a true AP and lateral image, the MIS-LLIF approach is much less safe, and not recommended [5].

M. T. Brown (✉)
Department of Neurosurgery, University of Tennessee, Memphis, TN, USA
e-mail: mbrow135@uthsc.edu

R. Cardenas · J. Fernandez (deceased)
Department of Neurosurgery, University of Tennessee, Memphis, TN, USA

Department of Neurosurgery, Semmes-Murphey Clinic, University of Tennessee, Memphis, TN, USA
e-mail: rcardenas@semmes-murphey.com

A. Arthur et al. (eds.), *Perioperative Considerations and Positioning for Neurosurgical Procedures*,
https://doi.org/10.1007/978-3-319-72679-3_12

Positioning the patient on the table is performed following intubation, induction of anesthesia, and placement of neuromonitoring electrodes. A bite block of rolled dressing sponges can be used to prevent tongue trauma if MEPs are to be used, though the use of monitoring, including MEPs, does not significantly change the positioning process for the elective patient. The patient is placed on the table in the lateral decubitus position; the upward facing side can be determined by the anatomy of the patient. If a scoliotic curve is present, the concavity is generally positioned upwards to both allow the maximum number of levels to be accessed with a single skin and fascial incision; this will also generally allow better access to the L4/5 disc space, when targeted. Some advocate for the convexity to be positioned upward for assistance in curve correction though this has not been routinely used in our adult practice of largely inflexible curves [6]. In degenerative cases, the more collapsed side of the disc space or the larger osteophyte is placed dependent in order to maximize the ease of disc space entry. If there is no curve or anatomic restriction, typically the right lateral decubitus position is preferred. Though the anatomic imaging study by Deukmedjian et al. does show a slight movement of the inferior vena cava (IVC) out of the operative field with left lateral decubitus positioning, this proved to have only millimeters of change and has not been felt to be practically advantageous in our experience. Instead, if a vascular injury were to occur, there is much greater ease in the repair of an arterial versus a venous structure [7]. We often use a shallow, inflatable beanbag beneath the patient that will not rise higher than midline upon deflation, as such practice would result in poor fluoroscopy projection. The beanbag is either covered with a flat sheet, or used without covering; no additional padding is present between the patient and the beanbag bolster. The patient is positioned on the table so that the iliac crest is overlying the break of the table. Historically, the table was angulated to a great extent to drop the iliac crest out of the operative field and increase visualization of the lower lumbar vertebrae. With institutional experience, and reports within literature of increased morbidity secondary to nerve strain, we have gradually decreased the degree of table break to the lowest amount that allows direct access to the operative level. An angle break of 40° has been shown to cause femoral nerve strain of 6–7%, which is typically considered sufficient to limit nerve perfusion and possibly result in neurapraxia [8]. Conventionally, postoperative hip flexor weakness has been attributed to dissection through the psoas muscle itself. A study by Molinares et al. in 2016 studied healthy individuals placed within the lateral decubitus position both with and without a table break of 25° for 1 h. The typical transient neurapraxia with hip flexor weakness and sensory disturbance was seen in all patients in the lateral jack-knife position, but not those in the lateral decubitus position. The L1, 2, and 3 nerve roots on the nondependent (would-be-operative) side experienced symptoms of neurapraxia with 10–60% decrease in hip flexion strength, and 38% still having diminished sensation even after 1 h of recovery following the positioning [9]. With this, lessening of the table break angle has decreased the postoperative neurapraxia seen in our patients. Additionally, hips and knees are both bent at 60° to relieve tension on the psoas and the lumbar plexus/femoral nerve.

Once lateral, several pressure points are identified and padded or supported accordingly. A pillow is generally used beneath the dependent knee to pad the peroneal nerve, two additional pillows are then placed between the knees to avoid an area of potential bony compression as well as to abduct the hip which further shortens the nondependent psoas muscle. The feet are similarly padded to avoid pressure along the medial and lateral malleoli. Peroneal nerve compression at the fibular head with resultant injury has been reported and can be identified early during the case by MEP monitoring that will show attenuation should nerve injury be ongoing [10, 11]. With proper padding, this has not been seen in our longstanding cohort of patients.

An axillary roll is also placed for decompression of the brachial plexus. Traditionally, this has included a rolled blanket or a wrapped liter bag of saline; with improvements in positioning aids, we currently utilize an appropriately sized gel roll based upon the patient's body habitus. Use of gel padding has been shown to more effectively reduce pressure under the patient's shoulder and produce a lower chest wall pressure than a bag of IV fluid [12]. We position the axillary roll beneath the chest wall, allowing for elevation of the shoulder and decompression of the plexus. This allows for extension of the dependent arm and forearm perpendicular to the operating table with appropriate padding of the ulnar nerve and makes available line access to the anesthesia team. Rarely, a long thoracic nerve injury can be seen with the chest wall pressure from the axillary roll, but this has not been seen in our experience [13]. The nondependent arm and forearm are similarly extended perpendicular to the table and rest on a Mayo stand padded with pillows to prevent areas of pressure. It is important to adjust the Mayo stand appropriately with any subsequent repositioning or elevation change of the operative table as table changes during the case can change the angle and stress placed on the resting extremities. The elevation of the chest wall will cause an elevation of the shoulders and cervical spine. Without additional support beneath the patient's head, cervical angulation would cause stretch on the brachial plexus and possible compression of dependent vasculature with concern for interruption of cerebral blood flow or venous congestion [14]. A large foam head holder is utilized with additional bolstering material to ensure a neutral position of the head and cervical spine. Reusable, inflatable pillows are commercially available and can serve as both axillary rolls and head elevators with improvement in shoulder and chest wall pressures. Implementation of these has not been necessary given the rarity of brachial plexus or cervical injuries during lateral positioning with our aforementioned arrangement [12].

Once basic patient positioning is established, securing the patient to the table is performed in a regimented, step-wise fashion, shown in Fig. 12.1. Three-inch wide silk tape is utilized to secure the patient and make small corrections in the rotation of the patient to achieve a true AP and lateral view during the case. First, a line of tape is run transversely across the iliac crest. This tape will wrap circumferentially around the patient and table. We ensure that the tape in contact with the patient is flat in order to reduce the risk of skin abrasions though direct skin contact is important to prevent motion of the patient intraoperatively [15]. This initial tape line will also initiate the process of orienting the patient perpendicular to the operating room floor. The second line of tape extends from the crest, at the site of the original tape line, caudally along the course of the thigh. This will extend distally from the knee to be secured to the table. This second tape is under subtle traction to bring the ipsilateral iliac crest down, enhancing visualization of the lower lumbar spine. A third tape line is then directed from the patient's knee distally along the leg, avoiding direct compression of the fibular head, again being secured to the table. A further line of tape is run circumferentially along the upper chest wall, care should be taken to avoid tape directly on the nipple or areola; this tape is placed with the assistance of fluoroscopy to align the vertebral bodies of the lumbar spine to further assist in obtaining a true AP and lateral view, with gentle rotation as necessary. The position of the C-arm fluoroscopy unit is then marked to allow for consistent angles with both lateral and under-table AP imaging throughout the case. The final line of tape retraces the first, making the last adjustment to the lower trunk rotation and to confirm appropriate visualization with C-arm fluoroscopy.

Once the patient is positioned and secured, the incision is planned using fluoroscopy. We utilize a cross-hair tool (Fig. 12.2) to assist in localizing the correct level. With lateral fluoroscopy, the crosshairs are aligned atop the center of the targeted disc space; an incision is then drawn along the diagonal overlying the disc space. In our experience, the most ergonomical and safest position is for the operating surgeon to stand on the dorsal aspect of the patient, with the C-arm base on the ventral side. This minimizes the distance to the operative field, particularly with obese patients. In our practice, this regimen of positioning for elective cases removes the need for caudal rib resection to enhance visualization.

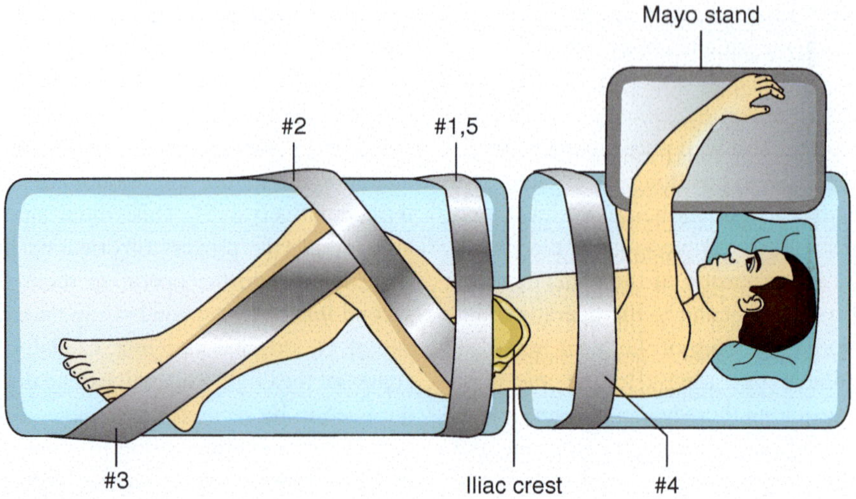

Fig. 12.1 The positioning and securing of the patient to the table with sequential placement of 3-in. silk tape bands

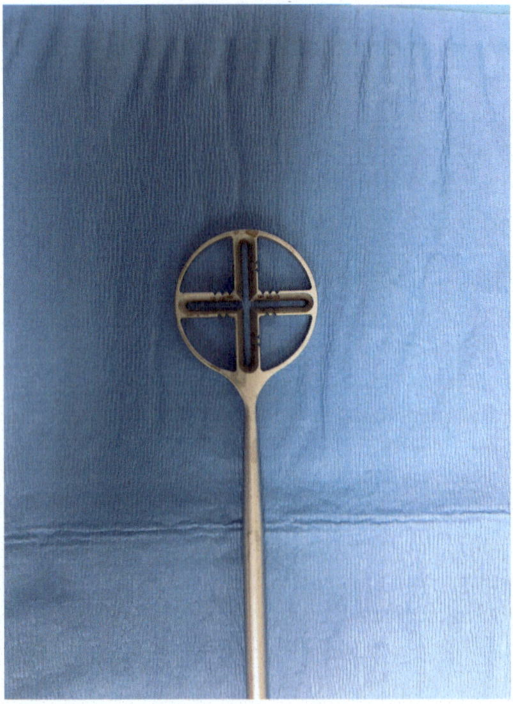

Fig. 12.2 The cross-hair tool to assist in incision planning over the localized, targeted disc space

Following typical preoperative preparation including local anesthetic and sterilization of the skin with appropriate draping, the procedure is carried out in accordance with the typical MIS-LLIF routine. Care is taken with the superficial dissection to avoid injury of the transiting nerves. The nerves particularly at risk of injury during the exposure include the subcostal nerve, the iliohypogastric nerve, and the ilioinguinal nerve. These nerves exit the lumbar plexus and are often encountered traveling inferomedially atop the fascia of the transversalis muscle, deep to the internal obliques [16]. Early identification of the nerves proves the best way for avoidance of inadvertent injury during the initial stages of dissection. Injury of these nerves can lead to pain, numbness, or abdominal wall paresis [17–19].

After developing and entering the retroperitoneal space, the psoas muscle is identified and the lumbar plexus becomes at risk during the next portion of the procedure. Traditionally, lateral fluoroscopy is used to place a guidewire into the operative disc space with active monitoring during serial advancement of dilators, culminating with a self-retaining retractor system. The anterior half of the disc space, within the sagittal plane, is the target of choice to allow for adequate discectomy and graft position while decreasing the risk of injury to the lumbar plexus. The lumbar plexus moves ventrally within the psoas muscle the more caudal the spine level; this places the neural structures within the psoas at a higher risk with lower targeted levels. With this in mind, the entry point is moved slightly ventral, up to the 2/3 point of the radiographic disc space at the L4/5 level (Fig. 12.3). Prior to placing the guidewire, we recommend direct visualization of the psoas muscle to ensure the genitofemoral nerve (often found running atop the muscle within the surgical corridor) is avoided; a Wylie retractor is extremely helpful in this endeavor [5, 16, 18]. Active nerve monitoring during dilation of the muscle proves very useful, particularly when directional. Rotating a directional probe during dilation can prevent inadvertent nerve injury, as well as ensures that the retractor is opened ventral to the plexus. When docking the retractors, inadvertent placement dorsal to the plexus could result in ventral nerve retraction leading to root stretch and injury [19]. Once the psoas is dilated, the retractor is placed and anchored, centered on the disc space. The discectomy can be performed with the plexus remaining in safety, posterior to the retractors.

In addition to neural structures, the lateral approach to the thoracolumbar spine also places vascular structures at risk. During the discectomy, the anterior longitudinal ligament (ALL) is maintained intact to preserve a protective barrier between the instruments and the abdominal/pelvic vessels. The introduction of instruments is done in such a way to minimize exposure of the vessels to injury. Pituitary and Kerrison rongeurs are advanced with the jaws directed dorsally to reduce inadvertent injury. The positioning of the patient places the structures at risk, but careful surgical technique can avoid pitfalls of iatrogenic injury.

Positioning for the Traumatic Spine

In addition to elective lumbar surgery, the lateral position is utilized within our practice for thoracolumbar trauma. Regional experience finds frequent thoracolumbar fractures from high-energy injuries that result in unstable burst fractures at the thoracolumbar junction. With neural canal compromise, or when posterior instrumentation does not fully stabilize the spine, a lateral approach to the fracture is indicated. This approach can successfully be utilized for pathology up to T10. In our experience, a combined procedure with general surgery exposure is ideal. An open exposure is preferred over minimally invasive due to the patient population and extent of the fractures encountered within our practice. For procedures on T12 and above, a dual-lumen endotracheal tube can be used to provide one-lung ventilation while deflating the ipsilateral lung. In the lateral position, one-lung ventilation can precipitate V/Q mismatch with pooling of

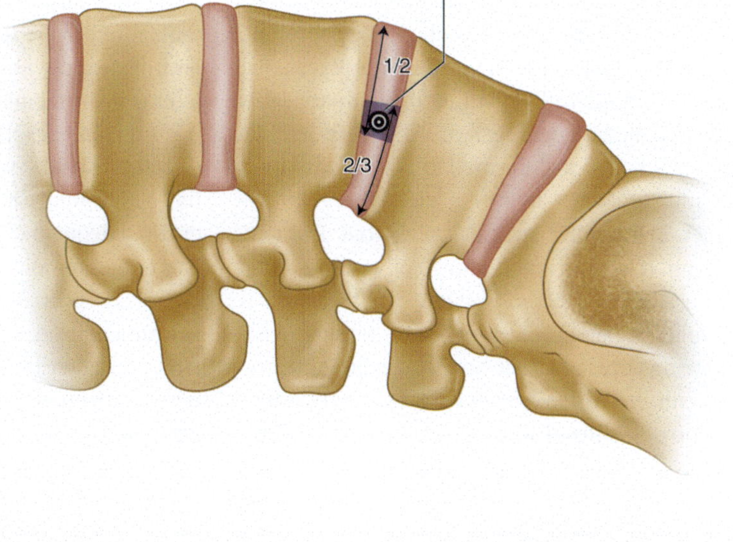

Fig. 12.3 The entry point should be placed within a "safe zone" within the disc between the midpoint and the ventral 1/3 of the operative disc space to minimize injury to the lumbar plexus

blood within the dependent vasculature. Though this does not preclude the practice, it is a consideration to be accounted for in preoperative evaluation [20].

In general, the patient is positioned in a similar manner to elective lumbar procedures. If MEPs are to be used, a baseline is obtained both before, and immediately after, positioning to ensure no loss of function in the setting of an unstable fracture or potentially compressive fragment. With unstable fractures, attention is also given to maintaining neutral alignment during the transition from the stretcher to the operative table. A slide board, log-rolling, and multiple assistants are often indicated to ensure safe alignment during positioning.

A standard flat-top bed is utilized with a beanbag with vacuum seal positioned beneath the patient and form-fit to maintain stability of the torso throughout the procedure. The lateral margin of the beanbag should remain below the level of the spine, so as to not obstruct AP fluoroscopy. The table can be left either flat, or with a slight break should a Skytron bed be utilized; the iliac crest is not an anatomic barrier for this level, and the break, if used, is generally for surgeon ergonomics. A right lateral decubitus position is preferred to avoid the obstruction of the liver at the surgical level, as well as to encounter arterial, rather than venous, anatomy on the surface of the spine. An axillary roll is appropriately positioned, and the patient is secured with traditional straps as well as tape. Without the crest as an anatomic obstruction, the full, regimented taping protocol of the elective thoracolumbar access is not required. Foam and pillow padding is placed over pressure points with attention to the ulnar nerves, the dependent peroneal nerve, between the patient's knees, and the malleoli of both ankles in a similar manner as during elective cases. The upper extremities are positioned out from the torso in a similar manner to elective cases. This, again, offers decompression of the plexus, peripheral nerves, and pressure points, while allowing access to lines by the anesthesia team.

With the patient secured, intraoperative fluoroscopy is utilized to identify the surgical level and to assist in planning of the surgical incision. In our practice, an experienced general or trauma surgeon is relied upon for the retroperitoneal access, with or without reflection of the diaphragmatic attachments; this also is of use in the event the vascular anatomy is obstructing direct access to the vertebral body [21]. A lateral transverse incision is used for initial skin opening. The access surgeon will perform the exposure in a retro- or transperitoneal approach as required by the patient condition, additional injuries, and nature of the procedure. The Bookwalter retractor system is generally preferred and remains in place following the exposure, but it is important to utilize radiolucent retractor blades to enable radiographic visualization during the spinal portion of the case.

Once the spine is properly exposed and the abdominal contents are out of the surgical field, the spinal portion of the procedure can begin. The lateral approach will expose the radicular arteries that travel circumferentially from the aorta, around the midportion of the vertebral body, before entering the spinal canal via the neuroforamina. As these vessels contribute to the vascular supply of the spinal cord, and the artery of Adamkiewicz can be found in the region, care must be taken when exposing the levels and performing vertebrectomies. If the vessel must be taken, it should be ligated and transected sharply. It is preferable to limit the arterial sacrifice, when possible, to unilateral and to no more than three segments to minimize the chances of cord ischemia and infarction [22–24].

With a large exposure, a traumatic injury of the spine can be repaired with appropriate bony and disc removal, graft or strut placement, and lateral instrumentation as necessary. The lateral position lends itself to harvesting iliac crest graft, if desired. Wide prep and draping during the initial positioning should take this into account to ensure adequate exposure to allow the harvest. It is not uncommon in our practice to supplement a lateral corpectomy for trauma with posterior instrumentation. The neural element decompression and anterior/middle column stabilization is best performed from the lateral approach, but with the forces often involved in these injuries, a cage and lateral plate is often insufficient to restore stability. For this, an additional posterior instrumentation, open, or often minimally invasive, is utilized to further regain structural stability and increase the chances of a solid fusion across the injury. Our current practice is to reposition for prone, posterior pedicle fixation, though other posterior instrumentation techniques from a lateral position have been described [25].

Physiologic Considerations

Lateral positioning changes several physiologic parameters that should be considered when planning for the anesthetic portion of the case. For respiratory considerations, the lateral position has been shown to decrease both vital capacity and tidal volume by 10% in awake subjects. This decrease is mitigated by the placement of an axillary roll in that a mildly suspended chest wall has improved compliance and decreases peak inflation pressures, possibly improving cardiac output and oxygenation that would be otherwise affected by positioning. The angulation of the table across the break has also been shown to decreased forced vital capacity when compared to flat lateral positioning due to decreased pulmonary compliance. Additionally, the lateral position can create a V/Q mismatch due to the vertical fluid static pressure gradient within the pulmonary vasculature. This becomes more important when single-lung ventilation is utilized in the thoracic spine [20].

In addition to pulmonary consideration, the vascular system is also affected by the lateral positioning. Significant venous pooling can occur within the dependent extremities which can create a type of "third-spacing" of the intravascular volume of up to 1 unit of blood. This can become more significant in patients with additional thoracic or abdominal pathology that can cause venous caval compression that can lead to hemodynamic instability. Further, the vertical gradient across the patient's body can also lead to changes in blood pressure readings in the dependent extremities. Due to fluid static pressure, the systemic blood pressure reading can change by 2 mmHg per in. of height difference across the body. With this in mind, it has been recommended that the blood pressure cuff be placed on the nondependent arm; this practice not only avoids incorrect measurements due to additional body weight compression, but also will read lower, so as to avoid any inadvertent hypotension that could potentially exacerbate a compromised cord vascular supply [20].

Complication Avoidance

The lateral position provides a direct surgical corridor to the thoracolumbar junction and thoracic spine, but does still present risk to the patient from the positioning itself. Many key positioning maneuvers have been developed from attempts at complication avoidance and assisting in surgical exposure. In addition to those listed previously, there are several positioning-related complications that can be avoided with careful attention to the patient prior to the skin incision.

Any prolonged surgical procedure can place the patient at risk for dependent decubitus ulcers. The lateral position, in particular, exposes several bony prominences to direct contact with the surgical table and support equipment. The lateral aspect of the ankle, knee, greater trochanter, iliac crest, chest wall, humeral head, and the parietal boss are all in line with the surgical table, and the upper extremities, when flexed at the shoulder, will also likely rest on solid support surfaces. Studies indicate that ulcers can develop following the first 1–4 h of positioning over bony prominences [26, 27]. For this, each bony prominence that is contact with a solid surface must be carefully checked and either padded or repositioned. A full-table load dispersing gel-pad is used as the base layer for our surgical beds, but additional foam or pillow padding is added for each pressure point on the patient. The axillary roll placed along the chest wall decompresses the plexus as well as the shoulder though it can increase the pressure measured at the chest wall [12]. For this, our institution has moved from use of a wrapped, liter bag of saline to gel rolls for reduction in local pressure; reusable, inflatable pillows have also been advocated for this purpose to further reduce chest wall pressure [12, 28, 29]. Attention at this stage of the procedure can prevent serious morbidity to the patient and should be a priority, regardless of the expected length of the procedure given the rapid nature of onset of ulcer formation.

Though the lateral position is typically utilized for thoracolumbar pathology, the upper extremities are of key importance during the positioning, and many nerves of the upper extremities are placed at risk, including the brachial plexus itself. The dependent shoulder is addressed with an axillary roll to reduce pressure on the joint and the bony prominence, but alleviating the pressure on the shoulder also reduces the risk of compression of the plexus by the humeral head. The placement of the axillary roll is crucial in that it can reduce the tension on the plexus by rotation of the arm out from beneath the chest, but the roll can also injure the plexus with direct compression if placed within the true axilla rather than along the superior chest wall. Compression of the long thoracic nerve from placement of an axillary roll has been reported though this is uncommon [13]. Attention to placement of the roll out of the axilla and, as suggested by Ameri et al., 10 cm distal to the axillary folds can avoid this rare complication. Overflexion of the shoulder should be avoided; we typically limit this to approximately 90°. Full supination and elbow extension can also stretch the descending nerves and should be avoided. As previously shown, peripheral nerve injury can occur with nerve stretch greater than 5–15% of baseline length [30]. In addition to the dependent arm and plexus, the nondependent upper extremity also faces positioning risk. Similar to the dependent arm, shoulder flexion greater than 90° and full elbow extension should be avoided to prevent nerve stretch. Over pronation also exposes the ulnar nerve to a greater chance of compression at the elbow. Cervical traction caused by lateral neck flexion can place stress on the nondependent plexus and should be mitigated by placement of a pillow to support the head [29].

Typically, the prone position raises the greatest concern for postoperative vision loss (POVL), but it has been reported in the lateral position. Posterior ischemic optic neuropathy (PION) is the most common cause of POVL, and most cases are associated with prolonged cases within the prone position [27, 30]. In reported cases performed in the lateral decubitus position, it is often felt that hypotension and anemia are causative factors. While in the lateral position, maintaining a stable blood pressure, avoiding overhydration with crystalloid, treating preoperative and intraoperative anemia, and minimizing operative time can reduce the risk of PION [31]. Further, the dependent eye can also be subject increased intraocular pressures; this can be mitigated by ensuring a neutral position of the neck with head support/pillow and maintaining the head at, or above, the level of the patient's heart during the procedure [27]. Direct compression of the dependent eye in the lateral position is less likely than while prone with use of a horseshoe head holder, but vigilance to ensure no globe compression can reduce the risk of causing a drop in ocular perfusion pressure. When PION does occur, asymmetric bilateral visual loss is seen, with more involvement of the dependent eye [31]. Additionally, postoperative visual disturbances and ocular pain can be seen secondary to corneal abrasion, most commonly in the dependent eye; in our experience, abrasions can be successfully avoided with tegaderm coverage overlying closed eyes and avoidance of any direct compression of the globe.

Another rare, but reported, complication of spine surgery while in the lateral decubitus position is unilateral parotid enlargement, otherwise known as anesthesia mumps. The complication is seen following surgeries in the prone or lateral decubitus position. Though the exact etiology is unknown, it is seen following prolonged cases and is often thought to be associated with intubation/extubation trauma to the parotid duct, external compression on the lateral face, or secondary to the use of certain anesthetic medications that predispose to stimulation of the salivary glands. Presenting with unilateral fullness and firmness of the parotid gland with painful sensations and lack of parotid secretions, the symptoms can last several minutes to several days. The condition is self-limiting and the treatment is supportive in nature, with NSAIDs, rehydration, and reassurance. To avoid this complication during spine surgeries in the lateral position, a soft, foam head-pillow is utilized to support the patient's face while avoiding extrinsic compression, and rotation of the neck is avoided to maintain good venous drainage. Premedication with anticholinergic drugs can also be considered to reduce secretions [32, 33].

Conclusion

Placing a patient in the lateral position for a spinal surgery provides many benefits. Some of these include access to the anterior columns of the spine with reduced approach morbidity, direct visualization of the vertebral body and disc space, and morbidity avoidance from muscle damage incurred during posterior exposures. With the benefits gained, the approach also places the patient at new risks from the unique positioning demands. The majority of these risks include proximity to abdominal and vascular structures during the procedure as well as the risk of nerve damage from stretch or direct injury. These risks can be successfully mitigated with careful attention to the positioning of the patient on the table and the joints and extremities with respect to the body. By correctly positioning, padding, and minimizing extremes, the lateral position can provide spine surgeons with an alternative and safe approach to treat various thoracic and lumbar spine pathologies.

References

1. Mayer MH. A new microsurgical technique for minimally invasive anterior lumbar interbody fusion. Spine. 1997;22(6):691–9.
2. McAfee PC, Regan JJ, Geis WP, Fedder IL. Minimally invasive anterior retroperitoneal approach to the lumbar spine. Emphasis on the lateral BAK. Spine. 1998;23(13):1476–84.
3. Ozgur BM, Aryan HE, Pimenta L, Taylor WR. Extreme lateral interbody fusion (XLIF): a novel surgical technique for anterior lumber interbody fusion. Spine J. 2006;6:435–43.
4. Davis TT, Hynes RA, Fung DA, Spann SW, MacMillan M, Kwon B, et al. Retroperitoneal oblique corridor to the L2-S1 intervertebral discs in the lateral position: an anatomic study. J Neurosurg Spine. 2014;21:785–93.
5. Billinghurst J, Akbarnia BA. Extreme lateral interbody fusion—XLIF. Curr Orthop Pract. 2009;20(3):238–51.
6. Lalonde NM, Villemure I, Pannetier R, Parent S, Aubin CE. Biomechanical modeling of the lateral decubitus posture during corrective scoliosis surgery. Clin Biomech. 2010;25:510–6.
7. Deukmedijian AR, Le TV, Dakwar E, Martinez CR, Uribe JS. Movement of abdominal structures on magnetic resonance imaging during positioning changes related to lateral lumbar spine surgery: a morphometric study. J Neurosurg Spine. 2012;16: 615–23.
8. O'Brien J, Haines C, Dooley ZA, Turner AW, Jackson D. Femoral nerve strain at L4-L5 is minimized by hip flexion and increased by table break when performing lateral interbody fusion. Spine. 2014;39(1):33–8.
9. Molinares DM, Davis TT, Fung DA, Liu JC, Clark S, Daily D, et al. Is the lateral jack-knife position responsible for cases of transient neurapraxia? J Neurosurg Spine. 2016;24:189–96.
10. Bhalodia VM, Sestokas AK, Tomak PR, Schwartz DM. Transcranial electric motor evoked potential detection of compressional peroneal nerve injury in the lateral decubitus position. J Clin Monit Comput. 2008;22:319–26.
11. Morgan KJ, Figueroa JJ. An unusual postoperative neuropathy: foot drop contralateral to the lateral decubitus position. A A Case Rep. 2016;7(5):115–7.
12. Della Valle AG, Salonia-Ruzo P, Peterson MGE, Salvati EA, Sharrock NE. Inflatable pillows as axillary support devices during surgery performed in the lateral decubitus position under epidural anesthesia. Anesth Analg. 2001;93:1338–43.
13. Ameri E, Behtash H. Omidi-Kashani. Isolated long thoracic nerve paralysis—a rare complication of anterior spinal surgery: a case report. J Med Case Rep. 2009;3:7366.
14. Jinnah AH, Mannava S, Plate JF, Stone AV, Freehill MT. Basic shoulder arthroscopy: lateral decubitus patient positioning. Arthrosc Tech. 2016;5(5):e1069–75.
15. Tatsumi RL. Lateral pressure and VAS pain score analysis for the lateral lumbar interbody fusion procedure. Int J Spine Surg. 2015;9(48):1–6.
16. Kim DH, Hudson AR, Kline DG. Atlas of peripheral nerve surgery. 2nd ed. Philadelphia: Elsevier Saunders; 2013. p. 185–9.
17. Dakwar E, Le TV, Baaj AA, Le AX, Smith WD, Akbarnia BA, et al. Abdominal wall paresis as a complication of minimally invasive lateral transpsoas interbody fusion. Neurosurg Focus. 2011;31(4):E18.
18. Moller DJ, Slimack NP, Acosta FL Jr, Koski TR, Fessler RG, Liu JC. Minimally invasive lateral

lumber interbody fusion and transpsoas approach-related morbidity. Neurosurg Focus. 2011;31(4):E4.
19. Yen C, Uribe JS. Procedural checklist for retroperitoneal transpsoas minimally invasive lateral interbody fusion. Spine. 2016;41(8S):S152–8.
20. Lawson NW, Meyer D Jr. Lateral positions. In: Martin JT, Warner MA, editors. Positioning in anesthesia and surgery. 3rd ed. Saunders; 1997. p. 127–152.
21. Dakwar E, Ahmadian A, Uribe JS. The anatomical relationship of the diaphragm to the thoracolumbar junction during the minimally invasive lateral extracoelomic (retropleural/retroperitoneal) approach. J Neurosurg Spine. 2012;16:359–64.
22. Ayhan S, Nelson C, Gok B, Petteys RJ, Wolinsky JP, Witham TF, et al. Transthracic surgical treatment for centrally located thoracic disc herniations presenting with myelopathy. J Spinal Disord Tech. 2010;23(2):79–88.
23. McCormick WE, Will SF, Benzel EC. Surgery for thoracic disc disease. Complication avoidance: overview and management. Neurosurg Focus. 2000;9:e13.
24. Vollmer DG, Simmons NE. Transthoracic approaches to thoracic disc herniations. Neurosurg Focus. 2000;9:e8.
25. Rhee JW, Petteys RJ, Anaizi AN, Sandhu FA, Voyadzis JM. Prosepective evaluation of 1-year outcomes in single-level percutaneous lumbar transfacet screw fixation in the lateral decubitus position following lateral transpsoas interbody fusion. Eur Spine J. 2015;24:2546–54.
26. Gefen A. How much time does it take to get a pressure ulcer? Integrated evidence from human, animal, and in vitro studies. Ostomy Wound Manage. 2008;54(10):26–8, 30-35
27. Shriver MF, Zeer V, Alentado VJ, Mroz TE, Benzel EC, Steinmetz MP. Lumbar spine surgery positioning comlications: a systematic review. Neurosurg Focus. 2015;39(4):E16.
28. Alfaz S, Sultan A, Iqbal M, Dhar SA. Lateral decubitus position in spinal surgery—current concepts. JK—Practitioner. 2007;14(2):110–2.
29. Kamel IR, Drum ET, Koch SA, Whitten JA, Gaughan JP, Barnette RE, et al. The use of somatosensory evoked potentials to determine the relationship between patient positioning and impending upper extremity nerve injury during spine surgery: a retrospective analysis. Anesth Analg. 2006;102:1538–42.
30. Kamel I, Barnette R. Positioning patients for spine surgery: avoiding uncommon position-related complications. World J Orthop. 2014;5(4):425–43.
31. Heitz JW, Audu PB. Asymmetric postoperative visual loss after spine surgery in the lateral decubitus position. Br J Anaesth. 2008;101(3):380–2.
32. Asghar A, Karam K, Rashid S. A case of anesthesia mumps after sacral laminectomy under general anesthesia. Saudi J Anaesth. 2015;9(3):332–3.
33. Liu FC, Liou JT, Li AH, Chiou H Jr, Day YJ. Acute unilateral parotid glands enlargement following endotracheal general anesthesia: report of two cases. Chang Gung Med J. 2007;30(5):453–6.

Spinal Procedures in the Prone Position

13

Prayash Patel and Christopher Nickele

Introduction

Spinal surgeries performed through a posterior approach include posterior decompression at any level, thoracolumbar pedicle screw instrumentation and fusions, cervical decompressions and fusions, and many lumbar interbody fusions. While the sitting position can be used for some posterior cervical decompression surgeries such as the foraminotomy, the prone position is used for most posterior spinal surgery given its practicality and ease of approach to the surgical target. However, spinal surgery in a prone position includes various technical considerations and complications of which surgeons must be cognizant. These considerations can vary from one procedure to the next depending on the pathology being treated and the location of the pathology.

P. Patel · C. Nickele (✉)
Department of Neurosurgery, Semmes-Murphey Clinic, University of the Tennessee Health Sciences, Memphis, TN, USA
e-mail: cnickele@semmes-murphey.com

Preoperative Assessment

By virtue of the physiologic impact of placing someone in a prone position, careful consideration must be given to the preoperative assessment of patients. Preoperative assessment should include attention to patient medical comorbidities, body habitus, breast and/or waist size, and length of the procedure. In spinal fractures, one should also consider the nature of the fracture and its stability or instability.

Positioning a patient face-down on the chest for prolonged periods of time requires attention to preexisting pulmonary conditions such as chronic obstructive pulmonary disease (COPD), bronchitis, restrictive pulmonary disease, and rib fractures. Preoperative pulmonary function testing should be considered for patients with significant pulmonary history, especially those with COPD. Similarly patients with significant cardiac history should also undergo a thorough preoperative assessment by a cardiac specialist. Prone positioning has been noted to result in significant hemodynamic and ventilation changes producing decreases in cardiac venous return as well as increases in systemic pulmonary and vascular resistance [1]. Such hemodynamic changes in conjunction with preexisting cardiac or pulmonary disease can significantly impact a patient's status in prone position.

A. Arthur et al. (eds.), *Perioperative Considerations and Positioning for Neurosurgical Procedures*,
https://doi.org/10.1007/978-3-319-72679-3_13

Patients with spinal cord compression and/or myelopathy must be carefully assessed for their ability to assume desired surgical position without becoming further symptomatic prior to surgery. Preoperative assessment for such patients should include an examination of the patient as they carefully and slowly extend their neck to determine whether any worsening of their condition or new symptomology is produced. If any degree of extension does produce new or worsening symptoms, then it is a clear indication that such maneuvers should be avoided during the intubation and anesthesia process. Specific considerations revolving around positioning with unstable fractures or severe spinal cord compression will be covered in a later section, when positioning in the setting of specific pathologies is discussed.

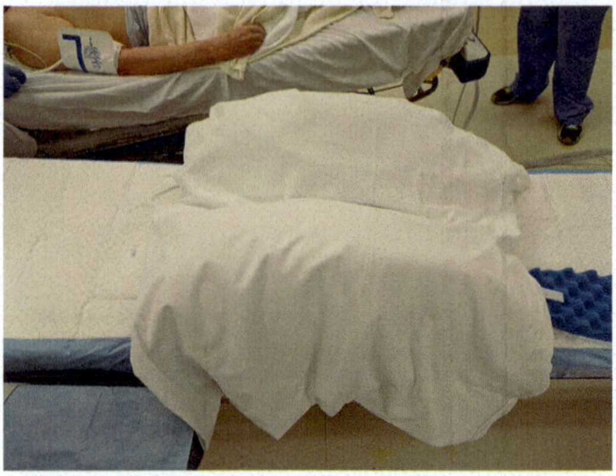

Fig. 13.1 A Wilson frame is placed on a Jackson table. The Wilson is covered with a bed sheet to protect the patient's skin and also to facilitate easier manipulation of the patient by utilizing the sheet to lift and adjust the patient's body

The Full Prone Position

Preparations

The ability of the cervical spine to sustain the manipulation necessary for laryngoscopy and intubation as well as the ability of the spine to sustain turning, all under conditions of muscle relaxation, should be clearly understood by all members of the surgical team.

After induction of general anesthesia and intubation steps are taken to ensure a safe and successful transfer of the patient from a supine position on the hospital bed to a prone position on the operative table. For preparation of the operating room table, we place a covering or bed sheets over the padding of the table. For Jackson tables in an open configuration, the chest, pelvic, and knee supports should be appropriately covered typically with pre-fit covers for the chest and pelvic pads and foam pads for the knee support plate. For Jackson tables in a closed or flat-top configuration or with other "closed" operative tables that do not allow the abdomen to hang free, prone position surgery will require either chest rolls or a support frame, typically a Wilson frame. Chest rolls may be conventionally available gel rolls or they can be constructed from blankets or sheets that are tightly rolled and secured with tape. The advantage of chest rolls constructed in this method is that they can be customized for the patient in both length and girth. When a Wilson frame is used, it should be covered with a bed sheet or other covering typically with generous overhang so as to allow operating room staff and surgeons to utilize this for manipulation of the patient's body after turning to a prone position (Fig. 13.1). If bed attachments are required for self-retaining or tubular retractions systems or other devices, these should be evaluated prior to draping and also evaluated to ensure that placement does not interfere with fluoroscopy.

If the surgical case may require rapid volume repletion, blood product transfusion, close arterial pressure monitoring, or close volume status monitoring, then appropriate catheters for central venous or arterial access should be placed prior to turning into the prone position. Similarly, leads for neurophysiologic monitoring should also be placed prior to turning the patient. All electrocardiogram (EKG) leads must be removed from the chest, or any place where they could end up compressed between the table support system and the skin or contribute to artifact on the X-ray once the patient is prone. Foley catheters should be placed prior to prone positioning, in cases that are anticipated to take longer than 2 h.

Sequential compression devices should be employed routinely and activated prior to induction of general anesthesia.

If a cervical spinal procedure is to be performed, the patient will most likely require placement of the Mayfield three-pronged head holder prior to turning. For adults, we utilize 50–60 pounds of force for the head clamp—more force can be used, but should never exceed 80 pounds. Prior to placing the head holder on the patient, the surgeon must ensure that the patient is adequately anesthetized to avoid significant changes in vital signs such a sudden increase in blood pressure or heart rate. The surgeon should always assess the Mayfield bed attachment as well, ensuring that it is securely attached to bed prior to turning the patient.

Types of Tables

Standard operative tables, such as the Mizuho Skytron table, do not provide an opening to allow the abdomen to hang freely, are the most commonly utilized operative tables. In prone position spinal surgery, these standard beds are often utilized for posterior cervical procedures and lumbar decompression or discectomies. These tables are not ideal for fusion procedures where the pedicles and other specific bony anatomy must be visualized in an anterior-posterior fluoroscopy view, as the bed construct is not radiolucent and significant obstructions will be encountered on intraoperative fluoroscopy—such as the pedestal in the middle of the table. When utilized for cervical procedures, the bed is often prepared with chest rolls as mentioned previously and three-pronged head holders such as the Mayfield head holder. One beneficial aspect of certain Skytron tables is the ability to slide the table surface either toward the head or feet. This improves ease of C-arm fluoroscopy positioning by allowing manipulation of the level of interest away from the table pedestal. It is always important to ensure that the table surface is positioned appropriately with regard to the table base which can impede C-arm movement.

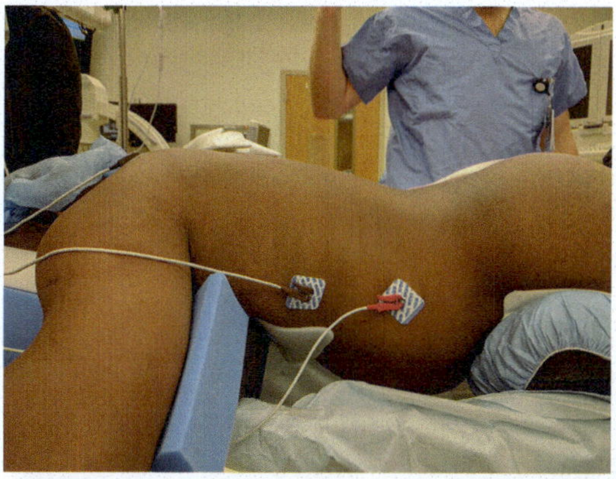

Fig. 13.2 An open configuration of Jackson frame allows the patient's abdomen to hang free assisting in reducing intra-abdominal pressure and in turn helps reduce venous pressure and bleeding

Fusion procedures in the prone position benefit from utilization of the Jackson operative table. The Jackson table is fashioned in one of two configurations for prone position spinal surgery. An "open" configuration allows the patient's abdomen to hang free without compression, reducing intra-abdominal pressure, which in turn reduces venous pressure in the thoracolumbar region allowing for reduced venous bleeding during the procedure (Fig. 13.2). This configuration is typically favored for transforaminal lumbar interbody fusions (TLIFs), posterior lumbar interbody fusions (PLIFs), and thoracolumbar pedicle screw fixations. The open configuration allows for natural lumbar lordosis, which is useful when the goal is fusion of the thoracolumbar spine in a natural alignment. The Jackson table is radiolucent allowing for unobscured fluoroscopy and anteroposterior imaging during instrumentation and interbody graft placement for thoracolumbar fusion procedures.

A "closed" or "flat-top" configuration is also utilized for thoracolumbar fusion procedures, especially where interbody placement is not required. Furthermore, it is often preferred in the setting of unstable thoracolumbar fractures where the additional abdominal freedom and consequent lack of support of an open configuration may result in worsening of the fracture. It serves to provide similar benefits in terms of radiolucency of the frame. When utilizing the Jackson table, one should always consider the position of the table ends which are adjustable and permit a change in the overall table height as well as allowing either a Trendelenburg or reverse-Trendelenburg positioning. There is a pin in place, holding each end of the table at its set height, and it should be confirmed that these pins are set appropriately prior to transferring the patient to the table (Fig. 13.3). For patient safety, these ends must be adjusted prior to transferring the patient to the table.

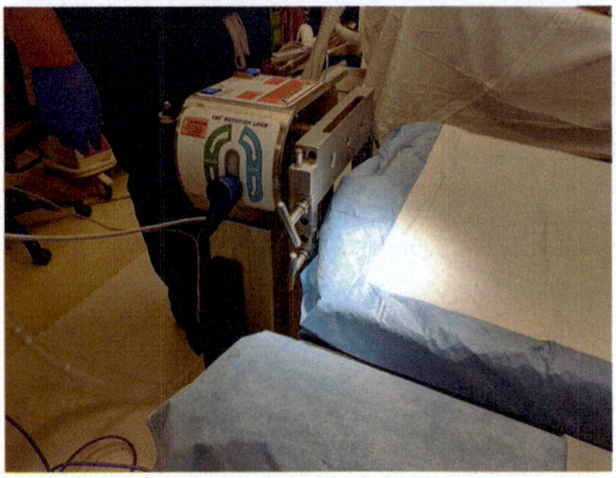

Fig. 13.3 Jackson tables can be adjusted as needed for either Trendelenburg or reverse-Trendelenburg by adjusting the large pins at the head and tail end of the table. Such adjustments must be done prior to transferring the patient to the table

The Wilson frame, the frame most commonly used by present authors, is radiolucent and when coupled with a closed Jackson table allows for unobscured fluoroscopy in both anteroposterior and lateral views. Wilson frames comprise two parallel bolster pads which can be widened or narrowed and are adjustable typically by a crank on the side of the frame which allows the arch of the pads to be raised or lowered. This manipulation of the pads is designed to allow the surgeon to alter the patient's sagittal lumbar alignment as desired for a procedure [2] (Fig. 13.4). In the setting of lumbar decompression and discectomy procedures, the Wilson frame is often utilized to allow for flexion of the torso and abdomen, increasing sagittal flexion of the lumbar spine, splaying the lamina, and enlarging the interlaminar operative corridor for these procedures. Care should be taken if any fusion procedure is done with the Wilson frame, as the same properties that are advantageous for decompression can cause problems with fusion. If instrumentation is performed with

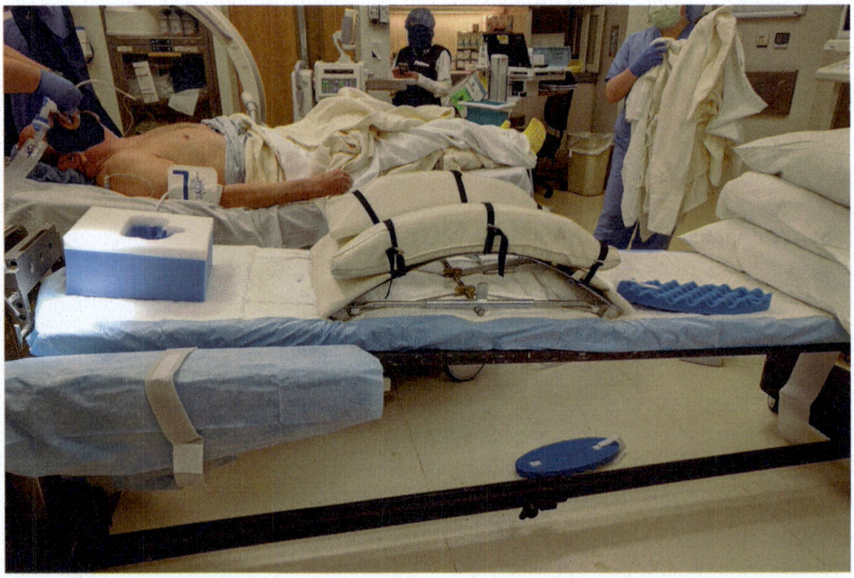

Fig. 13.4 The Wilson frame is seen here on a Jackson table. The Wilson frame comprises two parallel bolster pads which can be adjusted by utilizing the crank shaft on the side of the frame which allows the pads to be raised or lowered in effect allowing the surgeon to alter the patient's sagittal alignment as needed

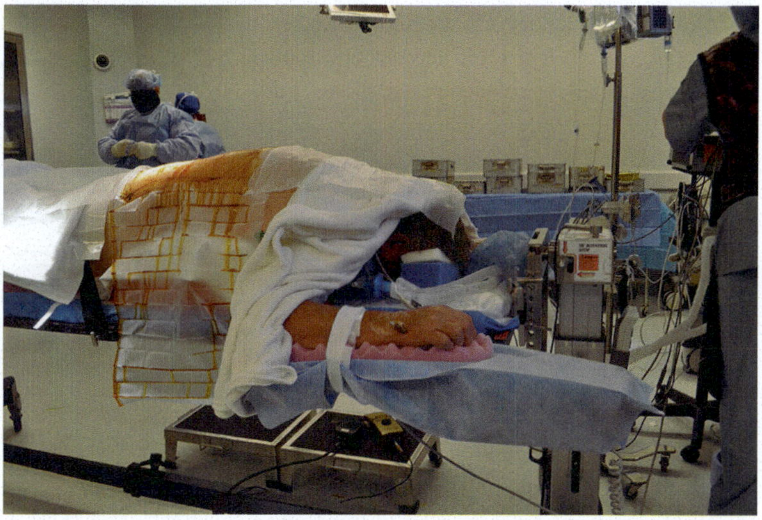

Fig. 13.5 The patient is being prepared to turn to a prone position on a Wilson frame. Note that the foam facial/head rest has already been placed on the face with the endotracheal tube within the designated recess (arrow). The patient's iliac crest should line up with the center of the Wilson frame for optimal positioning (dotted line)

the Wilson framed raised, it can cause fusion in a "flat back" alignment, with loss of the lumbar lordosis. Use of the Wilson frame has been associated with decreased cardiac output and reduced venous return with resulting effects on hemodynamics in prone position spinal procedures [3].

Turning the Patient Prone

After adequate preparations have been made for the patient to be turned prone on the selected operative table, careful cooperation is required for the actual act of turning the patient prone from a supine position. Turning the patient requires at least four people. It is recommended that at least two team members assist with the patient torso, one to push and turn and the other to catch the patient on the side of the operative table. A third person, generally the anesthetist, controls the patient's head. If the patient has an unstable cervical fracture, or if the patient's head is in pins, it is preferred that a surgeon control the head. A fourth member of the team should help with the patient's legs while positioning. All lines and catheters must be carefully prepared and transferred throughout this process. The endotracheal tube, once secured to the patient, must be disconnected during the turning process.

When the table is prepared as above, the team must level the hospital bed slightly higher than the operating table. The patient or bed should be slid so that the patient's chest is slightly closer to the head of the operating table than the chest pad or chest roll. The patient will travel a decent distance while being rolled prone, but if they are far from the operating table, they should be slid toward the table before rolling. When utilizing a Wilson frame or hip padding on an operative table, ensure that the patient iliac crest will line up with the center or apex of the frame and the superior aspect of the pad (Fig. 13.5). Often, a pad should be placed between the patient's arm and the frame of the operating table to avoid cutaneous injury during the flip. Elderly patients are at highest risk for these problems, such as degloving injuries.

Once everything is prepared, the team member responsible for the patient's head counts down before the turn. In this way, the patient's head, torso, and legs can be turned as a single unit. The team member responsible for catching the patient's torso should do so with one or both arms under the patient. This makes it easier to reposition the patient as needed. To help the surgical team avoid back injury, the operating table should be high enough so that the team members do not need to stoop over while positioning the patient. Extra lifting help should always be called for when positioning large patients.

Once turned onto the operative table, any adjustments that are necessary should only be made once all catheters are secured, the patient limbs and genitalia are safe, and the anesthetist has communicated continued control of the endotracheal tube.

Full Prone Position

One should ensure that breasts are positioned medially and/or inferiorly with the nipples free of compression when positioned on a Wilson frame or chest rolls. Patients with large or procedurally augmented breasts may pose a challenge for positioning and one should consider wide-based frames or chest rolls to accommodate large breasts. Foam padding should be utilized when necessary to ensure that any breast or abdominal tissue hanging laterally is appropriately protected from the bed frame. Similarly, the patient genitalia should be inspected to ensure that they are free of any compression. It is particularly important to ensure that both testicles and penis are free of compression when positioning male patients. Take care to ensure that the penis is hanging free with the testicles and is not compressed between a frame or table and the patient's leg. When the genitalia are in close vicinity to the bed frame, the temptation exists to place foam between the frame and the patient's anatomy. Care should be taken to be sure that this foam does not introduce a compression that did not previously exist. Generally, if there is no contact between the anatomy and the frame, foam is not required.

The arms are then positioned according to the procedure being performed and are typically placed inferiorly or superiorly on arm boards in a prone-surrender or "superman" configuration (Fig. 13.6) or are tucked to the patient's side. The use of oversized hip pads for a thin patient will sometimes allow the arms to be tucked to the sides, supported by the excess hip pads, even when using an open Jackson table. Foam padding is utilized under the arms where they contact the arm boards or table frame. If the arms are positioned superiorly on arm boards, they should appear relaxed and should not be abducted greater than 90° or overextended, as this has been associated with increased risk for brachial plexus injury [4]. Arms should be padded at the elbow to protect the ulnar nerve on the medial aspect, and also at the hand to keep the hand in a safety position as much as possible (Fig. 13.7). The axilla should be free of any compression. If it appears that the shoulder is unsupported or is coming in contact with the table frame, care should be taken to pad the shoulder and not place padding up into the axilla.

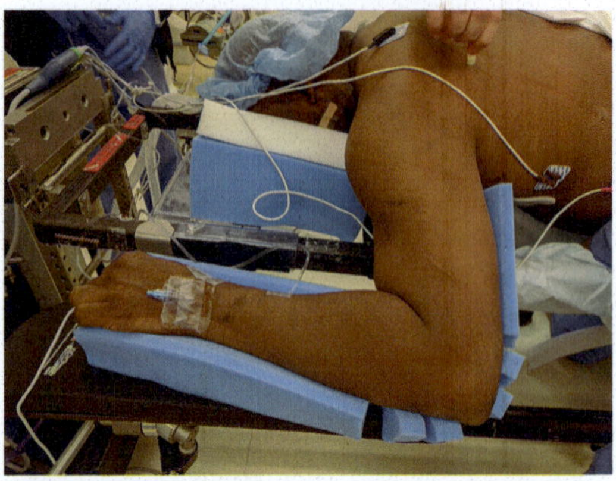

Fig. 13.6 The patient is placed in a prone position for a lumbar spinal procedure with his arms in a "superman" or prone-surrender position on arm boards. Foam padding is utilized to protect the skin and peripheral nerves

The head is placed into a foam head rest (face pillow) if a three-pronged head holder is not utilized. Often the foam head rest or face pillow will be placed over the patient's face prior to turning as it will allow from proper fitting of the facial structures and endotracheal tube and minimize head and neck manipulation once the patient has been turned to the prone position (Fig. 13.5). The patient's neck should be maintained in a neutral position and free of compression anteriorly while in the foam head rest with care taken not to overextend the neck. Significant flexion of the neck should also be avoided when possible as this can create problems to venous return, ventilation, as well resulting in decreased blood flow to the brain and spine due to effects on carotid and vertebral arteries [2].

The patient's chin should be inspected to ensure that it is free of constant external pressure or contact. The head and face must carefully be inspected as well to ensure that there is no compression of the nose, eyes, or other facial elements.

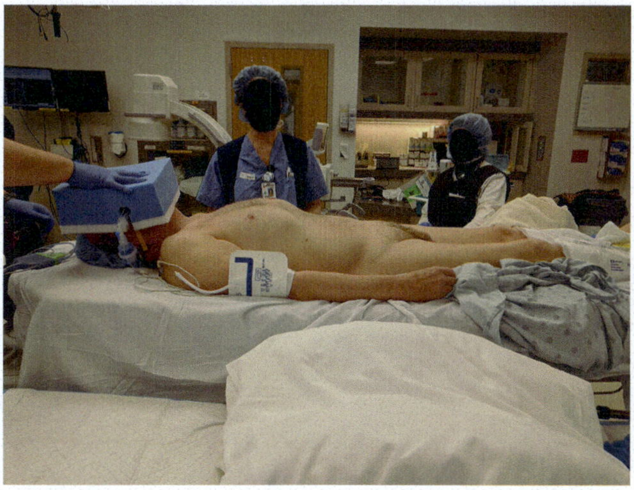

Fig. 13.7 The patient is placed prone on an open configuration Jackson table with arms in a "superman" or prone-surrender position. It is important to ensure that the arms are in a relaxed position and not overextended or abducted greater than 90°. Again foam padding should be utilized to protect the soft tissue from pressure injury and also the peripheral nerves, especially the ulnar nerve. Note that the axilla is also padded with foam to protect the brachial plexus

The lips and tongue must be inspected to ensure that they endure no compression, especially by the endotracheal tube, as the lips or the tongue can be pinched between the endotracheal tube and the teeth. A bite block is utilized to avoid pressure injury to the tongue when necessary. The patient's eyes should be taped closed with clear, thin tape or Tegaderm™ to protect the eyes from direct injury such as corneal abrasions or lacerations and from the possibility of chemical injury from skin sterilization agents. Alcohol and chlorhexidine gluconate will both cause corneal scarring and opacification if they reach the eye, but even detergents in scrub solutions can be problematic for the eye.

For all prone position surgeries, it is very important to ensure that the patient's eyes are completely free from any external pressure. Additionally, the patient's head should ideally be elevated above the level of the heart in an effort to prevent increased intracranial pressure and also increase intraocular pressure, which may rarely lead to ischemic injury and blindness. One advantage of placing the head in pins is to avoid ocular pressure, and one may consider utilizing the Mayfield even for lumbar cases for this reason. Although, there are studies that suggest that the complication of blindness in prone position surgery is as common in the setting of significant blood loss and low blood pressure as it is in the setting of direct compression of the globe [5, 6].

Foam or other padding is required where the knees contact the table. Knees should be flexed and the shins padded so that the toes are not under contact pressure. The patient's body should then be carefully secured to the operative table with straps extending across the torso when possible and also across the buttocks, ideally in a slight cranio-caudal direction as a sling-like support should the patient need to be put into a significant reverse-Trendelenburg position (Fig. 13.8). Foam padding is placed between the patient and the strap to protect the skin from direct compression by the straps and to keep the strap edges from cutting into the skin.

Cervical Spine Procedures in Prone Position

Spinal pathology for prone position surgery can be categorized as either degenerative, infectious, neoplastic, or traumatic. Although some of these pathologies may be glacially unstable, here we

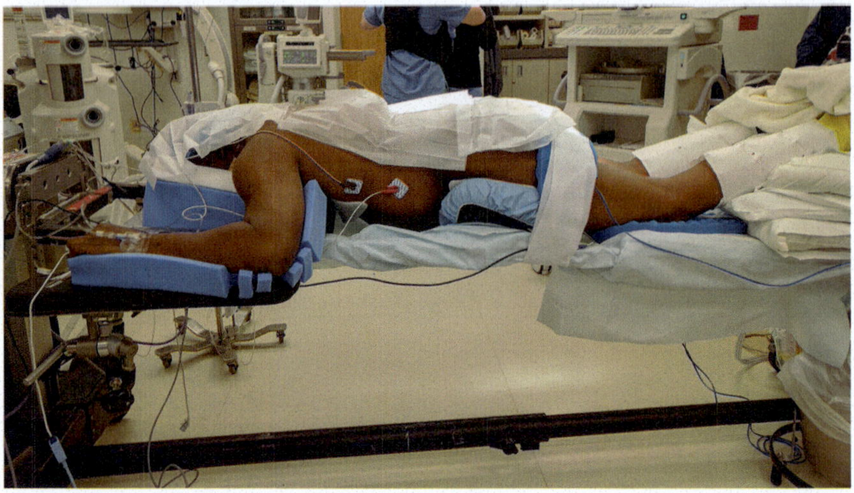

Fig. 13.8 The patient is positioned prone on an open configuration Jackson table. All pressure points are padded appropriately with foam padding. Note that the table is arranged in a reverse-Trendelenburg position by adjusting the head of the Jackson table (blue arrow). Also note that the patient has a padded strap placed around the buttock in a cranio-caudal direction as a sling-like support (yellow arrow). The patient's legs and feet are kept slightly elevated with pillows

will group degenerative, infectious, and neoplastic stable pathologies to describe considerations specific to this group with regard to prone positioning of the patient. Prone positioning for traumatic spinal fractures will be described for special considerations differentiating unstable and stable fractures.

Posterior cervical spinal procedures for degenerative pathology include cervical foraminotomies, laminectomies, and instrumentation and fusion procedures such as subaxial fusion, C1–2 fusion, and occipito-cervical fusion. Infectious pathologies that may require surgical intervention from a posterior approach include epidural infections and osteomyelitis causing deformity or instability. Neoplastic pathology in the cervical spine requiring prone positioning includes posteriorly located primary tumors of the neuraxis or axial skeleton, metastatic disease involving the cervical spine, and even anteriorly located pathology if the surgical goal is only posterior decompression. Neoplastic lesions may also result in instability requiring posterior fixation; however, positioning considerations for unstable pathologic fractures of both neoplastic and infectious etiology will be discussed more in depth later, in the section reviewing positioning management for unstable cervical fractures.

In patients with significant cord compression and acute myelopathy, every effort should be made to minimize extension of the patient's neck and keep the patient as neutral as possible. Awake, fiber-optic intubation may be the best option as it will allow for clinical assessment of the patient during and after intubation. Myelopathic patients are overall best served to have their necks kept inline and neutral during the intubation process with minimal manipulation. If the patient is examined preoperatively and has new symptoms with neck extension, then great care must be taken in the operating room with intubation and positioning. The surgeon should always be present to help keep the cervical spine held manually in a neutral position during the intubation process in such a setting.

A preoperative discussion between anesthesia and the surgeon should include the use of neurophysiologic monitoring, presence of myelopathy, and desired blood pressure parameters. Volatile anesthetics will suppress sensory evoked potentials to varying degrees and full paralytic dosing will cause loss of motor evoked potentials.

Maintaining mean arterial pressures greater than 85 mmHg has been thought to be related to improved outcomes in spinal cord injury patients [3]. Attempting to reduce epidural venous bleeding and ocular pressure by lowering venous pressure with reverse-Trendelenburg positioning can also impact venous return to the heart and arterial blood pressure causing hypotension and consequently reducing spinal cord perfusion [2, 7]. The surgeon should speak with anesthesia about anticipating such a drop in blood pressure when positioning for maximal venous drainage and the team must appropriately correct the arterial blood pressure according to the goals that have been set. Such considerations are particularly important in patients that are suffering from *acute* myelopathy.

Degenerative, neoplastic, and infectious cervical spine procedures are typically performed utilizing either a Skytron adjustable operative table or Jackson table. The latter is beneficial in cases involving the lower cervical or upper thoracic spine, or in patients with short or stout necks, where fluoroscopy could be challenging. The Jackson table is also preferred in any case requiring anteroposterior fluoroscopy. Most posterior cervical cases are best positioned with Mayfield Infinity three-pronged skull clamp system with appropriate table attachment—placement of the head clamp has been covered previously in the preparations section. Patients are typical placed neutral (fusions/instrumentation) or slightly flexed (decompression/foraminotomy) when no central compression or myelopathy is present (Fig. 13.9). Care must be taken to keep patients neutral while actively transferring them from a supine position to the prone position.

Patients in the prone position on a Skytron table are placed on chest rolls, detailed above in the preparations section. If the patient is flexed in pins, the surgeon must inspect the patient's chin to be sure that it does not contact the table. Arms should be secured to the patient's side and tucked with all pressure points appropriately padded as described previously. If done on a Jackson table, the arms boards should be down at the patient's sides. Fluoroscopy should be brought in at this point for lateral fluoroscopy if it is needed and

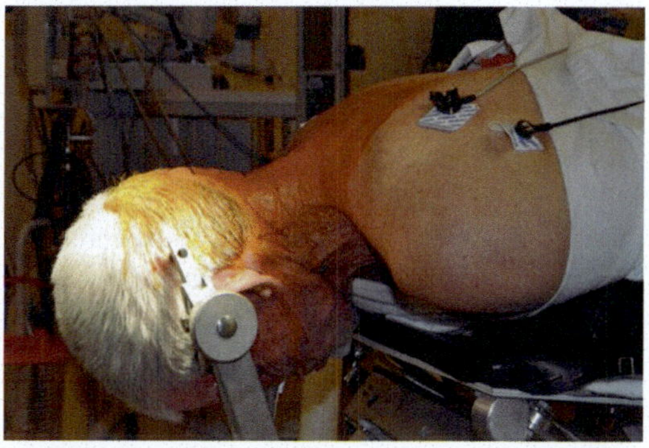

Fig. 13.9 Posterior cervical spinal procedures are often done utilizing the Mayfield three-pronged skull clamp for positioning. As seen here, it is important to keep the patient's neck in a neutral position or slightly flexed depending on the pathology being treated. Here, the patient is placed on a Skytron operative table on chest rolls with arms padded and tucked to the side

assess whether shoulder taping will be required to achieve sufficient lateral X-rays for the procedure. If shoulder taping is required, one must ensure that the tape does not involve any electrical leads or anesthesia lines. One should also avoid considerable posterior retraction of the shoulder or overly retracting the shoulder inferiorly as this may result in an injury to the upper trunk of the brachial plexus. When using a Jackson table, we place the head of the bed in one of the top three slots and the foot of the bed in the bottom slot prior to placing the patient on the bed to allow for a degree of reverse Trendelenburg. Regardless of the bed type, most posterior cervical procedures should be performed with the patient head above the level of the heart (reverse Trendelenburg) to provide a more physiologic state for the patient, better visualization in the operative field, reduced venous pressure and venous bleeding, and reduced intraocular pressure which can notably increase with prone positioning [8]. Arterial pressure changes must be accounted for and corrected appropriately when specific blood pressure parameters are required.

If neurophysiologic monitoring is to be utilized, this should be placed prior to positioning the patient prone. Pre- and post-positional SSEPs/MEPs should be performed to ensure that positioning has not created a significant change.

Care must be taken when utilizing neurophysiologic monitoring as intermittent stimulation can result in movement and twitching of arms and legs. As such, arms and legs must be secured well in anticipation of such movement. Furthermore, the tongue and lips must carefully be padded and protected typically with a bite block in place to keep stimulated contraction from resulting in bite-related injury.

Unstable Cervical Pathology

For cervical fractures deemed unstable, it should be communicated to the anesthetist that the patient have minimal manipulation of the neck during intubation. Consideration should be given to fiber-optic intubation, potentially with the patient awake to allow pre- and post-intubation neurologic examination. Patient transfer should occur with the patient's cervical spine supported with a rigid collar such as Miami J or Aspen and maintained in a neutral position with minimal manipulation. If the collar needs to be removed, the surgeon should be at the bedside to assist in keeping the neck supported and neutral. If the patient is positioned with a collar in place, it can be removed after the patient's head is fixed in the three-pronged head holder or in traction if appropriate. Patients with unstable pathology and spinal cord compression should also have strictly maintained blood pressure parameters throughout positioning and the procedure.

Often in the setting of fracture dislocations, manual reduction is needed to successfully reduce fractured vertebrae from an abnormal position prior to fixation. Surgeon, anesthetist, and OR staff should have a clear discussion about this prior to surgery and the steps involved for such a maneuver should be clearly outlined so that all parties are prepared for this stage of the procedure. When this is necessary, the primary surgeon or an assistant surgeon should be in charge of manipulation of the neck for reduction of the fracture. Such a reduction of a fracture or locked/perched facet joints is typically achieved by carefully releasing the Mayfield joints under the drapes to allow manual manipulation of the neck by the physician under continuous fluoroscopy at the appropriate stage of the surgery. Once the reduction maneuver has been accomplished, the Mayfield must be carefully tightened and secured again.

Thoracic and Lumbar Procedures in Prone Position

Thoracic and lumbar surgeries performed in the prone position include thoracic or lumbar laminectomies, lumbar foraminotomies, lumbar or thoracic discectomies, and thoracic and lumbar fusions—most often for degenerative pathologies. Other pathologies include neoplastic and infectious pathologies—osteomyelitis, discitis, and various bony or spinal neoplasms. Additionally, spinal deformity cases are performed either partially or entirely in the prone position.

Decompressive spinal procedures comprise the majority of spinal procedures in this region of the body. Patients are typically placed prone on a flat-top Jackson table or Skytron adjustable table often with a Wilson frame. For a purely decompressive surgery, the table choice is not critical although the Wilson frame, as described previously, allows for some flexion in the thoracolumbar region, essentially widening the corridor for decompression and providing better visualization for the operation. It must be noted that if AP fluoroscopic views are needed (such as with fusion or sometimes with foraminotomies), the Skytron bed is not typically radiolucent and may obscure AP X-ray images.

All pressure points are padded appropriately with foam padding. For thoracolumbar procedures, the arms will be positioned superiorly on arm boards as detailed in the full prone section. For patients with rotator cuff problems, the shoulders may not have full range of motion and the arm boards must be adjusted to accommodate for the patient's joints. Foam padding protects the knees from pressure, and pillows under the lower legs flex the knees and keep the toes from surface contact.

Lateral fluoroscopy can be brought into the field to ensure that adequate X-ray imaging can be achieved for localization given the current position. Spinal needle or blunt instrument localization should be performed as per usual to identify the appropriate level. As in posterior cervical cases, the head should ideally be kept slightly elevated if possible, especially for longer cases to avoid ocular pressure-related injuries. The abdomen should be kept free of significant compression to reduce venous congestion and bleeding. The breasts should be free of nipple compression and generally positioned down and in, relative to the chest pad or chest roll.

For patients requiring thoracolumbar instrumentation and fusion procedures such as pedicle screw fixation, transforaminal lumbar interbody fusions (TLIFs), or posterior lumbar interbody fusions (PLIFs), similar principles for prone positioning are utilized with some adjustments to assist with better visualization during fluoroscopy. For most fusion procedures, the radiolucent Jackson table typically in an open configuration is best as it allows for unimpeded visualization of bony anatomy on X-ray. As visualization of pedicles, interspaces, and vertebral body landmarks is crucial to adequate placement of instrumentation, fluoroscopy or another imaging modality is key to a successful spinal instrumentation or fusion case.

Always ensure that any wires, cables, tubing, or leads are not obstructing optimal visualization of necessary bony anatomy on fluoroscopy. In this sense, it is encouraged that the surgeon check both anteroposterior and lateral views of the work area to ensure that no significant alterations are needed to patient positioning or to remove obstructions prior to sterile draping. It is ideal for the fluoroscopy unit (typically C-arm) to be brought into the field and draped prior to incision and positioned either cranially out of the area of the operative incision or caudally distal to the surgical tech and mayo stand. If positioned cranially in the field, care must be taken to ensure that the patient's arms are free of contact with the machine, which rarely can be the source of peripheral nerve or myocutaneous injuries.

Spinal deformity correction cases are quite extensive, spanning multiple spinal levels, and requiring several hours of operative time. Given the degree of muscle dissection and bone drilling in deformity surgeries, one should expect and be prepared for significant blood loss and volume shifts. Such patients should be prepared with appropriate monitoring and IV access. Clear hemodynamic parameters should be set with blood products readily available. Special attention should be given in these cases to patient pressure points, face, eyes, breast, arms, and other potential sources of complications given the typical length of these procedures.

Unstable Thoracic or Lumbar Pathology

With unstable fractures of the thoracic or lumbar spine, care should be taken to avoid manipulation of the patient. These patients should be maintained flat unless otherwise indicated and controlled techniques should be utilized when patient transfer or manipulation is needed. Jackson frames in an open configuration should rarely be utilized in unstable fractures or pathology of the thoracic or lumbar spine as the absence of adequate abdominal support may exacerbate any displacement in the setting of instability. A closed or flat-top Jackson table is typically preferred for cases involving unstable thoracolumbar spine fractures. Chest rolls are utilized on these tables, and this allows for adequate patient support and radiolucency for imaging while avoiding overextension.

Conventional manual log-rolling techniques have thought to be the best suited for prone positioning of the unstable thoracolumbar spinal patient; however, recent cadaver studies have indicated that the utilizing a Jackson table-turn technique for prone positioning significantly reduces rotational and translational forces that could potentially worsen a fracture [9]. This technique involves the use of a Jackson table attachment which can allow for another table surface to be secured, and effectively "sandwiches" a patient securely between the two table surfaces. In this fashion, the patient is supine initially on the first Jackson table surface then the subsequent surface to be utilized for prone positioning is

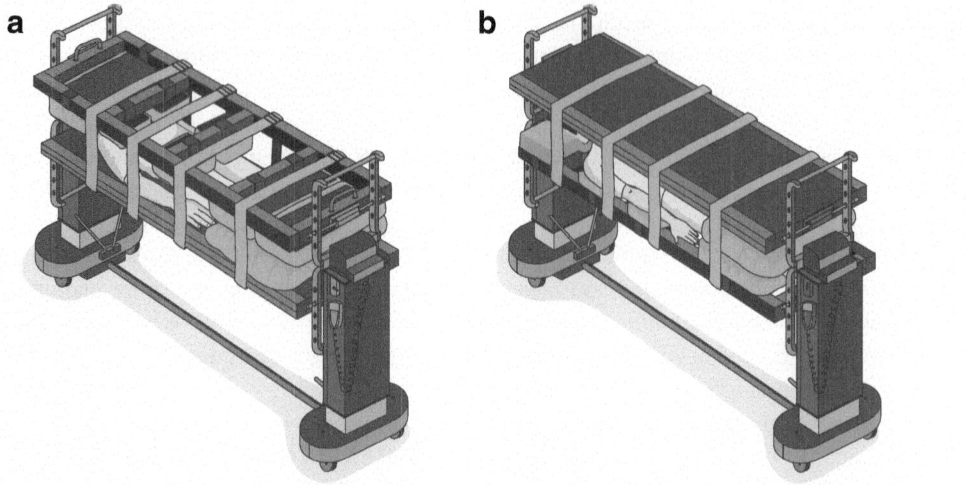

Fig. 13.10 The Jackson table sandwich technique requires a second table surface to be placed on top of the supine patient. After properly securing the patient (**a**) the bed can be rotated so that the patient becomes prone and the original table surface can be taken away (**b**)

secured above the patient carefully after the patient has been strapped into the first bed. The entire table is then rotated maintaining the patient rigidly fixed between the two table surfaces and allowing for minimal rotational or translational forces on the patient. Once rotated, the first bed utilized for supine positioning is removed leaving the patient prone on the second bed attached to the Jackson table frame (Fig. 13.10).

Special Considerations for Navigated Instrumentation

When using navigation that requires an intraoperative CT scan, the machine needs to be able to close around the patient. For fluoroscopy-based navigation, positioning is as it would be for instrumentation with live fluoroscopy.

Navigated instrumentation requires a radiolucent table. Thoracolumbar instrumentation is generally performed on an open configuration Jackson table for the sake of natural lumbar alignment in lordosis. This table is radiolucent and meets another requirement of navigated instrumentation—it lacks a pedestal in the middle of the table.

Placing the patient in the Mayfield three-pronged pins for head fixation causes additional concern, as the Mayfield connection extends below the normal table surface and is also quite wide. Again, for thoracolumbar fusions, this is not an issue, but for C1–2 fusions it can become difficult to close the intraoperative CT scanner around the patient. In this case, the Mayfield needs to be arranged so that inferior protrusion from the table is as little as possible, or a low-profile Mayfield adaptor needs to be used. Additionally, a radiolucent construct is available for the Mayfield head fixation system that can be utilized to avoid obstruction during radiography.

The patient's arms present the same concern that they must not be protruding in a way to block the CT scanner from closing. Generally, this does not require any change in positioning. If the arms are positioned so that the surgeon will be comfortable operating on the levels of interest, the CT scanner will also be able to close around those levels. For example, the patient's arms would be positioned up for a lower thoracolumbar fusion, but they would be positioned down for an upper thoracic fusion. Still, the scanner is broad, and care needs to be taken that it is not hitting against the arm boards when being brought in and out. In all cases, the navigation camera is traditionally positioned at the foot of the operative table.

Complications

Visual Complications

Visual complications following prone positioning were first reported in 1948, when a patient positioned improperly on a Bailey headrest suffered postoperative blindness [10]. Visual loss in the setting of spine surgery can occur at a rate ranging from 0.019 to 0.2% with higher rates seen in prone position surgery [11–13]. Risk factors described to be associated with higher rates of perioperative visual complications include diabetes mellitus, coagulopathy, neurologic disorders, and paralysis [11]. In general, ischemic optic neuropathy (ION) is described as the most common cause of visual loss postoperatively with up to 89% of such cases being attributed to this etiology [14]. Prone position surgery subjects patients to various factors that increase the risk for ION postoperatively. These risk factors include, often in combination, intraocular venous pressure, extensive blood loss (typically greater than 4 L), and hypotension intraoperatively [15]. Many of these risk factors can be avoided with careful attention during positioning and vigilance intraoperatively. Ischemic optic neuropathy may result in permanent visual loss; however, there may be some benefit obtained by utilizing corticosteroid therapy [16].

Central retinal artery occlusion is seen in this patient population in the setting of prolonged direct compression of the eye(s) resulting in increased intraocular pressure and thus reduced retinal perfusion, it can also occur from thromboembolic events in the perioperative period [17]. Avoiding pressure on the globes by ensuring patients' eyes are free if utilizing horseshoe headrests or even foam headrests can reduce the risk of this potential cause of visual loss. Immobilizing the head in a Mayfield can eliminate any direct pressure on the globes and thus significantly reducing this risk of potential postoperative complication. Cortical blindness as a result of ischemic damage to the visual cortex is another, albeit rare, complication of prone surgery that can result in postoperative visual loss. It is more commonly seen in deformity spinal surgery and procedures involving spinal fusion [11]. Typically, patients will improve over time, but complete recovery is rare [18]. Active monitoring and careful management of blood pressure as well as minimizing blood loss when possible will help reduce the risk of this rare complication.

Corneal abrasion are also possible in prone position spine surgery and are the most common eye complication amongst all spine surgeries [17]. General anesthesia can result in decreasing natural lubrication of the eye and, in combination with incomplete eye closure, can result in corneal abrasions. These are typically self-limiting but require postoperative ophthalmologic evaluation [17]. Adequate eye closure and protection with specialized goggles or Tegaderm™ after lubrication of the eyes after induction of anesthesia can help prevent such ocular injuries.

Peripheral Nerve and Brachial Plexus Injuries

Brachial plexus injuries, although rare, are known complications when performing prone position surgeries. The plexus courses over multiple bony structures such as the clavicle and the humeral head and in this course can be unintentionally stretched or compressed, risking injury to the nerves that can manifest as arm weakness and/or sensory deficits. Risk factors that increase the risk of such injury include diabetes mellitus, hypovolemia, and alcoholism [4]. When positioning prone, the most important factor to consider to prevent brachial plexus injury is the degree of abduction of the arms as they are placed on arm boards. Abduction at the shoulder greater than 90° puts the patient at risk of a lower trunk injury [4]. Aggressive taping of the shoulders with downward traction puts the patient at risk of an upper trunk injury. Significant extension and external rotation of the arm should be avoided as well as these arm positions have been associated with increased risk for brachial plexus injury—the elbows should be positioned below the level of the shoulders and the hands should be even with the elbows or lower [4]. The arms should be positioned in a relaxed nature on arm boards with appropriate ulnar and wrist padding and the axilla should be free and open. One retrospective review suggested that the prone-surrender or superman position with arm on arm boards superiorly was significantly higher risk for impending upper extremity nerve injury when compared to arms tucked at the patient side [19]. As such, it would be prudent to treat these cases as high risk for peripheral nerve injury for upper extremities and any neurophysiologic changes that are not corrected with conventional measures should be evaluated for repositioning maneuvers of the arms.

Ulnar nerve injuries have been reported in the setting of prone position spinal surgery and can be due to a variety of causes. The most commonly known sources of ulnar nerve injury are direct external compression of the nerve as it passes the cubital tunnel, malposition of the blood pressure cuff, excessive elbow flexion (>90°), or an arm falling off an arm board [4]. Obesity has also been described to be associated with increased risk for ulnar nerve injury in the setting of prone positioning [20].

Similar to ulnar neuropathy due to malpositioning, lateral femoral cutaneous nerves can also be injured if not properly cushioned or if the leg is inappropriately positioned. These patients can develop meralgia paresthetica resulting in pain and paresthesia of the anterior and lateral thigh. Direct external compression of the lateral femoral cutaneous nerve is usually the cause and such compression is more likely when pelvic bolsters are used for positioning, with such compression occurring in up to 24% of patients undergoing prone position spinal surgery [21].

Myocutaneous Complications

Myocutaneous complications are some of the most frequently encountered complications of prone position surgery [2]. They can occur from varied causes such as IV infiltration, cutaneous pressure over the course of a long procedure, or acute injury during the act of positioning. If an IV infiltrates while running a pressor or hypertonic solution, there is risk of damage to the limb. Pharmacy should be contacted to see if there is an antidote to be administered based on the solution that infiltrated. Also, plastic surgery consultation may be required if there is significant skin necrosis.

Plastic surgery consultation may also be required in the event of a degloving injury. When this occurs, it is usually caused during the positioning at the beginning of the case, or while positioning the patient back to supine on the hospital bed at the conclusion of the surgery. This can be avoided with proper foam padding under the downside arm during the flip to avoid direct contact to the bed frame. It is more common in elderly patients and patients taking long-term steroids, due to thinned skin.

Cutaneous injuries sustained from prolonged prone positioning are usually over the chest, hips, or knees, where the patient's weight is most concentrated on the padding. At the end of the case, these areas are likely to be red. If the skin blanches appropriately, the skin will not likely have any serious injury. If it does not blanch, or if it shows signs of blistering, it will need careful attention in the coming days and may require a skin care consult to optimize healing.

Pressure sores to breasts are also not uncommon, and female patients being positioned prone should always have their breasts carefully inspected and secured at the time of positioning. Patient with larger breasts obviously are at greater risk for such complications. Patients with a history of breast augmentation and implants can rarely develop rupture of their implants from prolonged prone positioning possibly resulting in breast necrosis [22].

Pressure-related injury to the head and neck are of concern for prone position surgery, and this risk increases with the length of the surgery as well as with volume replacement which can cause facial edema [23]. Appropriate use of padded headrests such as the ProneView® protective helmet system as well as elevation of the head has been shown to reduce the risk of pressure-related injury to the face [23, 24]. Use of the Mayfield three-pronged clamp has been described and utilized by surgeons to avoid pressure sores and cutaneous complications of the face [25].

Compartment syndromes in the setting of prone position surgery are quite rare. There are reports of lumbar spinal surgery being complicated by anterior thigh and tibial region compartment syndromes resulting in muscle necrosis and requiring fasciotomies in certain cases due to vascular compromise [26–28]. Factors that have been reported to increase the risk of limb compartment syndrome include muscular habitus, obesity, and lengthy surgical procedures [29]. Rhabdomyolysis can also occur in prone position surgery, often accompanying compartment syndromes, but can also rarely occur without any clear evidence of limb ischemia or external signs of compression such as skin changes [30]. In such cases, secondary injury due to myoglobinemia and myoglobinuria, especially renal injury, can occur and thus management must be appropriately tailored.

References

1. Toyota S, Amaki Y. Hemodynamic evaluation of the prone position by transesophageal echocardiography. J Clin Anesth. 1998;10:32–5.
2. Rozet I, Vavilala MS. Risks and benefits of patient positioning during neurosurgical care. Anesthesiol Clin. 2007;25(3):631–53, x.
3. Hadley MN, Walters BC, Grabb PA, Oyesiku NM, Pryzbylski GJ, Resnick DK, et al. Guidelines for the management of acute cervical spine and spinal cord injuries. Neurosurgery. 2002;50(Suppl 3):S1–S199.
4. Uribe JS, Kolla J, Omar H, Dakwar E, Abel N, Mangar D, et al. Brachial plexus injury following spinal surgery. J Neurosurg Spine. 2010;13:552–8.
5. Brown RH, Schauble JF, Miller NR. Anemia and hypotension as contributors to perioperative loss of vision. Anesthesiology. 1994;80:222–6.
6. American Society of Anesthesiologists Task Force on Perioperative Blindness. Practice advisory for perioperative visual loss associated with spine surgery: a report by the American Society of Anesthesiologists Task Force on Perioperative Blindness. Anesthesiology. 2006;104:1319–28.
7. Yokoyama M, Ueda W, Hirakawa M, Yamamoto H. Hemodynamic effect of the prone position during anesthesia. Acta Anaesthesiol Scand. 1991;35:741–4.
8. Carey TW, Shaw KA, Weber ML, DeVine JG. Effect of the degree of reverse Trendelenburg position on intraocular pressure during prone spine surgery: a randomized controlled trial. Spine J. 2014;14: 2118–26.
9. Prasarn ML, Zhou H, Dubose D, Rossi GD, Conrad BP, Horodyski M, et al. Total motion generated in the unstable thoracolumbar spine during management of the typical trauma patient: a comparison of methods in a cadaver model. J Neurosurg Spine. 2012;16:504–8.
10. Slocum HC, O'neal KC, Allen CR. Neurovascular complications from malposition on the operating table. Surg Gynecol Obstet. 1948;86:729–34.
11. Nandyala SV, Marquez-Lara A, Fineberg SJ, Singh R, Singh K. Incidence and risk factors for perioperative visual loss after spinal fusion. Spine J. 2014;14: 1866–72.
12. Stevens WR, Glazer PA, Kelley SD, Lietman TM, Bradford DS. Ophthalmic complications after spinal surgery. Spine (Phila Pa 1976). 1997;22:1319–24.
13. Patil CG, Lad EM, Lad SP, Ho C, Boakye M. Visual loss after spine surgery: a population-based study. Spine (Phila Pa 1976). 2008;33:1491–6.
14. Lee LA, Roth S, Posner KL, Cheney FW, Caplan RA, Newman NJ, et al. The American Society of Anesthesiologists Postoperative Visual Loss Registry: analysis of 93 spine surgery cases with postoperative visual loss. Anesthesiology. 2006;105:652–9.
15. DePasse JM, Palumbo MA, Haque M, Eberson CP, Daniels AH. Complications associated with prone positioning in elective spinal surgery. World J Orthop. 2015;6(3):351–9.
16. Hayreh SS. Ischemic optic neuropathies—where are we now? Graefes Arch Clin Exp Ophthalmol. 2013;251:1873–84.
17. Stambough JL, Dolan D, Werner R, Godfrey E. Ophthalmologic complications associated with prone positioning in spine surgery. J Am Acad Orthop Surg. 2007;15:156–65.
18. Nickels TJ, Manlapaz MR, Farag E. Perioperative visual loss after spine surgery. World J Orthop. 2014;5:100–6.
19. Kamel IR, Drum ET, Koch SA, Whitten JA, Gaughan JP, Barnette RE, et al. The use of somatosensory evoked potentials to determine the relationship between patient positioning and impending upper extremity nerve injury during spine surgery: a retrospective analysis. Anesth Analg. 2006;102: 1538–42.
20. Chung I, Glow JA, Dimopoulos V, Walid MS, Smisson HF, Johnston KW, et al. Upper-limb somatosensory evoked potential monitoring in lumbosacral spine surgery: a prognostic marker for position-related ulnar nerve injury. Spine J. 2009;9:287–95.
21. Cho KT, Lee HJ. Prone position-related meralgia paresthetica after lumbar spinal surgery: a case report and review of the literature. J Korean Neurosurg Soc. 2008;44:392–5.
22. Burdet L, Liaudet L, Schaller MD, Broccard AF. Bilateral breast necrosis after prone position ventilation. Intensive Care Med. 2001;27:1435.
23. Koreckij J, Price N, Schwend RM. Vectored cranial-cervical traction limits facial contact pressure from prone positioning during posterior spinal deformity surgery. Spine. 2011;36(15):E993–7.

24. Grissel M. Face tissue pressure in prone positioning: a comparison of three face pillows while in the prone position for spinal surgery. Spine (Phila Pa 1976). 2008;33(26):2938–41.
25. Goodwin CR, Recinos PF, Omeis I, Momin EN, Witham TF, Bydon A, et al. Prevention of facial pressure ulcers using the Mayfield clamp for sacral tumor resection. J Neurosurg Spine. 2011;14:85–7.
26. Dahab R, Barrett C, Pillay R, De Matas M. Anterior thigh compartment syndrome after prone positioning for lumbosacral fixation. Eur Spine J. 2012;21:554.
27. Ahmad FU, Madhavan K, Trombly R, Levi AD. Anterior thigh compartment syndrome and local myonecrosis after posterior spine surgery on a Jackson table. World Neurosurg. 2012;78:553.e5–8.
28. Geisler FH, Laich DT, Goldflies M, Shepard A. Anterior tibial compartment syndrome as a positioning complication of the pronesitting position for lumbar surgery. Neurosurgery. 1993;33:1117.
29. Kwee MM, Ho YH, Rozen WM. The prone position during surgery and its complications: a systematic review and evidence-based guidelines. Int Surg. 2015;100:292–303.
30. Foster MR. Rhabdomyolysis in lumbar spine surgery: a case report. Spine (Phila Pa 1976). 2003; 28(14):E276–8.

14 Special Considerations in Positioning for Neurosurgical Tumors: Spinal

Jason A. Weaver

Optimizing surgical positioning for the planned procedure can be critical in achieving the goals of the case and minimizing complications; however, it is easy to overlook this important aspect of the case for many reasons. Usually, as surgeons, we are extremely focused on the steps of the actual surgery. From a time perspective, we are often eager even somewhat rushed to get a case started. We dedicate just a small fraction of the overall time devoted to a patient on positioning, when considering the overall time spent on patient evaluation and selection, preoperative planning, imaging review, designing an appropriate approach or procedure, performing the case, and then managing the postoperative course. Although all of these aspects of the care of the patient are critical, and countless articles have been devoted to each, patient positioning is often only briefly mentioned in technique articles or altogether overlooked. Yet, when it comes to the successful surgical management of tumors involving the spinal cord, or spinal column, dedicating thought and time to optimizing positioning can profoundly affect outcome. In fact, a few extra moments spent on positioning can avoid an hour of struggling to get the last bit of tumor, save an extra half-liter of blood loss, prevent an ulnar neuropathy, or avert many other potential complications. We will consider such concerns unique to tumor surgery and discuss surgical positioning strategies that will help our patients, not to mention the entire surgical team.

Applying oncologic principles to surgical management of tumors along the spinal axis can be challenging. The surgical strategy can range from a simple biopsy to wide excisional en-bloc resection for benign or malignant tumors. First and foremost, preoperative knowledge of the tumor pathology dictates the oncologic goal. Second, detailed evaluation of the radiology to determine feasibility of that goal is also essential. The surgeon must consider many features unique to the spine, such as tumor location along the spinal axis and within the vertebral compartment (paravertebral, osseous, extra−/intradural, or intramedullary), as well as the effect of resection on stability. Balancing the extent of resection best suited for a specific pathology with the potential limitations imposed by the location highlights the unique challenges of the surgical management of spinal tumors. Consideration of a few key concepts can assist in defining surgical goals and optimizing patient positioning to achieve a result that maximizes oncologic resection and patient morbidity.

J. A. Weaver (✉)
Department of Neurosurgery, Semmes Murphey Clinic, University of Tennessee Health Sciences Center, Memphis, TN, USA
e-mail: jweaver@semmes-murphey.com

A. Arthur et al. (eds.), *Perioperative Considerations and Positioning for Neurosurgical Procedures*,
https://doi.org/10.1007/978-3-319-72679-3_14

Oncologic Terms Applied to the Spine

Before we can consider optimal positioning of our patient, we must first consider approach angles to tumor resection or a combination of approach angles. To determine approach angle, we must consider to what extent of resection is indicated with consideration of potential morbidity. This requires knowledge of the terminology and how each particular tumor pathology should dictate the extent of oncologic resection.

In an oft-quoted paper on surgical staging of primary tumors, Boriani et al. [1] provided strict definitions of oncologic terminology. When considering primary spinal column tumors, the definitions of surgical resections can be applied to any tumor whether benign or malignant, primary or metastatic, intradural, or intramedullary. A gross surgical resection will fall under one of the following three definitions: intralesional, en-bloc marginal, or en-bloc wide.

En bloc is the attempt to remove all of the tumor in one piece with a layer of healthy tissue. Gross and histologic studies then characterize further whether the resection was intralesional, marginal, or wide. When a surgeon attempts an en-bloc resection but cuts into a tumor, this is defined intralesional. If the surgeon successfully removes a tumor with the pseudocapsule intact, it is considered an en-bloc marginal resection. If the surgeon has removed all of the tumor with a continuous layer of normal tissue, it is considered an en-bloc wide excision or resection. Radical resections, often possible in orthopedic oncology, require removal of a tumor and its entire compartment, such as limb amputation. As Boriani et al. [1] pointed out, the existence of the epidural space, which extends from skull to coccyx, makes this impossible as applied to the spine. The authors further pointed out that terms such a vertebrectomy and spondylectomy, while describing what the surgeon did to the spine, carry no oncologic meaning and offer neither value in any discussion about surgical intent nor the actual degree of resection.

Palliative surgery is the partial removal of tumor (or surgery with no tumor removal) that serves a functional purpose, such as decompression of spinal cord, nerve root, or stabilization of the spine. Palliative surgery would often be performed for metastatic lesions.

The Importance of Pathology on Positioning

Although the descriptions of Boriani et al. [1] considered only primary tumors of the spinal column, the analysis is also a useful tool when applied to all spinal tumors, including benign and malignant tumors and those in other locations. Location can refer to both regions of the spinal column and compartments of the spine (i.e., intramedullary, intradural, extradural, intraosseous, or paraspinal). Preoperative diagnosis should dictate whether we attempt a palliative procedure or attempt gross removal of the tumor through intralesional or en-bloc resection. Once this is determined, we can then think about surgical approaches that, used solely or in combination, allow us to achieve our oncologic goal.

Primary Spinal Column Tumors

Enneking et al. [2] provided a useful correlation between biologic behavior of tumor and type of surgical resection with outcome. This system serves as a guide in the management of primary osseous tumors involving the spinal column. It uses radiography to categorize (benign v. malignant) lesions. Radiographic features predict biologic behavior and should therefore dictate operative strategy. Examples of benign primary spinal column tumors include eosinophilic granulomas, osteoid osteomas, osteoblastomas, osteochondromas, aneurysmal bone cysts, and giant cell tumors. Although benign histologically, not all such tumors behave in the same way and therefore some require a more aggressive approach. The staging system of Enneking et al. [2] serves as a useful guide in selecting aggressiveness of resection.

Stage 1 benign tumors (S1, latent, inactive) may be asymptomatic and usually are slow growing or do not grow at all. If treatment is required at all, it may be offered for palliative purpose or stabilization. Examples of such lesions include hemangiomas. Stage 2 benign tumors (S2, active) may grow slowly and thus over time cause progressive symptoms. Stage 3 benign tumors (S3, aggressive) may invade surrounding tissue and even have a thin discontiguous capsule. En-bloc resection should be considered for such lesions.

Although excellent tumor control rates are reported for intralesional resection of osteoblastoma, the recurrence rate is reported around 10% [3]. En-bloc resection may therefore be favorable when suitable for such lesions.

Likewise, aneurysmal bone cysts are often managed effectively with intralesional curettage. However, recurrence rates range from 10 to 25% [4, 5]. Intralesional removal can also lead to extensive intraoperative blood loss. Furthermore, iatrogenic instability associated with the removal of such large lesions often necessitates spinal stabilization. Such concerns have led to consideration of serial transarterial embolization as an effective treatment alternative [6]. Giant cell tumors are benign histologically but behave aggressively and can even produce pulmonary metastases [7]. A gross total intralesional resection offers long-term control in stage 2 giant cell tumors, whereas en-bloc resection is curative [8]. More recent studies have shown excellent control rates with stand-alone or adjuvant management with denosumab [9].

Primary malignant spinal column tumors are rare and often carry a dismal prognosis. In some cases, attempts at best oncologic resection can offer curative potential. In such cases, even planned morbidity associated with an approach may be acceptable in the overall management of the patient. Furthermore, given high rates of recurrence, there is often "one shot" at the surgical management of these cases. These cases highlight the utmost importance of detailed surgical planning and patient positioning.

The grading system of Enneking et al. [2] classifies low-grade primary malignant tumors into stages IA (tumor within the vertebral column) and IB (tumor invades outside the vertebral column) based again on radiographic features. En-bloc excision, when feasible, is the preferred treatment of choice. Similarly, high-grade malignancies are classified into stages IIA and IIB. Unlike stage IA and IB tumors, these tumors are highly aggressive and grow so rapidly that there is no continuous reactive tissue layer or pseudocapsule present. As such, micro-seeding of tumor nodules in surrounding tissue may present. For this reason, wide marginal en-bloc excision is indicated in these cases, again noting that radical resection is not possible in the spine [10].

Malignant primary spinal neoplasms that demand consideration for en-bloc resection include chordoma, chondrosarcoma, osteogenic sarcoma, and Ewing sarcoma. Given the extremely high recurrence rates for intralesional resection of such tumor versus the potential for a cure in select cases, the role of detailed surgical planning is emphasized. For example, recurrence is virtually guaranteed with intralesional resection of chordoma; however, the 50-year institutional experience reported by Boriani et al. [11] with both a retrospective and prospective analysis showed 12 of 18 patients treated with en-bloc resection experienced recurrence at an average of 8 years. All of these recurrences were either treated at another institution first and/or had contaminated margins. It is important to note that none of the seven patients treated initially with a successful wide marginal en-bloc resection demonstrated recurrence [11]. Similarly for chondrosarcoma, nearly 100% local recurrence was demonstrated with intralesional curettage, but with wide marginal en-bloc resection, the local recurrence dropped to 8% [12].

The Weinstein-Boriani-Biagini (WBB) Surgical Staging system was designed to assist in the nomenclature and planning of en-bloc surgical procedures (Fig. 14.1). It can therefore be useful in the planning of patient positioning in one- or two-staged procedures to achieve the oncologic goal. For example, the en-bloc resection can be achieved in three different ways, depending on the tumor location: vertebrectomy, sagittal resection, or resection of the posterior arch (Fig. 14.1). Because of the ring-shaped structure of the vertebral body, the authors [1] suggest that half of the vertebral structure should be disease free to allow for the removal of the healthy elements followed by en-bloc excision of the diseased portion in one piece.

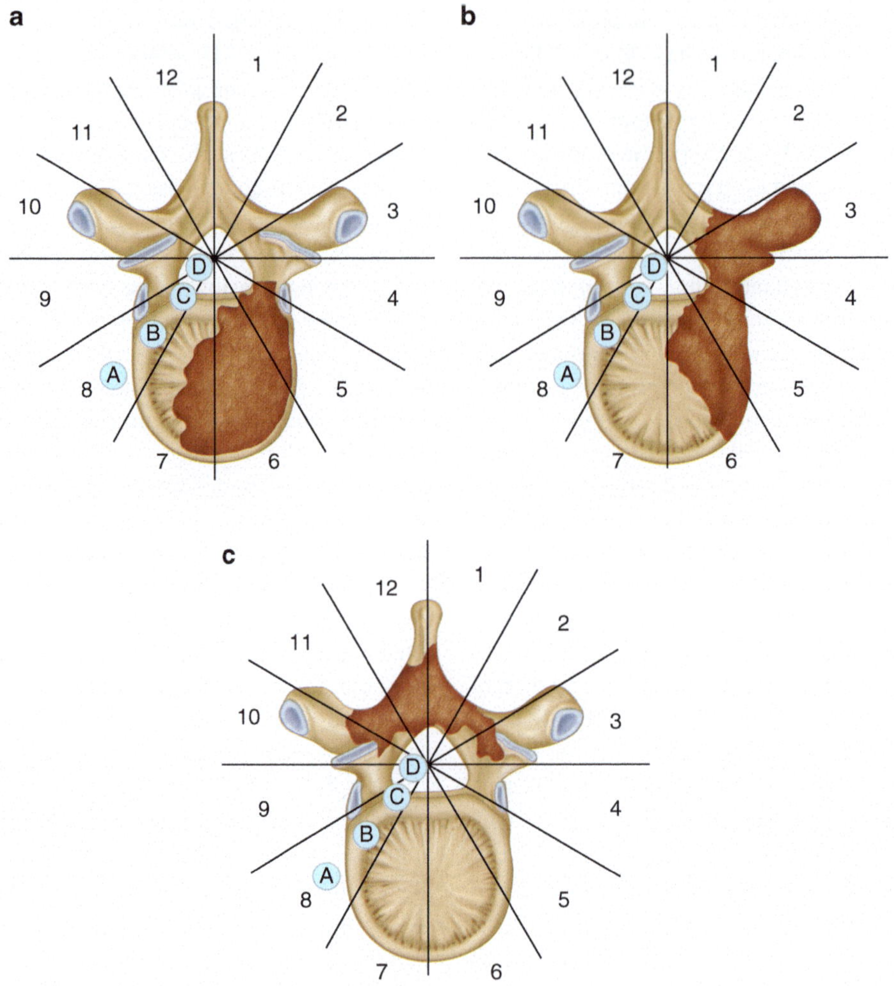

Fig. 14.1 Weinstein-Boriani-Biagini (WBB) Surgical Staging System: the numerals designate the radiating zones of the vertebral elements (1–12) and the letters designate concentric layers from outside to inside the vertebral column (A = extraosseous paravertebral to E = intradural). Possible types of en-bloc resection by WBB analysis. (**a**) vertebrectomy; (**b**) sagittal resection; (**c**) resection of the posterior arch

An en-bloc vertebrectomy, as described by Boriani et al. [1], is the removal of the vertebral body and the tumor, envisioned in the zones between 4 and 9 on the WBB system (Fig. 14.1a). This can be accomplished through a two-staged approach. In thoracic spine, where the nerve roots can be sacrificed, a one-staged approach with the patient in the prone position may be achievable in certain cases [13].

Case 1 shows a two-staged en-bloc resection of osteogenic sarcoma. The patient is a 33-year-old man with biopsy-proven osteogenic sarcoma. His metastatic workup is negative, and he has undergone four rounds of systemic neoadjuvant chemotherapy. Preoperative imaging demonstrates an Enneking stage IIA tumor confined to the osseous compartment, but also invading the right pedicle (Fig. 14.2). With >180-degree involvement of the vertebral structure, an en-bloc resection is challenging. In the first stage, the patient is positioned prone on an open-frame Jackson table (Mizuho OSI, Union City, CA), and through a standard midline exposure, the healthy dorsal elements are removed in piecemeal fashion. The right pedicle, which is involved with tumor, is removed with a single intralesional

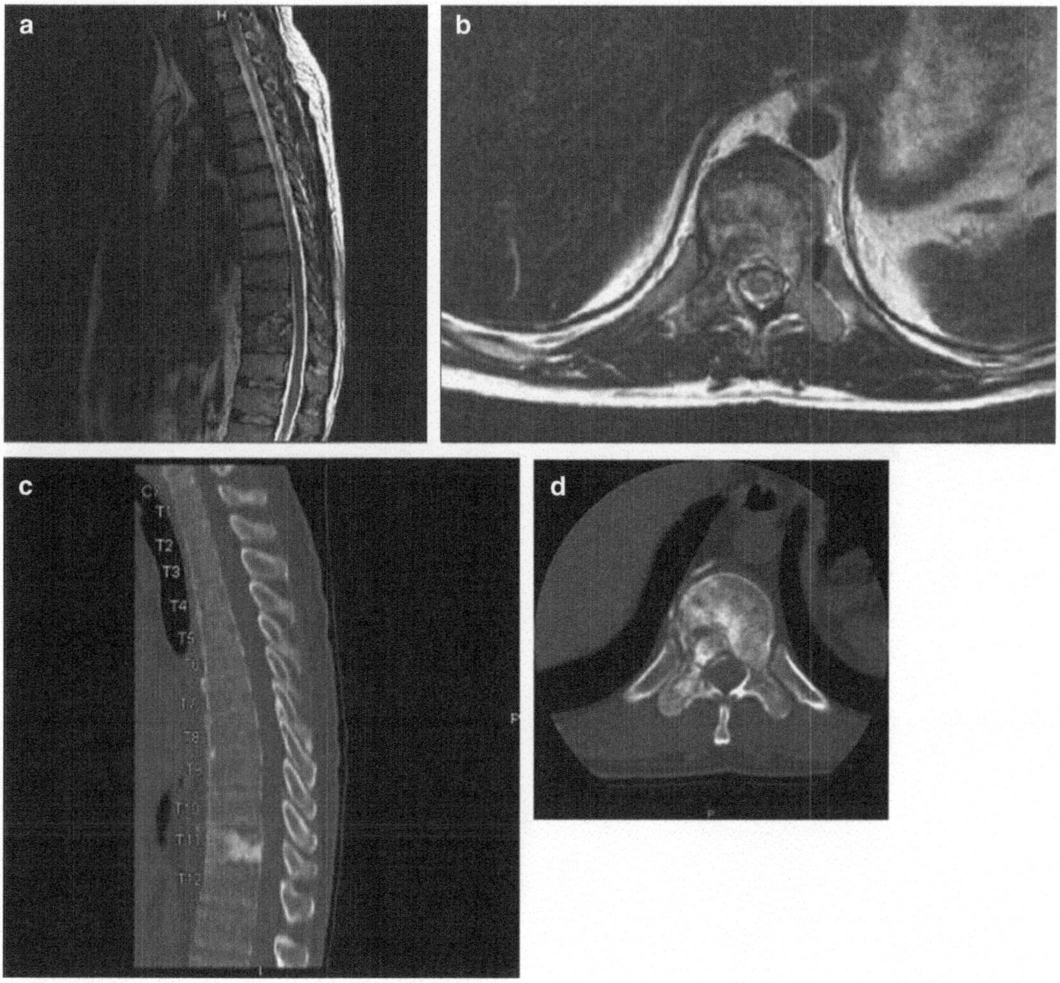

Fig. 14.2 Case 1. (**a**) Preoperative T2 W MRI and (**b**) CT demonstrating T10 lesion with marked reactive changes in the vertebral segment indicative of Enneking Stage IIA malignancy. (**c**) Sagittal CT demonstrating tumor confined to the T10 vertebral body and (d) Axial CT showing the unilateral involvement of the right pedicle making en-bloc resection challenging. Our approach was a planned intralesional resection of the involved pedicle to allow for removal of the vertebral body in an en-bloc manner

transection across the base of the pedicle. The posterior longitudinal ligament is transected across the entire disc space, and aggressive discectomies are performed above and below the diseased vertebral segment(s) (Fig. 14.3a, b). This allows mobilization of the anterior column, which will be delivered en-bloc during stage 2. Nerve root sacrifice, when feasible, is performed to facilitate resection. A silastic barrier is passed ventral to the dura to ensure complete detachment of the vascular structures and tumor pseudocapsule from the dura, and to provide a visual reference during the second stage. Pedicle screw stabilization is also performed (Fig. 14.4).

While a standard midline incision is an approach that all spine surgeons are comfortable with, positioning for this type of tumor surgery does deserve a critical analysis. Because blood loss can be extensive, we utilize an open-frame Jackson table (Mizuho OSI, Union City, CA) that allows the abdominal contents to rest freely unsupported below the patient. Proper positioning of the chest pad and hip/thigh pads allows adequate support to the patient's body, maintain a neutral spine

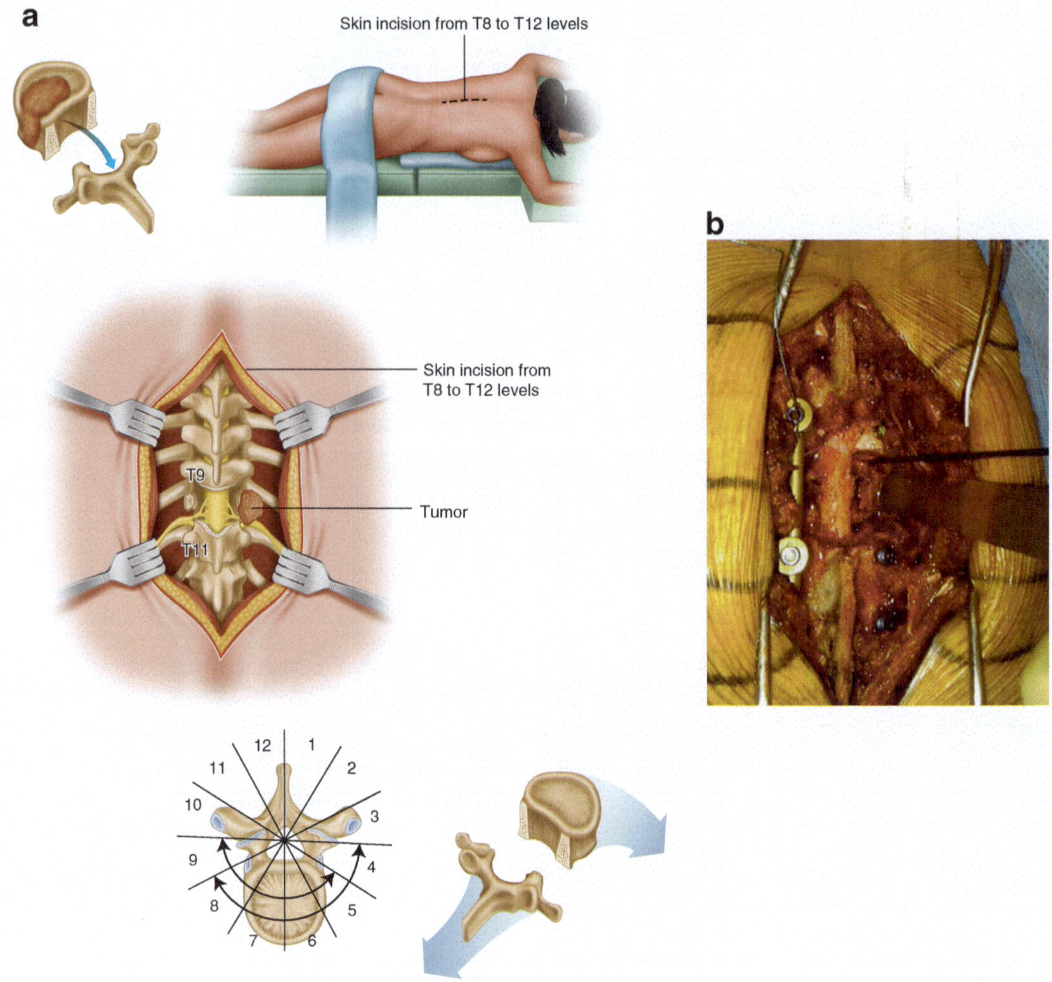

Fig. 14.3 Case 1: Stage 1: (**a**) Piecemeal removal of unaffected dorsal elements with planned unilateral pedicle transection. (**b**) Intraoperative photo demonstrates passage of a malleable retractor around the ventral aspect of the vertebral column ensuring adequate dissection and complete ligation of the segmental artery. In addition, complete discectomy with pituitary forceps is also demonstrated

position, in which the patient will be fused. Furthermore, because the abdomen is not compressed by the table, abdominal pressure is minimized and does not inadvertently transduce venous pressure. Proper placement of the chest pad across the mid-third of the sternum minimizes intrathoracic pressure and the need for high pressure positive ventilation, further reducing venous pressure. Such attention can markedly reduce blood loss during such lengthy cases with relatively large exposures, and potentially vascular tumor resections. Furthermore, less time spent on hemostasis can lead to a reduction in operative time.

The second stage is an anterior column approach performed from a transthoracic transpleural, retroperitoneal abdominal, or thoracoabdominal approach (Fig. 14.5). If tumor is extending into the paraspinous compartment on one side, an ipsilateral approach to the involved side is favored when anatomically possible. In our case, a right-sided approach with the patient in a left lateral decubitus position was taken because of the tumor involving the right pedicle. This requires the skill of the thoracic or general surgeon to take a nontraditional approach in which the liver and inferior vena cava, rather than the aorta, need to be mobilized. During

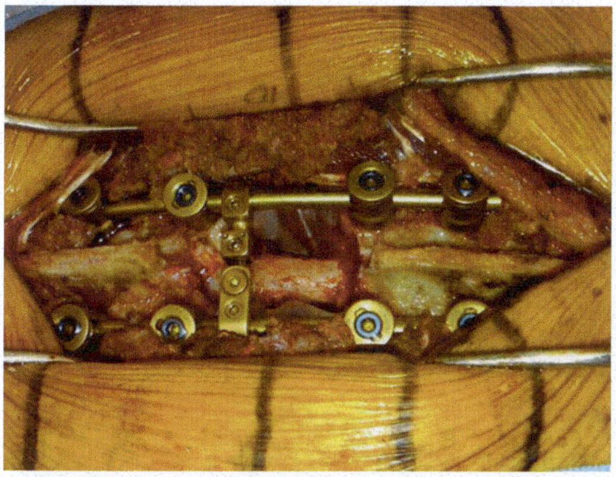

Fig. 14.4 Case 1: Completion of stage 1: The dorsal elements have been removed, the posterior longitudinal ligament transected, and discectomies performed at T9/10 and T10/11. A silastic barrier has been passed under the dura to ensure the tumor pseudocapsule has been completely freed from the ventral dura

this stage, the discectomies are completed, and the anterior segment(s) are delivered in en-bloc fashion (Fig. 14.6a–c) Tumor tissue is submitted for gross and microscopic examination to determine whether the resection was en-bloc (marginal or wide) or intralesional. Finally, the anterior column is reconstructed (Figs. 14.7 and 14.8a, b).

The en-bloc sagittal resection is performed when tumor involves zones 1–6 or 7–12 on the WBB system (Fig. 14.1b). Such a case may be performed in a combined anterior-posterior approach as described above or single-staged approach depending on tumor location. En-bloc resection of the posterior arch (Fig. 14.1c) is accomplished through a posterior approach with osteotomies through the pedicles or lamina as indicated by tumor location.

Case 2 represents a tumor in which the principles of both the en-bloc sagittal resection and

Fig. 14.5 Case 1: Stage 2: A right-sided transthoracic/transdiaphragmatic approach is preferred so that the affected pedicle is ipsilateral to the approach. The discectomies are completed, and the vertebral body is removed

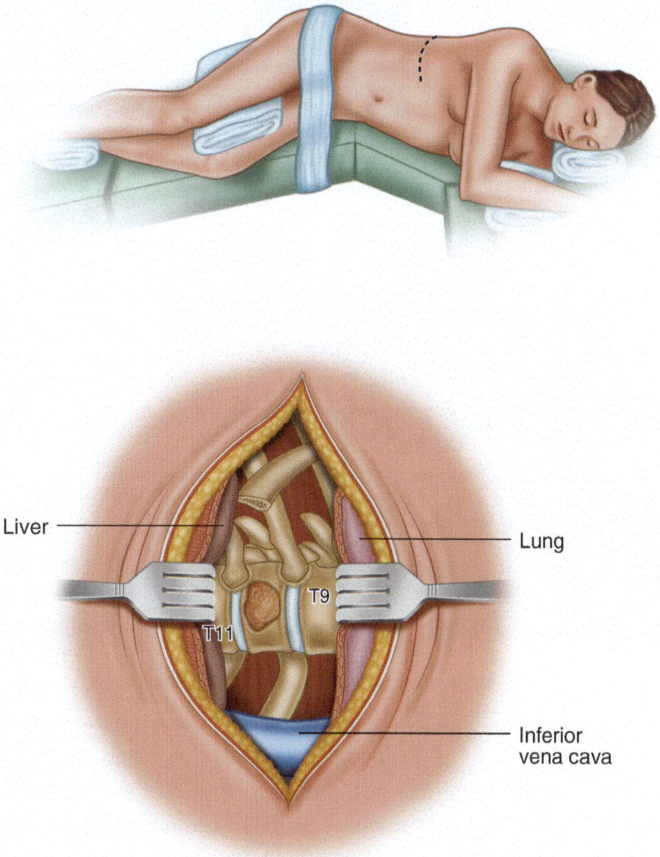

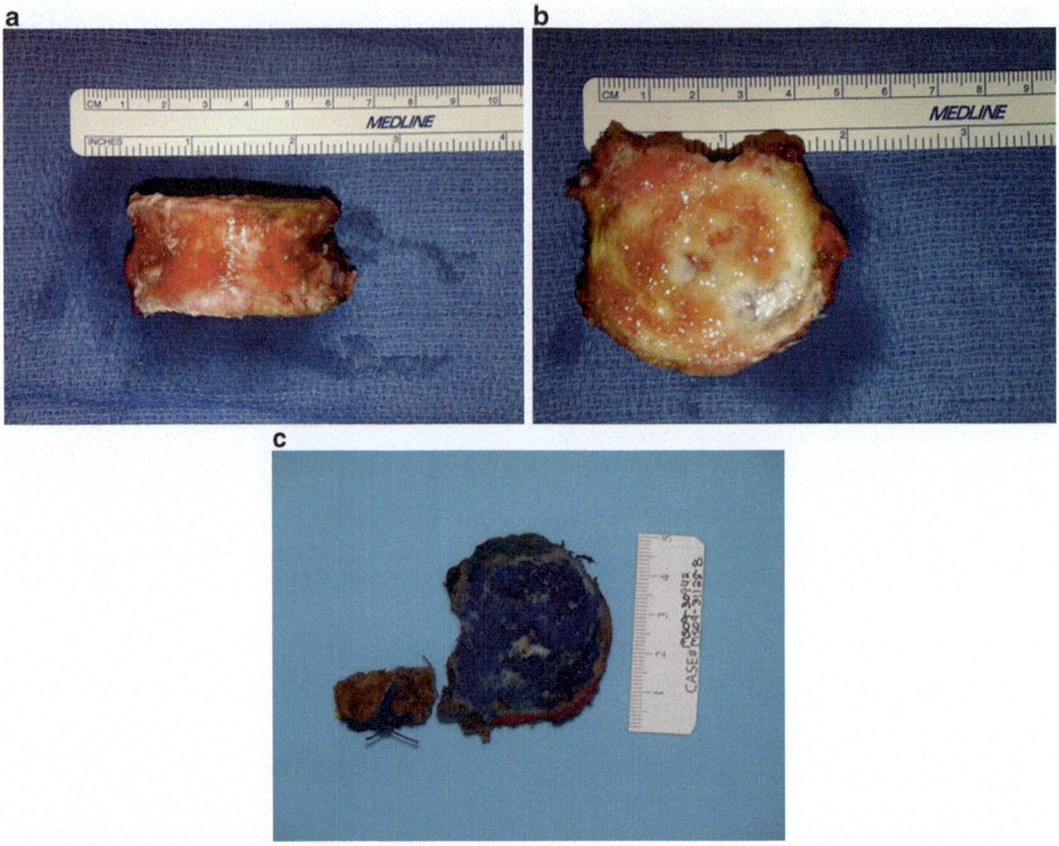

Fig. 14.6 Case 1: En-bloc specimen (**a** and **b**). Pathologic staining showing margins with the exception of the planned intralesional transection of the right pedicle (**c**)

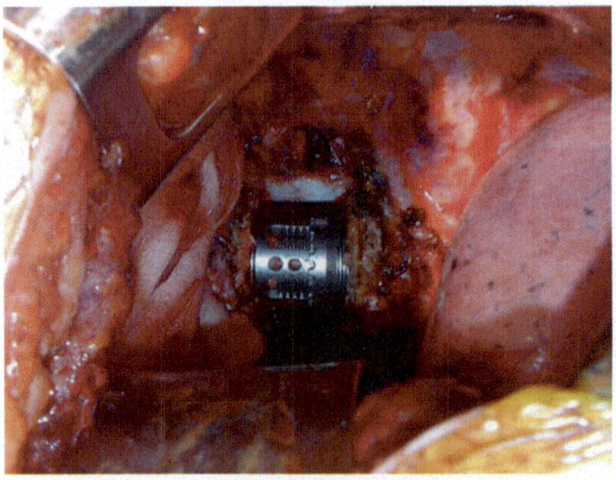

Fig. 14.7 Case 1: Anterior column reconstruction. The lung is on the right, and the liver is retracted and protected by a surgical sponge on the left of the image

resection of the posterior arch are applied successfully. This patient presented with imaging consistent with chondrosarcoma, without evidence of systemic disease. This tumor involved the posterior elements of T11-L1 in WBB zones 10–12 (Fig. 14.9). The patient is positioned prone on an open-frame Jackson table. Exposure is achieved over the dorsal aspect of the tumor with maintenance of a thin cuff of muscle over the tumor pseudocapsule (Fig. 14.10). Using intraoperative navigation with the Stealth system (Medtronic, Memphis, TN), osteotomies along the sagittal plane are created obliquely across the base of the spinous processes such that a split-thickness unilateral laminectomy would detach the base of the tumor from the affected segments (Fig. 14.11a, b). Not only does this allow removal of tumor with a margin of healthy tissue, but it spares exposing the epidural space to potential tumor seeding. A second set of navigated osteotomies is performed obliquely from lateral to medial along the rib heads and on the L1 transverse process to connect

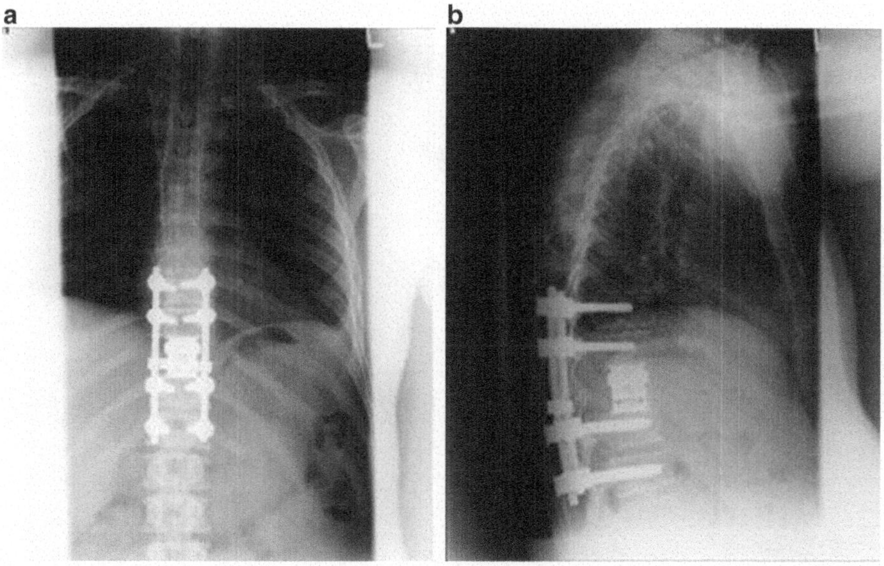

Fig. 14.8 Case 1: (**a**) Postoperative anteroposterior; and (**b**) lateral radiographs

with the first set of osteotomies, thus delivering the tumor en bloc. Pathological examination confirmed wide-margin en-bloc removal of a grade 1 chondrosarcoma (Fig. 14.12).

Extradural, Intradural, and Intramedullary Primary Tumors

Like primary tumors involving the spinal column, tumors involving the intradural and intramedullary spaces are often treated most effectively with gross total resection. Common extra- and/or intradural tumors include the nerve sheath tumors. Common intradural, extramedullary tumors include meningiomas. Common intramedullary tumors include astrocytomas, ependymomas, and hemangioblastomas. When surgical management is indicated, gross total resection minimizes local recurrence rates.

Nerve sheath tumors include schwannomas and neurofibromas. A recent multicenter review of surgically treated schwannomas through the AOSpine Multicenter Primary Spinal Tumors Database found recurrence in nine (5.32%) out of 169 patients, consistent with what has been reported historically [14]. Intralesional resection was associated with fourfold higher recurrence rate proportionate to those undergoing en-bloc removal. Location (intradural/extradural/or both) was not associated with a difference in recurrence rate. Although associated with lower rates of achieving gross total resection than with schwannomas, neurofibromas likewise show reduction in recurrence with gross total resection [15], and for malignant peripheral nerve sheath tumors (MPNST), negative margin status significantly impacts 5- and 10-year survival [16].

For meningiomas, complete resection is favorable. In a review of 62 patients, Nakamura et al. [17] used long-term follow-up to correlate recurrence rate with extent of resection. Complete resection (Simpson grades I and II) offered recurrence rates as low as 9.7%, with all recurrences noted for ventral meningiomas requiring Simpson II resection, and none for Simpson grade I. In the subset of Simpson grade II resections, a recurrence rate of 30% was noted, with mean time to recurrence at 12 years [17]. Incomplete resection (Simpson III and IV) was associated with 100% reoperation rate at 5 years for progression of tumor. This analysis underscores the importance of approach selection and patient positioning to

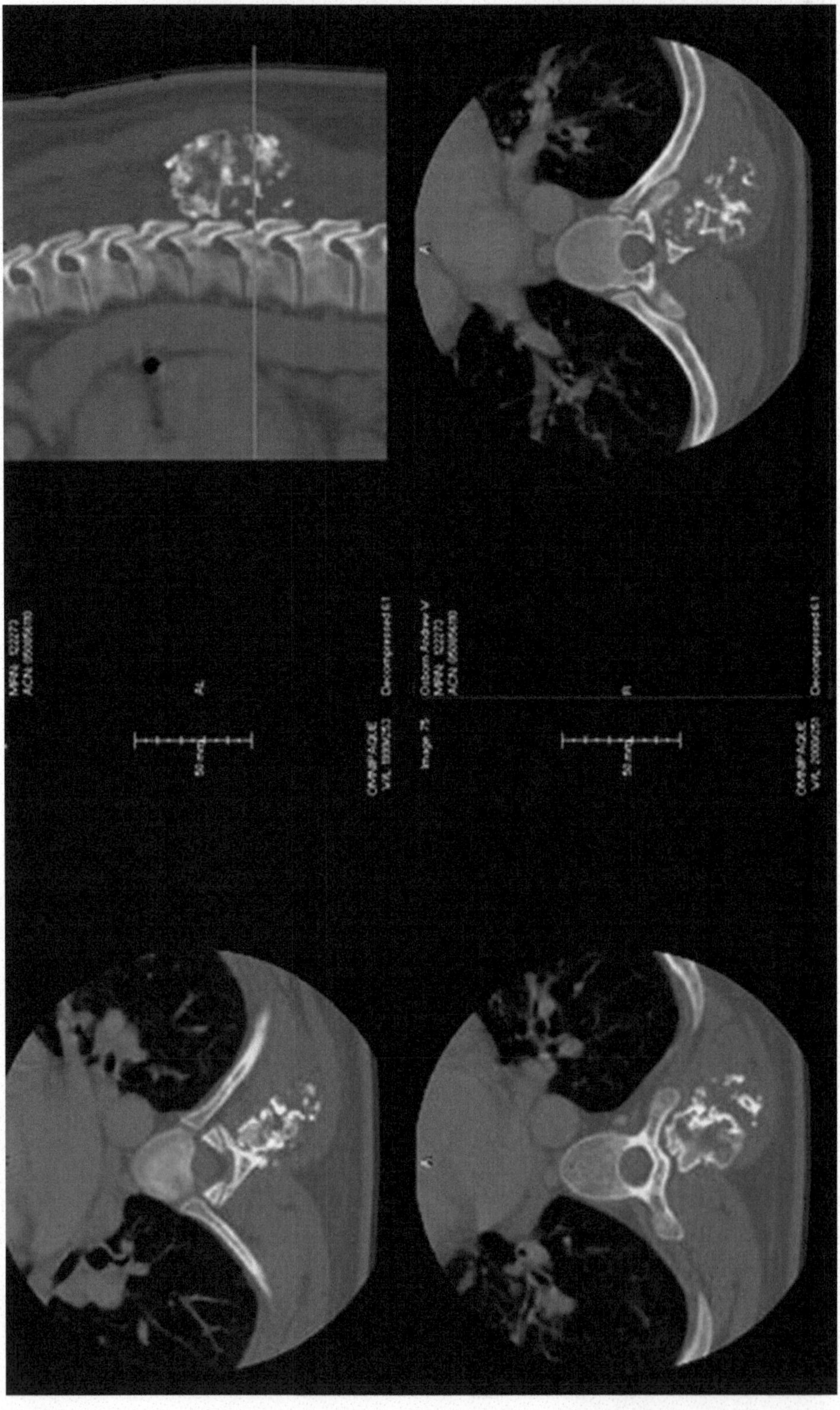

Fig. 14.9 Case 2: CT images demonstrating largely calcified mass arising from the left T12 transverse process but extending over T11-L1. Note the well-demarcated tumor capsule consistent with Enneking Stage IB lesion

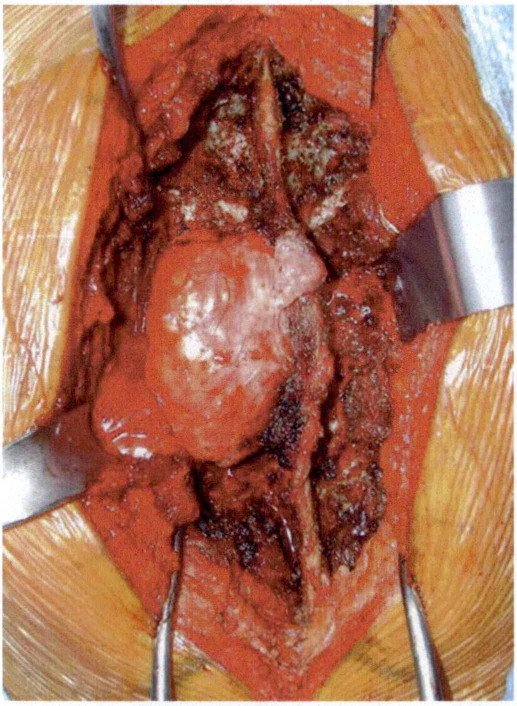

Fig. 14.10 Case 2: Intraoperative view of wide exposure of tumor. Note thin layer connective tissue over the tumor to allow for wide marginal en-bloc resection

achieve Simpson grade I resection when not limited by unacceptable morbidity.

Intramedullary tumors will most often be approached dorsally and the impact on positioning considerations is somewhat minimized in the subset of spinal tumors. Nonetheless, the low recurrence rate reported with gross total removal of spinal cord ependymomas—myxopapillary and anaplastic [18]—again underscores the dedication to careful preoperative planning. Because astrocytomas are infiltrating tumors, gross total resection is generally not obtainable. Therefore, the surgical goal may be to resect as much tumor as possible without adversely impacting neurologic function. No correlation has been demonstrated between extent of resection and recurrence [19]. There may, however, be an impact on overall survival with more radical resection of malignant astrocytomas. A retrospective study [20] demonstrated a survival rate of 78% among anaplastic astrocytomas that underwent a radical resection (defined as no residual postoperative enhancement on magnetic resonance imaging) contrasted with 38% for subtotal resection at 4 years.

Metastatic Spinal Tumors

With metastatic spinal tumors, like primary tumors, optimal surgical positioning depends on the goal of the procedure. Unlike with primary tumors, however, there is a wide array of considerations in treating a patient with metastatic disease to the spine [21]. The surgical management of metastatic disease can range from diagnostic only with percutaneous or open biopsy to en-bloc resection for complete eradication of disease. Surgical management of the vast majority of metastatic tumors will fall into an intralesional marginal excision and/or a palliative role: surgical stabilization of pathologic fracture, maintenance or restoration of neurologic function, and pain control. Surgery for oligometastatic disease has shown superiority to radiotherapy alone in all of these roles [22]. Thus, the goal of surgical resection dictates the surgical approach and the best position to yield optimal results. In certain circumstances, an en-bloc resection of metastatic tumor may best offer long-term palliation or potential for cure [9, 21, 23–25]. Such cases may include solitary sites of relapse or direct extension of the tumor, such as in superior sulcus tumors. Historically, a case for en-bloc resection has been made in patients with solitary sites of disease [26, 27], especially for tumors that were described as radio-resistant histologies or those resistant to conventional external beam radiotherapy.

Stereotactic radiosurgery and intensity-modulated radiation therapy (IMRT) for tumors of the spinal column has perhaps diminished the role of en-bloc resection in metastatic disease. Spinal IMRT and radiosurgery control rates even for classically described radio-resistant tumors, like renal cell carcinoma and melanoma, have been reported in the 75–87% at median follow-up of 37 months [28, 29]. Applying such control rates has led to a shift in management paradigm, allowing for less morbid surgical procedures, without

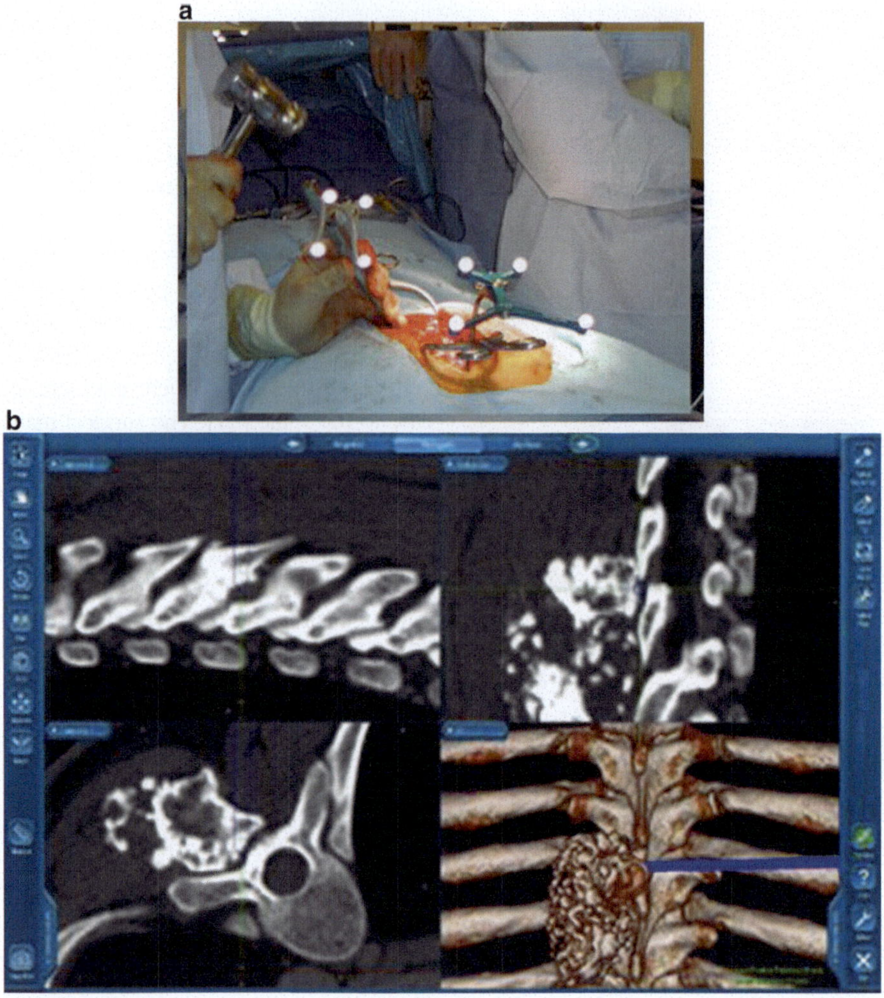

Fig. 14.11 Case 2: (**a**) Intraoperative image demonstrating stereotactic osteotomies to deliver the tumor en bloc. (**b**) Medtronic Stealth (Memphis, TN) navigation was utilized to register the osteotomes to the preoperative CT images

sacrificing local tumor control. For example, if we can spare the patient a second-staged anterior approach but still provide stabilization or palliation of pain or neurologic function, we can effectively meet all of the goals of management of metastatic disease to the spine with the least morbidity. This idea of combining surgical resection with stereotactic radiosurgery/radiotherapy has been termed "separation surgery." Like radiosurgery alone, durable local control rates have been shown as high as 90.7% at time of last follow-up [30]. In addition, the recent application of laser interstitial thermotherapy to reduce epidural compression in a minimally invasive manner has allowed the application of radiosurgery or IMRT to patients with high-grade epidural compression that might not be ideal surgical candidates [31]. Therefore, if we can reduce epidural compression, radiosurgery has been shown to offer effective long-term tumor control.

Case 3 involves a 35-year-old woman with recurrence of a superior sulcus tumor approximately 6 months after an upper lobectomy. She presented with severe local pain, right radicular pain, weakness in the right intrinsic hand muscles, and myelopathy. Imaging showed local

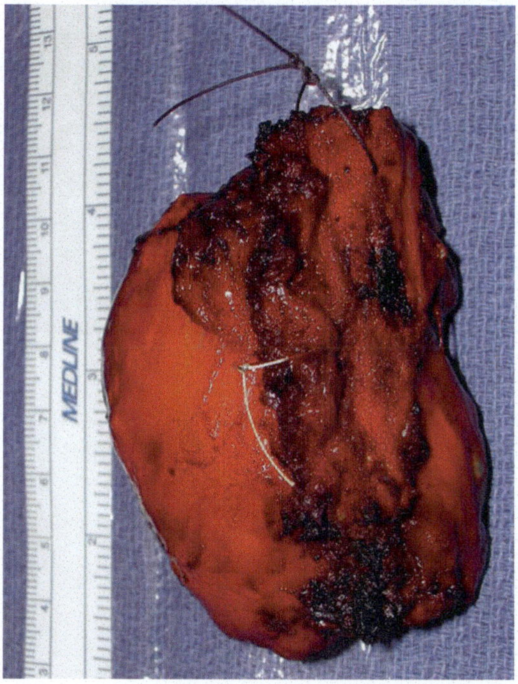

Fig. 14.12 Case 2: Pathological analysis confirms wide marginal en-bloc resection of grade 1 chondrosarcoma

invasion of the recurrence to the spinal column, involving segments C7-T3 with epidural compression of the spinal cord (Fig. 14.13a–e). Our approach was to combine surgical resection of the epidural disease and spinal stabilization with stereotactic radiosurgery (i.e., "separation surgery") to achieve the goals of pain and neurologic palliation, spinal stabilization, and durable tumor control. To effectively achieve durable control rates, we rely on radiotherapy rather than gross total resection. This requires resection of high-grade epidural compression to allow adequate margins between the spinal cord and tumor interface so that high-dose radiosurgery or radiotherapy (either in single-session or hypofractionated prescription) can be safely delivered to the spinal cord. This strategy can be accomplished through a single posterior approach, sparing the patient of another thoracotomy and anterior approach to the upper thoracic spine, with multilevel anterior column reconstruction.

The patient was positioned in a standard prone position with head fixed in the Mayfield apparatus to allow for neutral alignment across the cervical-thoracic junction. Through a midline incision, exposure of the spine was achieved and multi-level laminectomy was completed from C6 to T4. The epidural disease was radically resected and segmental stabilization was achieved through a lateral mass and pedicle screw construct extending from C4 to T7 (Fig. 14.14). Two weeks after surgery, the patient was treated with a single fraction of 22 Gy to the tumor. With effective resection of the epidural disease, creating at least a 2-mm margin between tumor and spinal cord (Fig. 14.15), the cord dose was maintained below 11 Gy, within published tolerance (Fig. 14.16) [32]. In this case, the patient maintained ambulatory function after treatment and died as a result of systemic metastatic disease rather than local progression at 14 months postoperatively.

Conclusion

Whether a tumor is an intramedullary, extra–/intradural, spinal column, or paraspinal tumor, optimizing surgical positioning first requires the surgeon to specifically define the goals of surgical resection. En-bloc resection is often indicated in the management of primary spinal tumors and perhaps even in select metastatic cases. Gross total resection is favored in the management of many intradural and/or intramedullary tumors. On the other hand, limited resection of disease may often be considered with new technology like stereotactic radiosurgery. Other adjuvant strategies, such as transarterial embolization, neoadjuvant chemotherapy, or chemotherapy alone, may further reduce the need for aggressive and often morbid surgical management. Thoughtful analysis allows us to select the best procedure and hence best positioning to limit morbidity without sacrificing goals of tumor control along with maintaining or restoring functionality, optimizing pain control, and providing spinal stabilization.

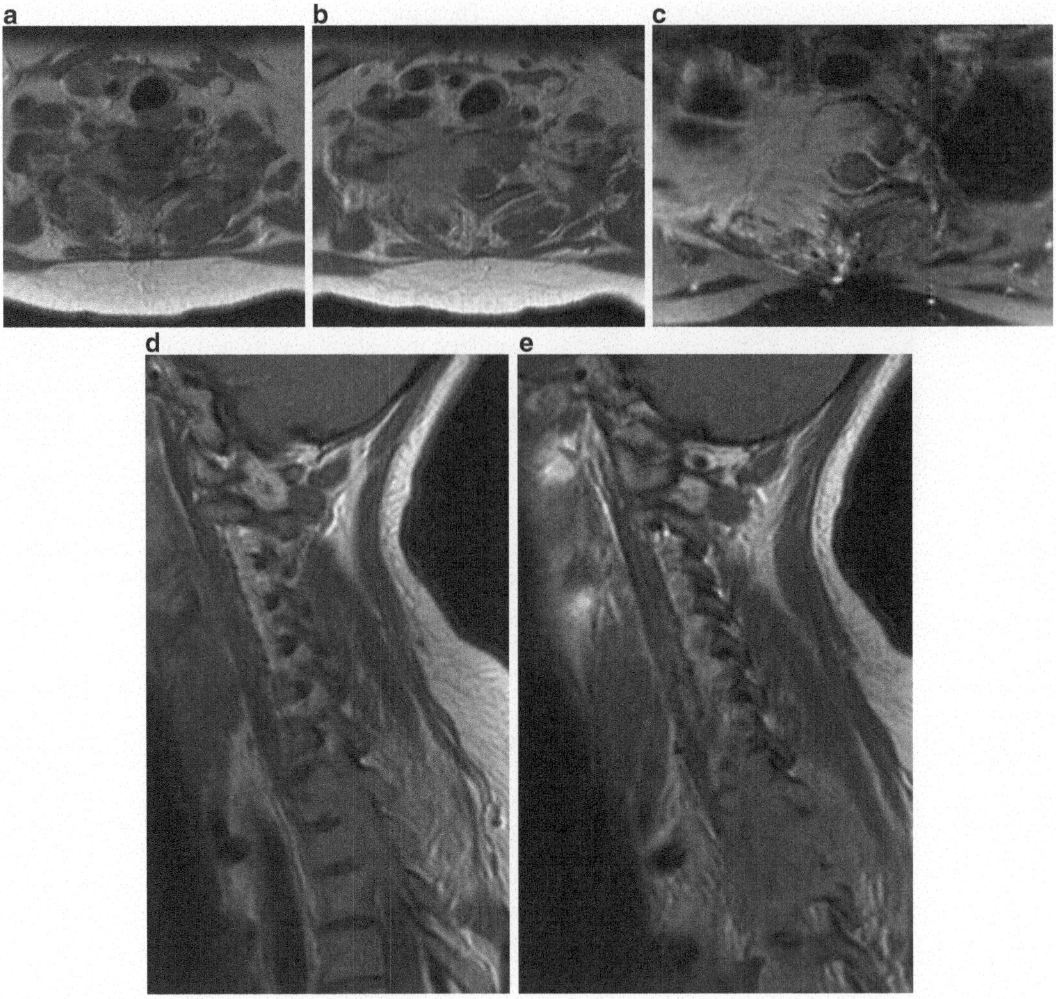

Fig. 14.13 (a–e) Case 3: Superior sulcus tumor involving vertebral segments C7-T3. Note the right transforaminal extension of tumor causing epidural compression

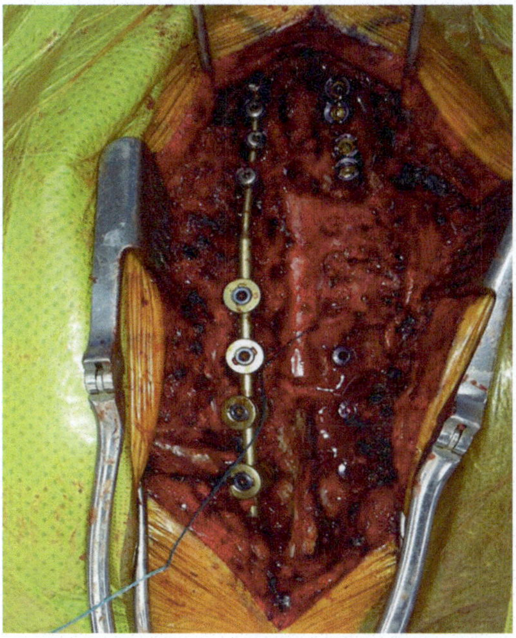

Fig. 14.14 Case 3: Intraoperative view demonstrating C6-T4 laminectomies with radical resection of epidural tumor and wide exposure of the right C7–T3 nerve roots. Posterior instrumentation with cervical lateral mass screws (C4-C7) and pedicle screws (T3-6) is performed to prevent iatrogenic instability

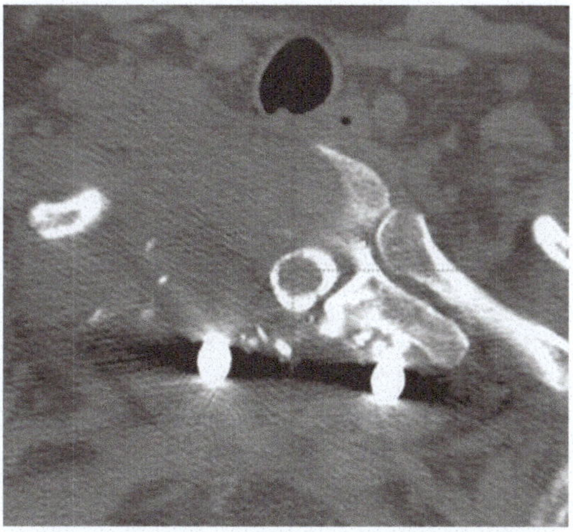

Fig. 14.15 Case 3: Postoperative CT myelogram is obtained to demonstrate adequate decompression of the spinal cord for safe and effective delivery of radiosurgery. MRI is not useful in the postoperative setting because artifact from the instrumentation causes inadequate visibility of the critical structures for safe radiosurgical planning. A margin of 2 mm is desired between tumor interface and spinal cord

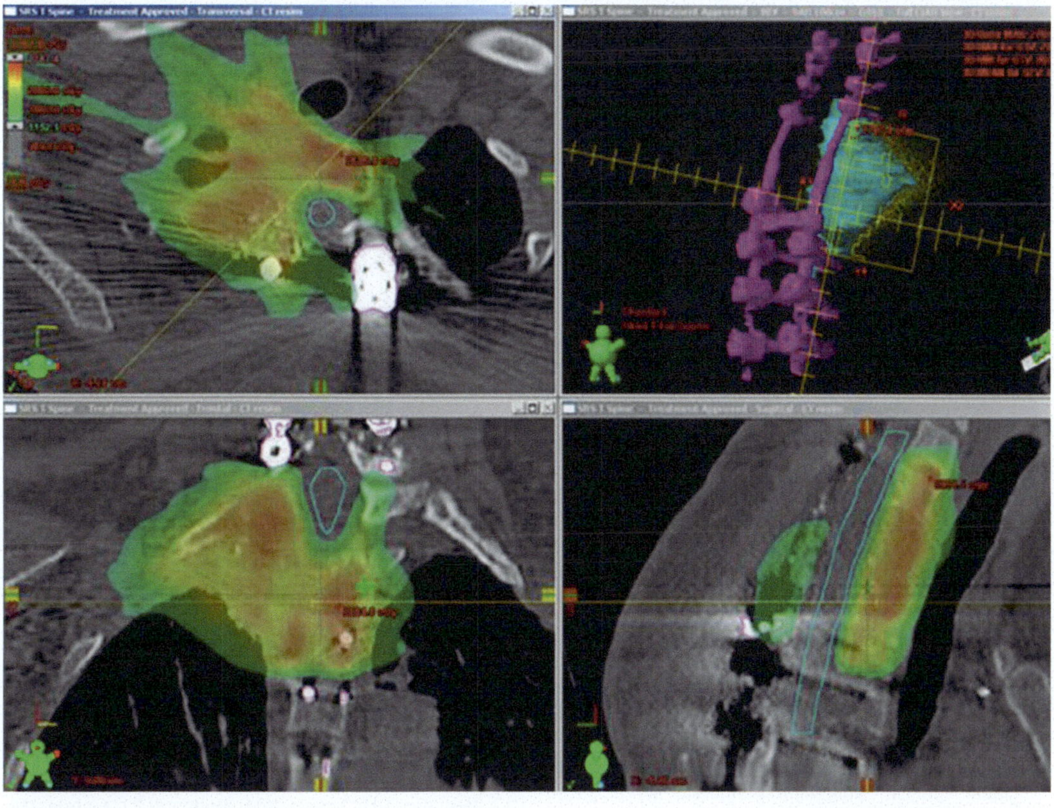

Fig. 14.16 Case 3: Single-fraction radiosurgery is delivered to the tumor at a dose of 22 Gy. The images demonstrate the color wash of dose distribution to the tumor volume and the rapid dose fall-off between the tumor and spinal cord, which received a max point dose of 11 Gy, well within spinal cord tolerance

References

1. Boriani S, Weinstein JN, Biagini R. Primary bone tumors of the spine. Terminology and surgical staging. Spine (Phila Pa 1976). 1997;22(9):1036–44.
2. Enneking WF, Spanier SS, Goodman MA. A system for the surgical staging of musculoskeletal sarcoma. Clin Orthop Relat Res. 1980;153:106–20.
3. Boriani S, Capanna R, Donati D, Levine A, Picci P, Savini R. Osteoblastoma of the spine. Clin Orthop Relat Res. 1992;278:37–45.
4. Capanna R, Albisinni U, Picci P, Calderoni P, Campanacci M, Springfield DS. Aneurysmal bone cyst of the spine. J Bone Joint Surg Am. 1985;67(4):527–31.
5. Hay MC, Paterson D, Taylor TK. Aneurysmal bone cysts of the spine. J Bone Joint Surg Br. 1978;60-B(3):406–11.
6. Doss VT, Weaver J, Didier S, Arthur AS. Serial endovascular embolization as stand-alone treatment of a sacral aneurysmal bone cyst. J Neurosurg Spine. 2014;20(2):234–8.
7. Boriani S, Weinstein JN. Oncologic classification of vertebral neoplasms. In: Dickman C, Fehlings M, Gokaslan Z, editors. Spinal cord and spinal column tumors: principles and practice. New York: Thieme; 2006.
8. Hart RA, Boriani S, Biagini R, Currier B, Weinstein JN. A system for surgical staging and management of spine tumors. A clinical outcome study of giant cell tumors of the spine. Spine (Phila Pa 1976). 1997;22(15):1773–82. discussion 83.
9. Goldschlager T, Dea N, Boyd M, Reynolds J, Patel S, Rhines LD, et al. Giant cell tumors of the spine: has denosumab changed the treatment paradigm? J Neurosurg Spine. 2015;22(5):526–33.
10. Sundaresan N, Boriani S, Rothman A, Holtzman R. Tumors of the osseous spine. J Neurooncol. 2004;69(1–3):273–90.
11. Boriani S, Bandiera S, Biagini R, Bacchini P, Boriani L, Cappuccio M, et al. Chordoma of the mobile spine: fifty years of experience. Spine (Phila Pa 1976). 2006;31(4):493–503.
12. Boriani S, De Iure F, Bandiera S, Campanacci L, Biagini R, Di Fiore M, et al. Chondrosarcoma of the mobile spine: report on 22 cases. Spine (Phila Pa 1976). 2000;25(7):804–12.
13. Tomita K, Kawahara N, Murakami H, Demura S. Total en bloc spondylectomy for spinal tumors: improvement of the technique and its associated basic background. J Orthop Sci. 2006;11(1):3–12.
14. Fehlings MG, Nater A, Zamorano JJ, Tetreault LA, Varga PP, Gokaslan ZL, et al. Risk factors for recurrence of surgically treated conventional spinal schwannomas: analysis of 169 patients from a multicenter international database. Spine (Phila Pa 1976). 2016;41(5):390–8.
15. Safaee M, Parsa AT, Barbaro NM, Chou D, Mummaneni PV, Weinstein PR, et al. Association of tumor location, extent of resection, and neurofibromatosis status with clinical outcomes for 221 spinal nerve sheath tumors. Neurosurg Focus. 2015;39(2):E5.
16. Wong WW, Hirose T, Scheithauer BW, Schild SE, Gunderson LL. Malignant peripheral nerve sheath tumor: analysis of treatment outcome. Int J Radiat Oncol Biol Phys. 1998;42(2):351–60.
17. Nakamura M, Tsuji O, Fujiyoshi K, Hosogane N, Watanabe K, Tsuji T, et al. Long-term surgical outcomes of spinal meningiomas. Spine (Phila Pa 1976). 2012;37(10):E617–23.
18. Lin YH, Huang CI, Wong TT, Chen MH, Shiau CY, Wang LW, et al. Treatment of spinal cord ependymomas by surgery with or without postoperative radiotherapy. J Neurooncol. 2005;71(2):205–10.
19. Houten JK, Cooper PR. Spinal cord astrocytomas: presentation, management and outcome. J Neurooncol. 2000;47(3):219–24.
20. McGirt MJ, Goldstein IM, Chaichana KL, Tobias ME, Kothbauer KF, Jallo GI. Extent of surgical resection of malignant astrocytomas of the spinal cord: outcome analysis of 35 patients. Neurosurgery. 2008;63(1):55–60. discussion 60-1.
21. Tomita K, Kawahara N, Kobayashi T, Yoshida A, Murakami H, Akamaru T. Surgical strategy for spinal metastases. Spine (Phila Pa 1976). 2001;26(3):298–306.
22. Sundaresan N, Steinberger A, Moore F, Sachdev V, Krol G, Hough L, et al. Indications and results of combined anterior-posterior approaches for the spine tumor surgery. J Neurosurg. 1996;85(3):438–46.
23. Patchell RA, Tibbs PA, Regine WF, Payne R, Saris S, Kryscio RJ, et al. Direct decompressive surgical resection in the treatment of spinal cord compression caused by metastatic cancer: a randomised trial. Lancet. 2005;366(9486):643–8.
24. Sundaresan N, Rothman A, Manhart K, Kelliher K. Surgery for solitary metastases of the spine: rationale and results of treatment. Spine (Phila Pa 1976). 2002;27(16):1802–6.
25. Bilsky MH, Vitaz TW, Boland PJ, Bains MS, Rajaraman V, Rusch VW. Surgical treatment of superior sulcus tumors with spinal and brachial plexus involvement. J Neurosurg. 2002;97(3 Suppl):301–9.
26. Tomita K, Kawahara N, Baba H, Tsuchiya H, Nagata S, Toribatake Y. Total en bloc spondylectomy for solitary spinal metastases. Int Orthop. 1994;18(5):291–8.
27. Yao K, Boriani S, Gokaslan Z, Sundaresan N. En bloc spondylectomy for spinal metastases: a review of techniques. Neurosurg Focus. 2003;15(5):1–6.
28. Gerszten PC, Burton SA, Ozhasoglu C, Vogel WJ, Welch WC, Baar J, et al. Stereotactic radiosurgery for spinal metastases from renal cell carcinoma. J Neurosurg Spine. 2005;3(4):288–95.
29. Gerszten PC, Burton SA, Ozhasoglu C, Welch WC. Radiosurgery for spinal metastases: clinical experience in 500 cases from a single institution. Spine (Phila Pa 1976). 2007;32(2):193–9.
30. Laufer I, Iorgulescu JB, Chapman T, Lis E, Shi W, Zhang Z, et al. Local disease control for spinal metastases following "separation surgery" and adjuvant hypofractionated or high-dose single-fraction stereotactic radiosurgery: outcome analysis in 186 patients. J Neurosurg Spine. 2013;18(3):207–14.
31. Tatsui CE, Stafford RJ, Li J, Sellin JN, Amini B, Rao G, et al. Utilization of laser interstitial thermotherapy guided by real-time thermal MRI as an alternative to separation surgery in the management of spinal metastasis. J Neurosurg Spine. 2015;23(4):400–11.
32. Benedict SH, Yenice KM, Followill D, Galvin JM, Hinson W, Kavanagh B, et al. Stereotactic body radiation therapy: the report of AAPM Task Group 101. Med Phys. 2010;37(8):4078–101.

15 Special Considerations for Intracranial Tumors

Pascal O. Zinn and Ganesh Rao

Introduction

In this chapter, we will focus on special considerations when positioning the patient for intracranial tumor surgery for the most common approaches and most frequently encountered tumor pathology. Although tumor location plays an important role in positioning, tumor histopathology (i.e., vascularization), potential for brain swelling, blood supply, venous drainage, and the use of neuro-navigation should also be considered when planning the approach and positioning.

Intracranial tumors can be categorized in numerous ways. Tumors may be within the brain parenchyma (i.e., intra-axial) or may originate in structures outside the parenchyma (i.e., extra-axial). Intra-axial tumors may be primary (i.e., originating from the brain) or metastatic (arising from other organ systems and spreading to the brain). Extra-axial tumors include those arising from the meninges or skull which may compress or invade the brain.

P. O. Zinn
Baylor College of Medicine and The University of Texas MD Anderson Cancer Center, Houston, TX, USA
e-mail: Zinn@bcm.edu

G. Rao (✉)
Department of Neurosurgery, The University of Texas MD Anderson Cancer Center, Houston, TX, USA

Regardless of the complexity of positioning, basic patient safety considerations must be considered prior to surgery. Beginning surgery with a patient in the ideal position is a key part to preparing for a successful neurosurgical operation.

This chapter provides special considerations when positioning patients for intracranial tumor surgery, particularly focusing on neoplastic lesions and highlights "tricks of the trade," pitfalls, and common mistakes. Positioning in neurosurgery is often an afterthought in textbooks and on daily teaching rounds; however, we cannot emphasize enough the importance of patient positioning to our field. Bearing in mind those special considerations and integrating key information such as patient comorbidities, patient positioning such as based on tumor location and presumed pathology lays the foundation for a safe and successful surgery.

Perioperative Considerations

In neurosurgery, there are five basic patient positions used to perform most procedures: supine, lateral, prone, three-quarter prone, and sitting position. For every position, there are slight variations; and inherent to every position, there are certain advantages and caveats that must be considered, such as changes in circulatory and respiratory physiology that may affect gas exchange and both body and cerebral hemodynamics [1]. The latter basic five patient positions

A. Arthur et al. (eds.), *Perioperative Considerations and Positioning for Neurosurgical Procedures*,
https://doi.org/10.1007/978-3-319-72679-3_15

are discussed as part of specific craniotomy approaches in this chapter.

Proper positioning serves two major purposes. First, providing patient safety during long surgeries with padding of all pressure points prevents skin decubiti ulcers and nerve damage (i.e., ulnar nerve palsy). Second, positioning, in particular the head position, is crucial for the neurosurgical exposure and trajectory to the site of interest within the brain or skull [2]. There are two main modalities for head positioning in neurosurgery: fixed (i.e., in a Mayfield head holder) or unfixed ("doughnut" or "horseshoe" head holder). For elective brain tumor surgery, the Mayfield head holder is the preferred way as a fixed head increases safety and is often necessary to use frameless stereotactic navigation systems. The duration of a brain tumor craniotomy surgery is commonly beyond 2–3 h, thus fixation to decrease head motion and to prevent scalp pressure ulcers is beneficial. Pin placement in the skull is a critical consideration as portions of the skull (the frontal and mastoid sinuses and squamosal temporal bone) are quite thin and may fracture when pressure is applied. Pins should be positioned well away from the eyes and ears. In patients with shunts, care must be taken to avoid pinning the valve and distal tubing as this may result in a shunt malfunction that can affect the outcome of the procedure. In children, smaller pins (and less pressure) should be used. An ideal position also takes into account the trajectory to access the lesion of interest: preferably it should minimize the amount of traversed healthy brain and eloquent cortex, as well as leveraging gravity to minimize brain retraction (i.e., malar eminence at highest point so frontal and temporal lobes are slightly pulled away by gravity to better access a deep lesion through the Sylvian fissure) and increase venous return to minimize bleeding and decrease intracranial pressure. Body and head positioning during a neurosurgical case can have lasting impact on postoperative care. Proper positioning is a key component of postoperative complication avoidance due to decreasing the incidence of pressure ulcers, peripheral nerve palsies, and rhabdomyolysis which in return decreases length of stay and postoperative rehabilitation times [3–6].

Intracranial Tumor Pathology

Intra-Axial Tumors

Intra-axial tumors are part of the brain and arise from precursor cells located within the brain parenchyma or from cells metastasizing to the brain parenchyma. The most common intra-axial primary brain tumor is a glioma (i.e., astrocytoma, oligodendroglioma, ependymoma) presumed to arise from the non-neuronal lineage and making up around 80% of all primary brain tumors in adults [7, 8] (Fig. 15.1). Standard of care for symptomatic gliomas is most often surgical resection and if higher grade is found on histopathology subsequent radiation and chemotherapy is recommended [9, 10]. The resection of solitary brain metastases, particularly large ones, is associated with increased survival and when coupled with postoperative radiation, has improved local control [11, 12] (Fig. 15.2). Metastasectomy is

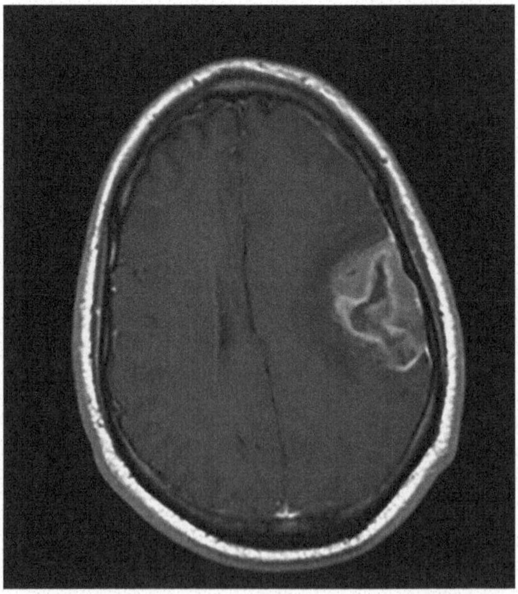

Fig. 15.1 MRI scan of a primary brain tumor, a left posterior frontal glioblastoma

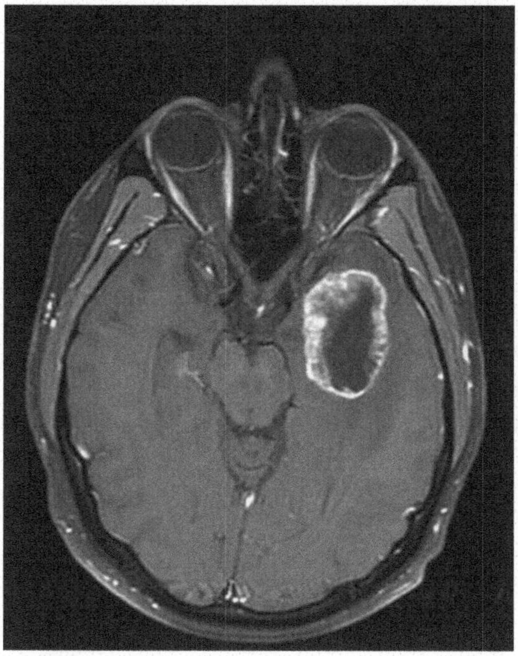

Fig. 15.2 MRI scan of a metastatic brain tumor, a left temporal sarcoma

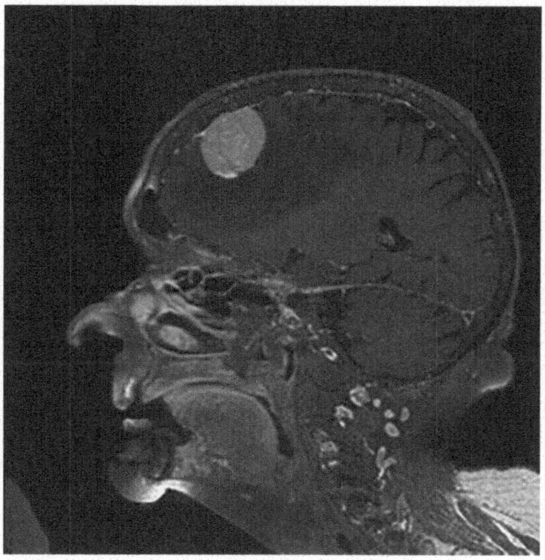

Fig. 15.3 MRI of an extra-axial meningioma. This secretory meningioma has significant perilesional edema

one of the most commonly performed procedures in neurosurgical oncology.

Even superficial lesions on the cerebral cortex require considerable thought with respect to positioning and the placement of an incision. Positioning is key when planning for a corridor to a deeper seated intra-axial mass while protecting eloquent brain. The trajectory is particularly important when considering adequate illumination from either a head light or microscope into the depth of the resection cavity. Adequate head position of the patient is of essence for gravity to open a natural corridor to the site of interest to minimize brain retraction. An elevated head position generally reduces parenchymal edema caused by brain irritation from retraction and surgical manipulation, often more so with intra-axial higher grade lesions since they are intimately associated with the brain and may be causing significant amounts of perilesional edema and inflammation and growth often occurs in a highly invasive fashion. Intra-axial metastases often cause significant amounts of edema due to displacement and compression of the brain parenchyma and possibly draining veins. Thus, for positioning for intra-axial highly invasive or inflammatory lesions, head elevation above the heart to support venous return and reduction of brain edema by reversing fluid extravasation, as well as leveraging gravity to minimize brain retraction is key. However, with too much rotation, venous drainage can be compromised by occlusion of the jugular veins. Care must be taken to ensure that venous obstruction is minimized in these situations.

Extra-Axial Tumors

Extra-axial intracranial tumors are located within the skull or at the skull base and reside outside the brain parenchyma, if deeper seated and arising from the skull base these can be some of the most challenging lesions to be surgically treated. In this paragraph, we will discuss the most common pathologies for extra-axial non-skull base tumors. These are most commonly masses arising from the meninges and dural based metastases and less frequently masses stemming from the bony skull. These types of tumors often displace the brain and rarely significantly invade the brain. Thus, they can cause significant edema and mass effect (Fig. 15.3). It is particularly challenging when those masses are adherent to the dural sinuses and/or compress major draining veins (i.e., veins going to the superior sagittal sinus, or the anastomotic veins of Labbé or Trolard). Interrupting a draining vein during surgery can cause rapid parenchymal swelling and cause venous hemorrhagic strokes resulting in major neurologic deficits and even death. Preoperative identification of veins is crucial as to identifying the best possible head position to obtain a corridor as to avoid those critical structures. Dural based masses often receive blood supply from dural vessels, thus identifying major feeding arteries early and to bipolar and cut them reduces intraoperative bleeding and operative time; however, feeding arteries must be identified on preoperative imaging and when positioning, this must be kept in mind as to have early feeding artery access.

Skull Base Tumors

Skull base tumors are often particularly challenging to operate on since they are adherent to vital structures (i.e., cranial nerves and vessels) passing through the skull base. Nerves and vessels intimately associated with bony canals are often fixed and adherent to the bone and fibrous tissue and thus minimal retraction can cause major injury. Typical skull base pathology encountered frequently in neurosurgery includes meningiomas (i.e., planum sphenoidale, tuberculum sellae, or petro-clival location) in all three cranial fossae as well as schwannomas (i.e., vestibular schwannoma or lower cranial nerve schwannomas), and frequently we encounter either primary or metastatic carcinomas of the skull base and nasopharyngeal cavities eroding the skull base and possibly invading the dura and brain. The skull base can be accessed in a 360-degree fashion (i.e., trans-sphenoidal from the front and below, far lateral for lesions of the foramen magnum or lower cranial nerves) with approaches tailored to every specific lesion and its relationship to the safest surgical trajectory. Special considerations for positioning for each of the major skull base approaches will be discussed in this chapter. Similar to intra- or extra-axial non-skull base lesions, the previously described general rules for positioning apply. In addition, for skull base tumor surgery, while positioning, extra thought must be given to adequate padding of the body due to the longer duration of skull base cases given their complexity. For example, the lateral position requires adequate axillary support with an axillary shoulder roll to avoid shoulder dislocation and postoperative arm pain and particular attention must be paid to padding of common nerve pressure points, such as median, ulnar, and peroneal nerves. During prolonged surgeries, the patient is also at greater risk for extremity deep venous thromboses and pulmonary embolisms. Thus, it is recommended to elevate the extremities whenever possible to support venous return and avoid pooling of blood in the large venous systems (i.e., lower extremities).

Comorbidities

As mentioned, metastatic brain tumors are the most common intracranial tumor diagnosed. These patients often present with comorbid conditions that warrant consideration during positioning. For example, patients with advanced metastatic disease will present not only with brain metastases, but also extensive lung metastases (or in the case of lung cancer, a primary tumor that is progressing) (Fig. 15.4). Compromised

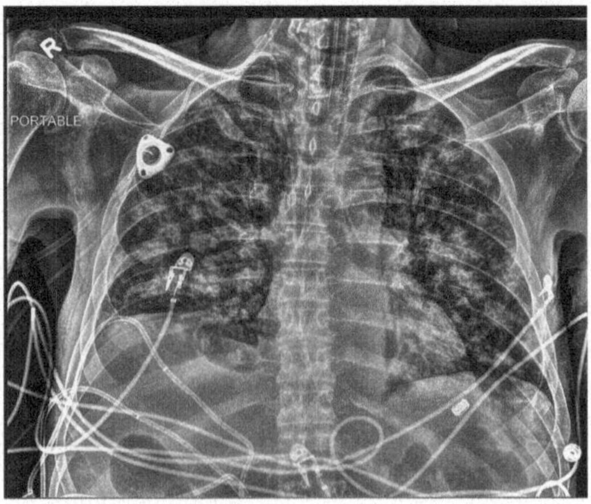

Fig. 15.4 Chest X-ray of patient with metastatic cancer demonstrating significant pulmonary involvement

lung function may require additional ventilatory support but may also affect patient positioning. For example, a patient with tenuous respiratory status may not tolerate prone positioning given the increase in peak pressures. This may require lateral positioning with head rotation to access an occipital or cerebellar lesion, for example.

Patients with primary or metastatic tumors may also be corticosteroid dependent. These lesions present with significant perilesional edema requiring the use of steroids for symptomatic relief. Steroids are associated with significant side effects however, and can include immunosuppression which can compromise wound healing. As such, care must be taken to ensure adequate wound closure given the risk for wound healing complications. In general, we advocate the use of antibiotic-impregnated irrigation during the closure and the maintenance of sutures in place for at least two weeks before removal.

Patients may also require repeat surgery for the management of recurrent tumors. In this circumstances, systemic infections have been reported to occur at a higher rate in these patients as well after second craniotomy for recurrent tumors [13]. Planning for repeat craniotomy is not often considered for brain tumor surgery, but the value of re-resection for recurrent disease has been reported [14, 15]. Therefore, preoperative planning regarding the size of the incision and underlying craniotomy should be considered with the possibility of recurrent tumor and subsequent surgery.

Positioning for Common Approaches: Tricks of the Trade and Pitfalls

General considerations for every approach and position must include patient safety and room setup. Securing the patient to the operating room table is critical as patients may be rotated (tilted) in either direction and thus are at risk of falling off the table. Another important point is to fully position the patient before locking in the Mayfield as any partial operating table adjustment will cause pulling or pushing and may dislodge the Mayfield pins causing scalp or skull injury. During induction, paralytic agents can be used which may facilitate exaggerated head positions because of pharmacologically induced muscle laxity. However when these paralytics wear off, increased pressure on the head may result as muscle contractions resume, resulting in slippage and scalp lacerations. Once the patient is locked in position, it is best to use Trendelenburg (to lower the head) and reverse Trendelenburg (to raise the head) as this will avoid dislodging the pins. Placement of the neuro-navigation camera in the room and attachment of the three-point fixation head holder to the bed to leave ample room for attaching the navigation reference frame is critical. If the reference frame is blocked by the draping, nurse's Mayo stand, or the surgeon, it is rendered effectively useless. Operating room table selection is also a key consideration. Most tables allow for Trendelenburg and reverse Trendelenburg movement which is critical for various approaches but also to facilitate venous drainage (i.e., head elevation in the setting of significant cerebral edema). Similarly, most tables allow for tilting (left and right, also called "airplaning"). Care must be taken to ensure the patient is secured to the table as it is possible for a patient to fall off the operating table if too much tilt is used.

Supine Position

This is the most frequently used patient position in neurosurgery and carries minimal risks from anesthesiologic and neurosurgical perspectives as it is easily achievable and does not involve any awkward positioning of the anesthetized patient [1]. The face and endotracheal tube are accessible to the anesthesiologist. Placing the patient in the supine position assists the surgeon in maintaining orientation (Fig. 15.5). There is a slight risk with significant head rotation which decreases venous return and causes increased bleeding and intracranial pressure elevation. There is also a slightly increased risk of aspiration as compared to the lateral or prone position [16]. As a rule of thumb for supine positioning,

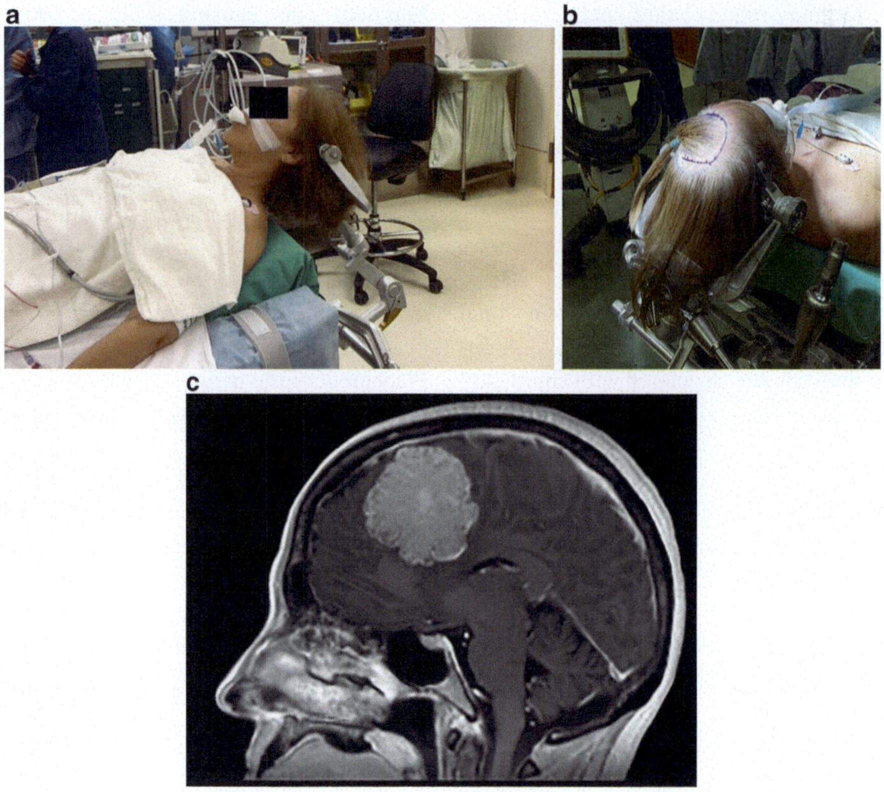

Fig. 15.5 Supine position (**a** and **b**) of patient undergoing a craniotomy for a lesion in the left frontal lobe depicted in the MRI (**c**)

the head of the patient is elevated, the hips in flexion and legs elevated as to prevent deep venous thromboses. Bony prominences (i.e., elbows, heels) and peripheral nerve pressure points (i.e., ulnar and peroneal nerves) must be adequately padded and "seat belt" or adhesive tape fixation prevents sliding of the patient when the operating table is tilted. There are circumstances for which the supine position may be preferred even if it does not give the best access to a particular intracranial lesion. In the setting of metastases, this may be preferred due to the fact that patients may present with concurrent lesions in the lung or mediastinum that may make ventilation more difficult (i.e., prone or lateral positions). Coordination with the anesthesiologist is critical to ensure proper patient care and mitigation of positions that may compromise adequate ventilator support.

Trans-Sphenoidal

Trans-sphenoidal approaches are more frequently being performed trans-nasal and less frequently sublabial. This is the primary approach for sellar pathology including functional or nonfunctional pituitary adenomas, Rathke's cleft cysts, craniopharyngiomas, and other anterior skull base pathologies including meningiomas. We use the Mayfield head holder with most commonly two pins on the left side and one pin on the right, about two finger breadths above the pinna, although others have described positioning the patient on a horseshoe head holder. Depending on the exact location and extent of the lesion that needs to be accessed, the head position varies; however, as a rule of thumb we position the head very minimally turned to the operator (5–10°), minimally extended and translated up in almost neutral or horizontal position. The neuronavigation camera is most often positioned at the head of the patient, thus the Mayfield attached to the surgical table from the inside. We position the head of the patient slightly elevated above the heart to minimize bleeding and support venous return, this is particularly important when working around the cavernous sinus in a trans-sphenoidal approach.

For trans-sphenoidal approaches to the clivus and posterior fossa slight head flexion (15-degree flexion of the forehead-chin line) [17] is recommended to maximize the angle of exposure, it follows that exposure of the anterior skull base from a trans-sphenoidal route (i.e., tuberculum sella meningiomas) requires the patient's head to be positioned in slight extension (10–15° extension of the forehead-chin line) [18] to obtain a more anterior trajectory and thus preventing the endoscope and surgical instruments from hitting the thorax of the patient [19].

Frontal/Trans-Frontal Sinus Approach

Most frequently, a bi-coronal or extended bi-coronal incision is used to access lesions via a frontal or trans-frontal sinus approach with or without removal of the orbital rim. This approach offers excellent exposure for large midline lesions extending lateral bilaterally (i.e., large anterior skull base meningiomas), as well as for lesions of the medial orbits or lesions involving the frontal sinus (i.e., nasopharyngeal carcinomas), particularly if a lateral orbito-zygomatic osteotomy or classic pterional approach is expected to provide insufficient exposure towards the contralateral side. Prior to final positioning some surgeons may place a lumbar drain given difficulty for CSF drainage for brain relaxation using this approach. The patient is positioned supine with the head above the heart. The three-point fixation pins are commonly placed behind the ears as not to interfere with the incision. The head is translated up and slightly flexed on the chest and slightly extended on the neck [20], and this varies depending on the exact location of the surgical site of interest. Care must be taken not to drape towels right above the eyebrows to avoid downward pressure to the eyes when the forehead skin flap is elevated and retracted anteriorly.

Orbito-Zygomatic and Pterional Approaches

The orbito-zygomatic osteotomy (OZO) is an extended pterional approach and can be performed in one- or two-piece fashion [21]. OZO is most frequently used in skull base and vascular neurosurgery; however, it is the preferred approach as well for neoplastic lesions located in the petro-clival and spheno-orbital areas [22], as well as tumors located in the vicinity of the basilar apex (Fig. 15.6). The patient is positioned supine on the operating table, an ipsilateral small shoulder roll can be placed if higher degree rotation is needed, and the patient's neck is not supple enough; and the head generally rotated 30–60° to the side contralateral to the pathology. While rotation is increased for tumors located in the anterior and middle cranial fossae, rotation is reduced for lesions involving the clivus and posterior fossa. The head is slightly extended towards the floor, this together with the rotation will bring the malar eminence to the most supe-

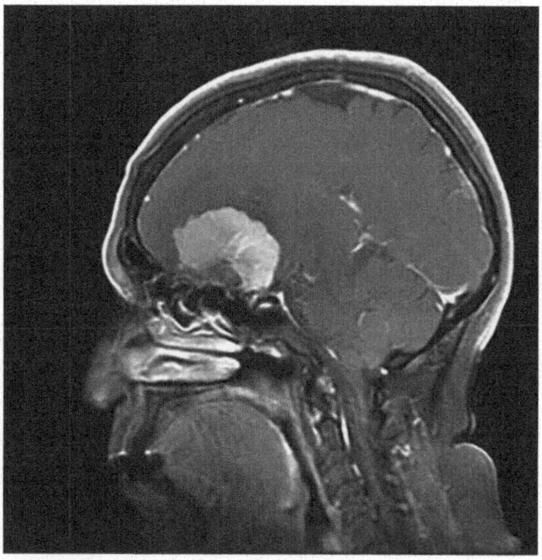

Fig. 15.6 MRI scan of a spheno-orbital meningioma that may be approached with an orbito-zygomatic approach

rior point in the operative field [22, 23]. This is identical to the classic pterional craniotomy and positioning, and having the malar eminence highest in the operative field is an indirect measure for the location of the Sylvian fissure and will take advantage of gravity to allow both the temporal and frontal lobes to naturally fall away, thus minimizing the need for retraction and thus retraction-associated injury.

In addition to the combined pterional/OZO approach, the pterional (frontotemporal) craniotomy alone is one of the most frequently used craniotomies in neurosurgery and is the work horse approach for internal carotid and middle cerebral artery aneurysms and a wide range of neoplastic lesions of the frontal and temporal lobes, Sylvian fissure or deeper lesions such as sphenoid ridge, tuberculum sellae, or third ventricular locations. The head is generally slightly extended and turned 30° away from the site of interest.

Temporal

For approaching a temporal lesion either a transtemporal or subtemporal route can be chosen; the patient is positioned supine with a shoulder roll behind the ipsilateral back to allow for 60–80-degree head rotation towards the contralateral side. Often a straight or slightly curved incision above the ear is chosen. For subtemporal approaches, a higher degree of head tilt is recommended and thus often lateral patient position is chosen. The approach to a temporal tumor, particularly one that requires access to the mesial temporal lobe is facilitated by placing the head with slight vertex towards the floor. This helps the surgeon reach the mesial temporal structures including the uncus. For subtemporal approaches, particularly those to the brain stem, placement of a lumbar drain is sometimes helpful to assist with superior retraction of the temporal lobe. Considerations for the lateral position will be discussed in the following paragraph.

Lateral Position

The lateral position is used for patient requiring subtemporal, skull base (including approaches to the apical portion of the petrous bone), peripetrous, and posterior fossa approaches. For supratentorial brain tumors, particularly those in the parasagittal location just lateral to midline, the lateral position can be very helpful. We find that having the tumor side dependent (i.e., towards the floor) can facilitate brain retraction as gravity will naturally let the ipsilateral hemisphere retract away from the falx (Fig. 15.7). General risks include brachial plexus injury, stretch injuries (axillary trauma), and pressure palsies (i.e., suprascapular nerve injury), and direct compromise of upper extremity perfusion caused by compression

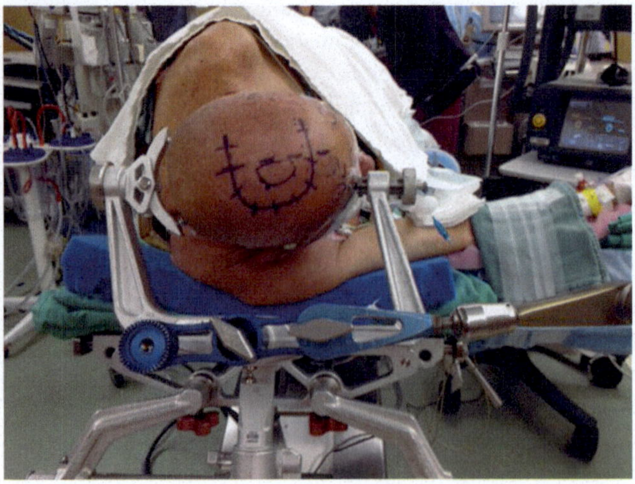

Fig. 15.7 Tumor on the right side of the falx is approached with the tumor side down. The patient is positioned in the right lateral decubitus position

by an axillary roll. From the anesthesiology standpoint, ventilation-perfusion mismatch can occur [1]. Lateral, as compared to supine, positioning may lead to decreases in mean arterial pressure, venous return, stroke volume, and cardiac output; it may also decrease total lung capacity and the jugular venous resistance. In return, heart rate, systemic vascular resistance, and V/Q mismatch may increase [1]. Thus, particularly with significant neck flexion, intracranial pressure may increase dramatically. Attention is required for positioning the patient's lower arm due to potential injury to brachial plexus and axillary artery. We place an axillary roll under the upper chest as to alleviate the axilla from direct pressure and the dependent arm is positioned below the operating table on a low arm board or pillow padded on the three-point fixation extension which connects to the table. The upper arm is positioned on a pillow or high arm board and is taped to the body and operating table. Proper functioning of intravenous and arterial lines after positioning must be ensured and nonfunctional arterial lines of the dependent arm can indicate that the axillary roll was incorrectly placed. A pillow is placed between the legs and as a rule, also for the lateral position, a V-shaped body configuration must be aimed for as to elevate the head above the heart and support venous return from the lower extremities as to minimize risk for deep venous thromboses.

Retrosigmoid

The retrosigmoid approach is commonly used for lesions of the cerebellopontine angle (e.g., vestibular schwannomas, epidermoid cysts, meningiomas) [24]. Some surgeons advocate supine or sitting position; however, most frequently a lateral or three-quarter prone position is chosen as to minimize head rotation. Mayfield three-point fixation is used and generally three movements for head positioning are performed: first, contralateral rotation for positioning the temple parallel to the floor; second, contralateral bending so the vertex is slightly tilted towards the floor; and third, slight neck flexion as to open the cervical-suboccipital angle [25]. This also minimizes the soft tissue depth over the foramen magnum and will allow for more direct access for CSF drainage. As described above, attention must be paid to adequately pad the dependent axilla and correctly placing an axillary roll as well as taping down the superior shoulder towards the patient's legs without causing brachial plexus stretch injury. In addition to using a bean bag, we suggest placing at least two belts or using silk tape to secure the patient, which is performed in anticipation of tilting the operating table during the procedure to maximize visualization of the lesion.

Far Lateral

The far lateral approach is an extension of the retrosigmoid approach. The patient position is commonly lateral (park bench) or three-quarter prone and is best suited for lesions lateral and anterior to the brain stem, foramen magnum, and jugular foramen region [26]. The patient's head is tilted slightly towards the floor and also slightly translated superiorly to open up the space between the edge of the mastoid and the transverse process of the atlas [26]. Lesions requiring a far lateral approach are often near cranial nerves (i.e., lower cranial nerves for jugular foramen pathology) and thus, if neuromonitoring is used, attention must be paid to properly test and secure electrodes before starting the case. Electrodes often get dislodged if the patient is repositioned or signals can be lost if the patient is not properly positioned (i.e., compression of the axillary artery by direct pressure from an improperly placed support roll for axilla and shoulder). Thus, careful electrophysiology baseline assessments and testing of the hardware is key prior to starting the case.

Parieto-Occipital

Parieto-occipital areas in the brain can commonly be approached with the patient in either prone or three-quarter prone position. For the latter patient position, similar principles apply as for the lateral position. Either a bean bag or sufficient padding is required and extra attention must be paid to the dependent arm and adequate shoulder support using a properly placed axillary roll. If the lesion approached is close to midline even with a three-quarter prone position, the head must be significantly turned and this is best used for patients with a sufficiently supple neck. Careful attention must be paid to pinning the patient's head, whereas the single Mayfield head clamp pin goes to the ipsilateral lateral forehead avoiding the supratrochlear nerve and vessel bundle; the dual pin side of the clamp goes to the contralateral mastoid region as far off midline as possible. This will avoid blocking a skin incision past midline for lesions that are attached to midline structures (i.e., superior sagittal sinus) or crossing midline. Of note, particularly when pinning in the retro-auricular or mastoid region, ventriculo-peritoneal shunt catheters passing the region must be avoided.

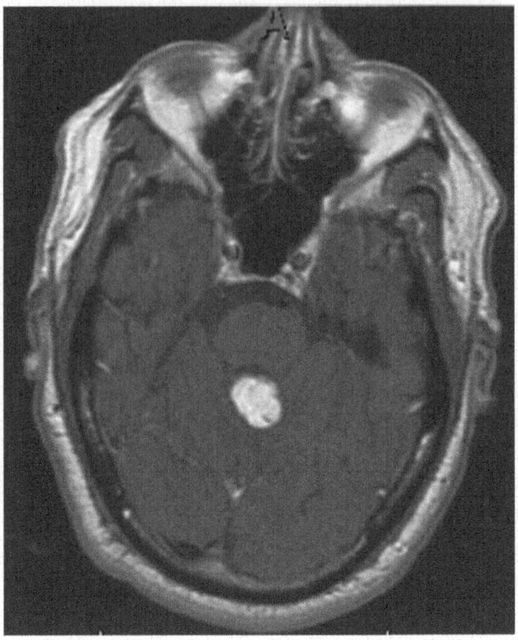

Fig. 15.8 MRI scan of a patient with a hemangioblastoma in the midline involving the cerebellar vermis

Prone and Sitting Position

Suboccipital

The suboccipital craniotomy is most often performed with the patient in prone position, less frequently a sitting position can be used. This is surgeon preference and guided by specific safety and monitoring concerns with sitting position (i.e., venous air embolism and need for precordial Doppler monitoring). In this paragraph, we will focus on the classic prone position and also discuss the sitting position.

Prone position is generally the choice for approaches to the posterior fossa, suboccipital region, and posterior approaches to craniocervical junction and spine in neurosurgical oncology (Fig. 15.8). These approaches include tumors in the vermis, medial aspect of the cerebellar hemispheres, and dorsal or dorsolateral lesions at the foramen magnum or craniocervical junction. Prone position provides excellent exposure for the abovementioned regions without having an increased risk for venous air embolisms as compared to the sitting position [1]. Prone position is one of the more challenging positions in neurosurgery from the standpoint of our anesthesia colleagues since it requires disconnecting the intubated patient from the circuit and rotating the patient prone onto the operating table. Positioning an intubated patient prone challenges hemodynamics as well as simple physical logistics such as keeping in place venous and arterial lines, Foley catheter, the endotracheal tube, and possible neuromonitoring electrodes amongst others. Other caveats are access to patient's airway, pressure sores, vascular compression, restrictive pulmonary compromise (i.e., overly tight taping of the patient to the operating table), brachial plexus injuries, and blindness [1, 27]. Turning the patient prone from the supine position increases intra-abdominal pressure, decreases venous return to the heart, and may increase systemic and pulmonary vascular resistance [28]. Although the cardiovascular responses to positioning prone mostly have been characterized in the setting of acute respiratory distress syndrome [29], yet, data suggest that left ventricular ejection fraction and cardiac index may decrease and thus causing hemodynamic instability [30]. Tissue oxygenation, however, may improve with prone positioning because of improved matching of ventilation and perfusion [1, 29, 31]. The patient is anesthetized in the supine position, and then turned prone with the head in neutral position onto soft chest rolls, a special frame, or operating table (e.g., Wilson frame, Jackson table). Cranial tumor procedures may benefit from the assistive positioning devices providing support to the patient's chest while reducing pressure to the abdomen, which in return improves ventilation, avoiding hypercapnia and decreasing bleeding by optimizing venous return [32]. For patients who are morbidly obese, operating room tables that can accommodate these patients may be used. For prone position patients, care must be taken to use wide gel rolls or padding in order to ensure that a large pannus is not compressed as this may increase intrathoracic pressure and make ventilation more difficult.

The sitting position was commonly used for posterior fossa surgery and for posterior cervical approaches; however, many neurosurgeons are shifting away from sitting position due to the additional risk of hemodynamic instability and venous air embolisms [33, 34], which in return requires additional monitoring such as precordial Doppler and possibly a right atrial central venous catheter to aspirate air emboli. The sitting position provides little benefit over the prone position, except significantly lower cranial venous pressure and thus decreased risk of bleeding [32]. The sitting position can help with retraction, particularly for infratentorial supracerebellar approaches. However, lower venous pressure and pooling of blood in the lower extremities carries significant additional risk for hypotension, venous air embolism, and lower extremity deep venous thromboses [35]. Sitting position also increases the risk for pneumocephalus and subdural hematoma [36], thus most surgeons may consider the sitting position to carry greater risks than benefits. The mechanisms of venous air embolism include negative venous pressure and exposure of veins and venous sinuses to air during surgery. A large venous air embolism may decrease cardiac output by creating a right ventricular outflow air trap [37] and provoke acute right heart strain and significant myocardial ischemia. The incidence of venous air embolism in the sitting position may be estimated at 20–50% when precordial Doppler monitoring is used for detection [33], and 76% when transesophageal echocardiography is used for detection [38]. A patent foramen ovale should be excluded before every case [39], as it is a source of paradoxical air embolism and stroke [40]. In addition to standard monitoring, such as pulse oximetry and end tidal carbon dioxide, precordial transthoracic Doppler is used for early detection of venous air embolisms [41]. If a Doppler is not available, attention must be paid to acute decreases in end tidal carbon dioxide concentrations in the presence of hypotension as a warning sign for venous air embolism. In case of a venous air embolism, the surgical wound must be extensively irrigated, the site of venous air entry must be lowered relative to the patient's heart (usually by placing the patient in Trendelenburg), the patient has to be placed in left lateral decubitus position (left side down) to potentially untrap the right atrial outflow tract, if possible air can be aspirated from the right atrium via a central venous catheter, and cardiovascular support with vasopressors must be initiated in case of hypotension [42].

Despite the associated risks, sitting position is the preferred position for many neurosurgeons to access the posterior fossa and posterior cervical spine, bearing the pathophysiology and diagnostic signs of venous air embolisms in mind, as well as being prepared to respond in case of such an emergency, will create a safe environment to carry out the operation.

Awake Craniotomies

Awake craniotomies deserve special discussion due to the unique requirements. We typically employ the lateral or supine with a bump behind the ipsilateral shoulder. Significant care is taken to ensure that the patient is comfortable prior to intubation. For patients in the supine position, we will place a gel roll underneath the ipsilateral shoulder so that the patient is lying at a 45-degree angle. The head is then rotated further to the contralateral side. In our experience, patients will complain during the procedure of pain in the dependent hip and the dependent shoulder. We place a pillow between the legs. Recently, we have employed the technique of placing a sequential compression device stocking underneath the gel padding directly under the dependenthip. The device inflates and deflates during the procedure and this has provided significant relief to our patients during surgery. After the patient verifies that he or she is not experiencing any discomfort in our preferred position, we then place the patient under anesthesia using a laryngeal mask airway (LMA). The LMA technique has proven valuable to us because it is not as uncomfortable as an endotracheal tube and it allows us to proceed with the portions of the procedure prior to exposure of the brain with efficiency as the patient is unlikely to feel discomfort or pain. Care is taken during draping to ensure that the anesthesiologist has access to the patient's face. The head may be slightly extended to allow for easy placement and removal of the LMA. A neutral position is also favorable; however, we try to avoid flexion as this position makes it difficult to place the LMA. We use three-point fixation for our awake craniotomy patients and the single pin is positioned such that the patient's vision is minimally obstructed. Once the brain is exposed, we then ask the anesthesiologist to proceed with removal of the LMA. This is generally a very smooth process. Once the LMA is removed, the patient is given time to wake up and cooperate with testing. We generally try to keep the patient awake for testing no more than 2 h as fatigue will set in and the patient will have difficulty cooperating. When having the patient awake is no longer necessary, the anesthesiologist will typically replace the LMA after sedating the patient. The LMA remains in place until the operation is completed.

Summary

Positioning for procedures in neurosurgical oncology has special considerations. Proper positioning has direct implications to safety and efficiency of the actual surgery, perioperative care, and has lasting implication on postoperative morbidity and long-term follow-up. Many patients will present with increased intracranial pressure from their tumors. Thus, positioning to minimize cerebral edema is a key consideration. Taking advantage of gravity (placing the patient and tumor in a dependent position) may be helpful. Positioning the head such that the tumor is most accessible (often at the highest point of the field) is also useful for tumor resections. The location of the tumor is key to proper positioning and should dictate the approach. Unlike other neurosurgical procedures that have potentially predictable locations of pathology (e.g., temporal lobectomy for mesial temporal sclerosis), slight variations in tumor location can significantly alter the positioning and approach.

Patient positioning in neurosurgery, frequently under-emphasized in the literature, is a key part of neurosurgery and an absolute necessity to safely conduct and perfect the neurosurgical operation. The most fundamental neurosurgical principles such as immobilizing the patient's head in a head holder, properly registering the neuronavigation, illumination of the surgical field, exposure of the brain tumor leveraging gravity to reduce brain retraction, hemostasis, CSF drainage, and brain relaxation as well as optimizing hemodynamics and creating an environment for safe anesthesia all depend on proper positioning of the patient and careful preoperative planning by the neurosurgeon.

References

1. Rozet I, Vavilala MS. Risks and benefits of patient positioning during neurosurgical care. Anesthesiol Clin. 2007;25(3):631–53.
2. St-Arnaud D, Paquin MJ. Safe positioning for neurosurgical patients. AORN J. 2008;87(6):1156–68. quiz 69-72. PubMed PMID: 18567169.
3. Winfree CJ, Kline DG. Intraoperative positioning nerve injuries. Surg Neurol. 2005;63(1):5–18.
4. St-Arnaud D, Paquin MJ. Safe positioning for neurosurgical patients. Can Oper Room Nurs J. 2009;27(4):7–11. 6, 8–9 passim. PubMed PMID: 20131710.
5. McEwen DR. Intraoperative positioning of surgical patients. AORN J. 1996;63(6):1077–9.

6. Bostanjian D, Anthone GJ, Hamoui N, Crookes PF. Rhabdomyolysis of gluteal muscles leading to renal failure: a potentially fatal complication of surgery in the morbidly obese. Obes Surg. 2003;13(2):302–5.
7. Behin A, Hoang-Xuan K, Carpentier AF, Delattre J-Y. Primary brain tumours in adults. Lancet. 2003;361(9354):323–31.
8. Ostrom QT, Gittleman H, Liao P, Rouse C, Chen Y, Dowling J, et al. CBTRUS statistical report: primary brain and central nervous system tumors diagnosed in the United States in 2007–2011. Neurooncology. 2014;16(suppl_4):iv1–iv63.
9. Stupp R, Brada M, van den Bent MJ, Tonn JC, Pentheroudakis G. High-grade glioma: ESMO Clinical Practice Guidelines for diagnosis, treatment and follow-up. Ann Oncol. 2014;25(suppl_3):iii93–iii101.
10. Stupp R, Mason WP, van den Bent MJ, Weller M, Fisher B, Taphoorn MJB, et al. Radiotherapy plus concomitant and adjuvant temozolomide for glioblastoma. N Engl J Med. 2005;352(10):987–96. PubMed PMID: 15758009.
11. Patchell RA, Tibbs PA, Walsh JW, Dempsey RJ, Maruyama Y, Kryscio RJ, et al. A randomized trial of surgery in the treatment of single metastases to the brain. N Engl J Med. 1990;322(8):494–500. PubMed PMID: 2405271.
12. Patchell RA, Tibbs PA, Regine WF, Dempsey RJ, Mohiuddin M, Kryscio RJ, et al. Postoperative radiotherapy in the treatment of single metastases to the brain: a randomized trial. JAMA. 1998; 280(17):1485–9.
13. Chang SM, Parney IF, McDermott M, Barker FG 2nd, Schmidt MH, Huang W, et al. Perioperative complications and neurological outcomes of first and second craniotomies among patients enrolled in the Glioma Outcome Project. J Neurosurg. 2003;98(6):1175–81. PubMed PMID: 12816260.
14. Bloch O, Han SJ, Cha S, Sun MZ, Aghi MK, McDermott MW, et al. Impact of extent of resection for recurrent glioblastoma on overall survival: clinical article. J Neurosurg. 2012;117(6):1032–8. PubMed PMID: 23039151.
15. Oppenlander ME, Wolf AB, Snyder LA, Bina R, Wilson JR, Coons SW, et al. An extent of resection threshold for recurrent glioblastoma and its risk for neurological morbidity. J Neurosurg. 2014;120(4):846–53. PubMed PMID: 24484232.
16. Drakulovic MB, Torres A, Bauer TT, Nicolas JM, Nogué S, Ferrer M. Supine body position as a risk factor for nosocomial pneumonia in mechanically ventilated patients: a randomised trial. Lancet. 1999; 354(9193):1851–8.
17. Jho HD, Ha HG. Endoscopic endonasal skull base surgery: Part 3—the clivus and posterior fossa. Minim Invasive Neurosurg. 2004;47(01):16–23.
18. Jho HD, Ha HG. Endoscopic endonasal skull base surgery: Part 1—the midline anterior fossa skull base. Minim Invasive Neurosurg. 2004;47(01):1–8.
19. de Divitiis E, Cavallo LM, Esposito F, Stella L, Messina A. Extended endoscopic transsphenoidal approach for tuberculum sellae meningiomas. Neurosurgery. 2007;61(suppl_5):ONS229–ONS38.
20. Chi JH, Parsa AT, Berger MS, Kunwar S, McDermott MW. Extended bifrontal craniotomy for midline anterior fossa meningiomas: minimization of retraction-related edema and surgical outcomes. Neurosurgery. 2006;59(suppl_4):ONS-426–ONS-34.
21. Tanriover N, Ulm AJ, Rhoton ALJ, Kawashima M, Yoshioka N, Lewis SB. One-piece versus two-piece orbitozygomatic craniotomy: quantitative and qualitative considerations. Neurosurgery. 2006;58(4):ONS-229–ONS-37. PubMed PMID: 00006123-200604002-00006.
22. Zabramski JM, Kiriş T, Sankhla SK, Cabiol J, Spetzler RF. Orbitozygomatic craniotomy. J Neurosurg. 1998; 89(2):336–41. PubMed PMID: 9688133.
23. Lemole GM Jr, Henn JS, Zabramski JM, Spetzler RF. Modifications to the orbitozygomatic approach. J Neurosurg. 2003;99(5):924–30. PubMed PMID: 14609176.
24. Samii M, Gerganov V, Samii A. Improved preservation of hearing and facial nerve function in vestibular schwannoma surgery via the retrosigmoid approach in a series of 200 patients. J Neurosurg. 2006;105(4):527–35. PubMed PMID: 17044553.
25. Elhammady MS, Telischi FF, Morcos JJ. Retrosigmoid approach: indications, techniques, and results. Otolaryngol Clin N Am. 2012;45(2):375–97.
26. Ma L, Shrestha BK, You C, Hui X-h. Revisiting the far lateral approach in the treatment of lesions located at the craniocervical junction—experiences from West China hospital, Sichuan University, Chengdu. Interdiscip Neurosurg. 2015;2(3):133–8.
27. Edgcombe H, Carter K, Yarrow S. Anaesthesia in the prone position. Br J Anaesth. 2008;100(2):165–83.
28. Toyota S, Amaki Y. Hemodynamic evaluation of the prone position by transesophageal echocardiography. J Clin Anesth. 1998;10(1):32–5.
29. Jolliet P, Bulpa P, Chevrolet J-C. Effects of the prone position on gas exchange and hemodynamics in severe acute respiratory distress syndrome. Crit Care Med. 1998;26(12):1977–85. PubMed PMID: 00003246-199812000-00023.
30. Yokoyama M, Ueda W, Hirakawa M, Yamamoto H. Hemodynamic effect of the prone position during anesthesia. Acta Anaesthesiol Scand. 1991;35(8):741–4.
31. Guérin C, Reignier J, Richard J-C, Beuret P, Gacouin A, Boulain T, et al. Prone positioning in severe acute respiratory distress syndrome. N Engl J Med. 2013;368(23):2159–68. PubMed PMID: 23688302.
32. Harrison EA, Mackersie A, McEwan A, Facer E. The sitting position for neurosurgery in children: a review of 16 years' experience. Br J Anaesth. 2002;88(1):12–7.
33. Porter JM, Pidgeon C, Cunningham AJ. The sitting position in neurosurgery: a critical appraisal. BJA. Br J Anaesth. 1999;82(1):117–28.

34. Standefer M, Bay JW, Trusso R. The sitting position in neurosurgery: a retrospective analysis of 488 cases. Neurosurgery. 1984;14(6):649–58. PubMed PMID: 00006123-198406000-00001.
35. Rath GP, Bithal PK, Chaturvedi A, Dash HH. Complications related to positioning in posterior fossa craniectomy. J Clin Neurosci. 2007;14(6):520–5. PubMed PMID: 17430775.
36. Di Lorenzo N, Caruso R, Floris R, Guerrisi V, Bozzao L, Fortuna A. Pneumocephalus and tension pneumocephalus after posterior fossa surgery in the sitting position: a prospective study. Acta Neurochir. 1986;83(3):112–5.
37. Durant TM, Long J, Oppenheimer MJ. Pulmonary (venous) air embolism. Am Heart J. 1947;33(3):269–81.
38. Papadopoulos G, Kuhly P, Brock M, Rudolph KH, Link J, Eyrich K. Venous and paradoxical air embolism in the sitting position. A prospective study with transoesophageal echocardiography. Acta Neurochir. 1994;126(2):140–3.
39. Fathi AR, Eshtehardi P, Meier B. Patent foramen ovale and neurosurgery in sitting position: a systematic review. Br J Anaesth. 2009;102(5):588–96.
40. Mammoto T, Hayashi Y, Ohnishi Y, Kuro M. Incidence of venous and paradoxical air embolism in neurosurgical patients in the sitting position: detection by transesophageal echocardiography. Acta Anaesthesiol Scand. 1998;42(6):643–7.
41. Hitselberger WE, House WF. A warning regarding the sitting position for acoustic tumor surgery. Arch Otolaryngol. 1980;106(2):69.
42. Mirski MA, Lele AV, Fitzsimmons L, Toung TJK. Diagnosis and treatment of vascular air embolism. Anesthesiology. 2007;106(1):164–77.

16 Special Considerations for Pediatric Positioning for Neurosurgical Procedures

Michael DeCuypere

Abbreviations

CSF Cerebrospinal fluid
VP Ventriculoperitoneal

Introduction

The proper positioning of infants and children undergoing neurosurgical procedures presents special challenges to the neurosurgeon, anesthesiologist, and operating room care team. This is a direct result of age-related differences in surgical lesions, as well as anatomical and physiological differences in children. With this being said, there are many similarities in regard to general positioning guidelines of adult patients undergoing neurosurgery. This chapter will focus only on special considerations when positioning pediatric patients for the most commonly encountered procedures.

M. DeCuypere (✉)
Department of Neurosurgery, University of Tennessee Health Science Center, Memphis, TN, USA

LeBonheur Children's Hospital, Memphis, TN, USA

Semmes-Murphey Neurologic and Spine Institute, Memphis, TN, USA
e-mail: mdecuypere@semmes-murphey.com

Age Terminology

Children undergo a wide range of neurosurgical procedures, from elective to emergent and life saving. When considering optimal positioning, the care team should always take into account the patient's chronological age and developmental level. While most procedures are performed within dedicated pediatric medical centers, a significant number are found in adult centers, underscoring the importance of recognition of the special needs of each pediatric age group. The most commonly used terms for discussing pediatric age groups are:

- Premature newborn—born prior to 37 weeks gestation
- Newborn—less than 72 h of age
- Neonate—first 28 days of life
- Infant—neonate to 12 months of age
- Toddler—13 to 24 months
- Childhood—2 years to 11 years of age
- Adolescence—12 to 18 years of age (some sources 21 years of age [1])

The special needs of each age group will be mentioned as necessary in the following sections. If no age group is specifically mentioned, it can be assumed that the particular principle will apply to all age groups.

A. Arthur et al. (eds.), *Perioperative Considerations and Positioning for Neurosurgical Procedures*,
https://doi.org/10.1007/978-3-319-72679-3_16

General Principles of Pediatric Positioning

As is the case with adults, careful preoperative planning is essential to allow adequate access to the patient for both the surgeon and anesthesiologist. During pediatric procedures, a small neonate or infant may quite literally disappear under the surgical drapes. Therefore, the anesthesiologist must ensure an unobstructed view of the child during surgery. This includes access to the airway and all lines (arterial lines, intravenous lines, urinary catheter, and ventriculostomy/lumbar drain tubing).

The endotracheal tube should be secured carefully and intuitively based on the procedure. The patient's airway should always be accessible during the procedure. When drapes are applied to the face area, care should be taken to avoid attaching them to or around the endotracheal tube. This is especially important when using sterile adhesive drapes commonly found in pediatric medical centers.

All pressure points should be padded and peripheral pulses checked or prevent compression or injury. Bed sheets or disposable bed linen is commonly used for tucking and securing upper extremities to the bed. If bed rotation is anticipated, padded straps are secured across the patient and bed maneuver testing is carefully performed prior to sterile drape application. It is imperative to prevent skin and soft tissue injury due to improper contact with objects such as instrument stands (if utilized) and grounding wires.

Several physiologic effects of body and head position should be considered during preoperative planning and utilized as needed. In most cases, the body habitus of children is much more amenable to changes of positioning given there smaller size. However, some older adolescents may approach or even surpass adults in weight and height. Head elevation (in either supine or prone position) will offer enhanced cerebral venous drainage and decreased overall cerebral blood flow. This position may also cause increased venous pooling in the lower extremities and postural hypotension in children, however. Conversely, the head down position will increase cerebral venous and intracranial pressure. This position may be beneficial during venous sinus injury, but will also result in decreased functional residual capacity and lung compliance. The prone position, one of the most common utilized in pediatric neurosurgery, often results in venous congestion of the face and neck, as well as venocaval compression. Head flexion should also be mentioned here, as this position is sought in many prone procedures.

Extreme flexion, however, should be avoided as this may lead to brainstem compression in those patients with certain mass lesions of the lower posterior fossa. This may also cause endotracheal obstruction from kinking or displacement to the carina or main stem bronchus. Likewise, extreme head rotation may impede venous return via the jugular veins and lead to increased intracranial pressure, impaired cerebral perfusion and venous bleeding.

Thermal Homeostasis

Maintenance of normothermia, with avoidance of both hypothermia and hyperthermia, is the goal of intraoperative thermoregulation. Neonates and infants are especially susceptible to hypothermia during surgical procedures due to their large surface area-to-weight ratio. Large head size relative to body size, thin skin, lack of subcutaneous fat, and limited compensatory mechanisms puts these patients at risk for rapid heat loss [2].

Hypothermia can be prevented warming the room to at least 23 °C (73.4 °F), ensuring the patient's temperature is at least 36 °C (96.8 °F) at surgical start and using warmed intravenous fluids. Patient insulation, forced-air warming devices, and circulating water mattresses are additional methods of preventing surgical hypothermia. It is vital to remember the importance of normothermia for adequate emergence from anesthesia, and the time required for rewarming even a mildly hypothermic child, especially a neonate or infant.

Head Immobilization Devices and Pediatric Patients

Head immobilization devices, such as the Mayfield skull clamp (Integra LifeSciences, Plainsboro, New Jersey), serve to immobilize the head during surgery and support pressure from surgical manipulation. While widely utilized in adult neurosurgery, immobilization device use in pediatrics is lower and remains a function of surgeon preference. Despite common availability, there are few reports of complications in the literature and virtually no guidelines for their safe usage in children. This has led to wide operational variability amongst surgeons, even within the same institution. Most commonly, infants under the age of 1 are not immobilized with a pinning device and pediatric size pins are utilized in patients under the age of 10. However, there is wide variability of practice in the pediatric neurosurgical community regarding the size of pins and torque screw reading (lbs) applied [3]. At our institution, for instance, immobilization devices are not utilized in patients less than 1 year of age and adult pins are used in all children who are placed in immobilization devices. The typical torque screw reading is variable, but we start at 10 lbs per year of age up to 50 lbs.

Due to weaker (thinner) bones of the skull, children are felt to be more susceptible to complications associated with head immobilization devices than adults [4]. Some complications of immobilization devices in children have been reported in the literature and include depressed skull fractures, epidural hematomas, pneumocephalus, and venous air embolism [5, 6]. It appears, however, that the overall rate of complications associated head immobilization device use is low. A recent, large retrospective study of MRI-compatible head immobilization device use in children revealed a complication rate of 0.7%, while conventional head immobilization device use yielded a 0.2% complication rate [7].

The presence of prolonged increased intracranial pressure tends to predispose children to complications while placing a head immobilization device. Prolonged increased intracranial pressure, typically chronic and on the order of months, can lead to decreased thickness of the cranial vault and thus higher incidence of pin-plunging with application, event at low torque screw pressures [8–10]. As a general guide, caution should always be observed while applying a head immobilization device in pediatric patients. Whenever possible, one should avoid using pin-type immobilization devices, if possible, and opt for a padded horseshoe-shaped headrest instead. While applying a device, certain warning signs should prompt one to stop and re-assess the safety of the patient (including neuroimaging). These include pins going too deep within the scalp/skull (pin plunge), cracking sounds, or a torque screw not reading properly or losing pressure.

Prone Positioning in Children

The prone position is frequently utilized in pediatric neurosurgery, most commonly for posterior fossa and spinal surgery. A spectrum of stretch injuries and compression issues can be associated with this position, in addition to the above-mentioned physiologic sequelae. Optimal prone position of a toddler is depicted in Fig. 16.1. This section will examine this position in detail.

Anesthesia is induced and all vascular access is obtained while the patient is in the supine position. A urinary catheter is placed if the procedure is expected to last longer than 2 h or if urinary output measurement is needed. It requires a careful and combined effort to flip the patient into the prone position, paying special attention to keep all lines and tubes intact. Typically, this maneuver is led by the anesthesiologist, with all members of the operating room team assisting. It should be noted that small body size does not always make for easier supine-to-prone transition, especially in neonates.

As mentioned above, the choice of head immobilization device is made on a case-by-case basis and a padded "U" shaped or horseshoe head holder should be utilized whenever possible. When using this immobilization device, care should be taken to avoid unnecessary compression

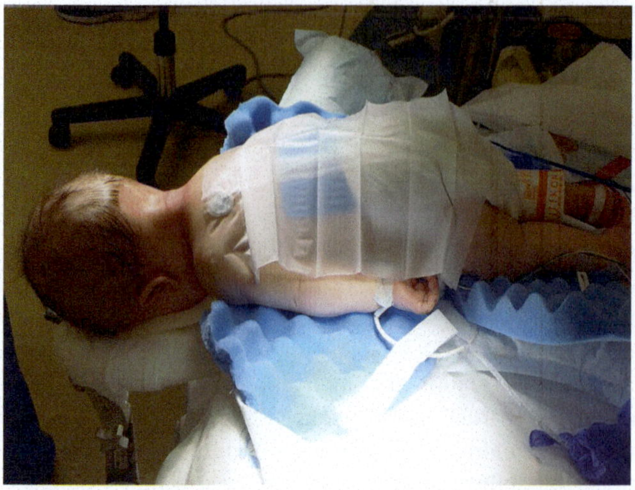

Fig. 16.1 Infant positioned prone on the horseshoe headrest. Note the supplementary padding added to the face area

of the eyes bilaterally. This is achieved by adjusting the width of the device and padding the face with additional foam as needed. With proper utilization, the horseshoe head holder can easily maintain a flexed head position without causing any untoward compression of the eyes or face. As mentioned above, care should be taken to avoid over-flexion of the head during prone positioning, which can lead to endotracheal tube issues and compression of the chin on the chest. Typically, at least one finger's breadth of clearance is needed between the chin and chest area. Over-flexion for extended periods can also lead to tongue edema due to blockage of venous or lymphatic drainage, which may cause post-extubation airway obstruction.

Padding is placed under the chest and pelvis to support the torso and minimize any increase in abdominal or thoracic pressure. This can be achieved in a variety of ways. In neonates and infants, two transverse-oriented padded rolls are fashioned from foam and sized appropriately to support the weight of the child. In children and adolescents, parallel-oriented chest rolls can be utilized as in adults. Ensuring free abdominal wall motion is imperative in either case, as increased abdominal pressure can lead to impaired ventilation, venocaval compression, and increased epidural bleeding.

Supplemental padding should be used liberally and placed under the elbows (prior to arm tucking, if necessary) and knees. It is important to remember thermoregulatory issues, and blankets and warmers can be added as necessary after padding is complete (Fig. 16.1).

Special Circumstances in Pediatrics

Neonatal Surgery

Most surgery on neonates is performed on an urgent basis and, as such, neonates tend to have higher perioperative morbidity than other pediatric age groups. Uncovering congenital anomalies, particularly of the heart and lungs, in the operating room may manifest as hypoxia and hemodynamic instability. This underscores the importance of easy access of the anesthesia team to the patient and should be planned for during positioning.

In particular, closure of a myelomeningocele presents unique problems for the operating room team. Tracheal intubation with the child in supine position may lead to rupture of membranes covering the exposed spinal cord (Fig. 16.2). However, supine intubation can be performed safely by supporting the child on "doughnut" or ring-shaped padding with the myelomeningocele in the center. Sometimes, for instance in the case of a large myelomeningocele, the lateral decubitus position can be utilized for intubation. Excision and repair of the myelomeningocele is performed in the prone position and can be

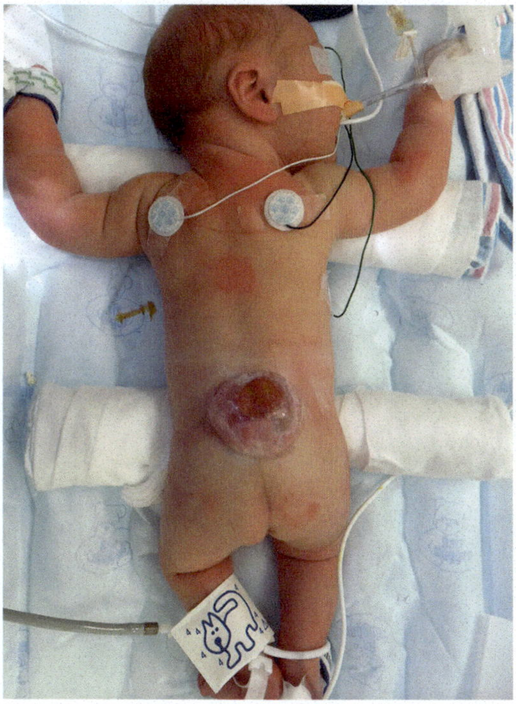

Fig. 16.2 Neonate positioned supine for myelomeningocele closure

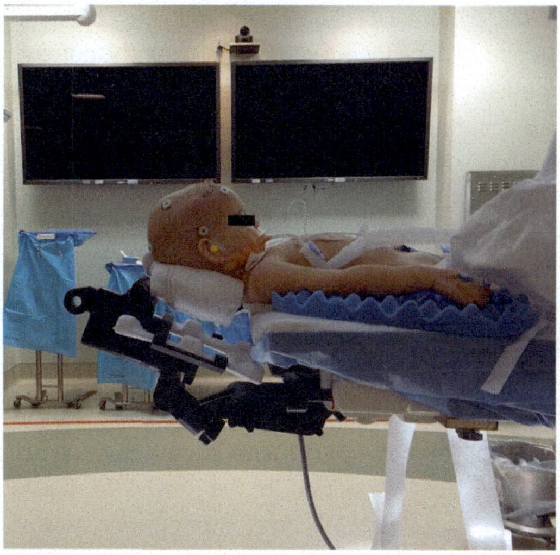

Fig. 16.3 A child positioned supine on the horseshoe headrest for an endoscopic procedure

combined with insertion of a ventriculoperitoneal shunt for hydrocephalus afterward in the supine position [11].

Hydrocephalus and Shunt Procedures

Hydrocephalus refers to an increased volume of CSF due to either over production or reduced uptake within the brain. The urgency of surgical intervention is related to several factors, most commonly raised intracranial pressure. The surgical management of hydrocephalus is CSF diversion from the ventricles to another body cavity, such as the peritoneum, pleural space, or right atrium. The placement of a VP shunt is the most commonly performed pediatric neurosurgical procedure. Alternatively, CSF diversion can be accomplished endoscopically, by performing a third ventriculostomy.

Preparation for VP shunt placement typically requires skin exposure from the head to the lower abdomen. As such, heat conservation strategies should be utilized, especially in premature newborns and neonates. The patient is positioned supine with the head turned to the opposite side of the proximal shunt. A padded roll is typically placed under the shoulders to elevate the torso for ease in tunneling the distal shunt tubing. The surgeon may need to manipulate the patient's head during the procedure (for instance, during ventricular cannulation) and the anesthesia team should be notified and prepared during this maneuver. The anesthesiologist may even want to manually hold the endotracheal tube in place under the surgical drapes. Intraoperative tunneling of the shunt tubing may be particularly stimulating, and the anesthesia team should be notified when this part of the procedure is happening to provide additional pain control.

Endoscopic third ventriculostomy surgery can be performed with the patient's head in a pin-type immobilization device or in a horseshoe headrest based on surgeon preference (Fig. 16.3). Frameless image navigation now makes rigid head fixation unnecessary.

Sometimes children present with severe, chronic hydrocephalus, with gross enlargement of the head (macrocephaly). This will present challenges to positioning, but also with airway management. The head may be a large proportion of the patient's body weight and thus must be supported appropriately when moving the patient. Intubation may need to be performed in the lateral decubitus position to avoid unnatural craniocervical manipulation. Otherwise, standard positioning approaches are utilized with emphasis on robust padding for the head.

Pediatric Brain Tumors

Brain tumors are the most commonly encountered solid tumor of childhood, and the majority of these lesions occur in the posterior fossa. Surgery for these lesions, therefore, almost always requires the prone position. At our institution, we have virtually eliminated the use of the sitting position for posterior fossa surgery in children. Rotation and elevation of the operating room bed may be required during the procedure and thus rigid head immobilization in pins is frequently used. All possible bed positions should be carefully tested prior to starting surgery to ensure patient safety, especially when multiple corridors of surgical approach are anticipated (Fig. 16.4).

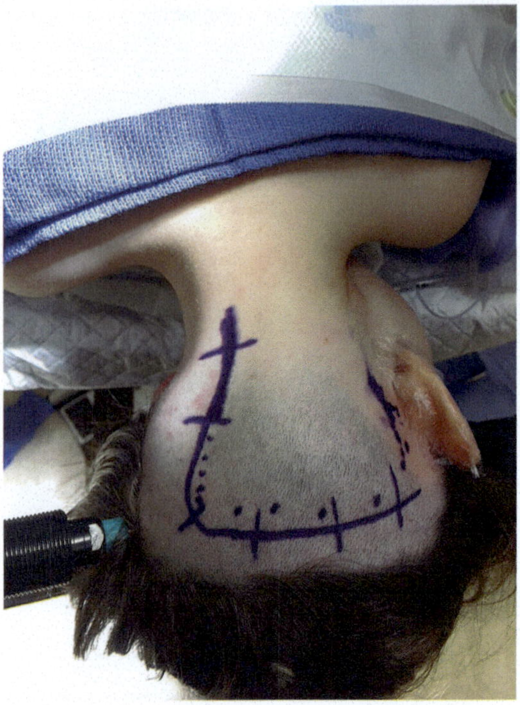

Fig. 16.4 A child positioned prone in a head immobilizer for brain tumor resection. Note the planned incision includes a midline posterior fossa approach in combination with a retrosigmoid approach. This approach is utilized for large ependymomas. This will require significant lateral operative bed mobility

Surgery for Craniofacial Abnormalities

Craniosynostosis is defined as the premature closure of one or more skull sutures and usually occurs in otherwise healthy children. The best results are obtained if surgical repair is performed early in life, usually before 12 months of age. Surgery for cranial remodeling is varied and involves the removal of the part(s) of the skull vault by a neurosurgeon, followed by refashioning by craniofacial plastic surgeons. Typically, the patient is positioned supine with some degree of head flexion. The use of a horseshoe head holder may be useful and the chin should be padded between contact areas with the chest. Ocular lubricant should be placed in the eyes and eyelids taped shut (if possible) as the upper face may fall into the surgical field during these procedures. It is important to inspect all tape or occlusive dressings of the face below the orbital rim to avoid excessive facial edema. These procedures are associated with a significant loss of blood volume and perioperative transfusion is invariable required. Thus, ready access to all vascular lines is paramount.

Epilepsy Surgery

The surgical treatment of medically intractable epilepsy is common in children and may range from focal cortical resection, corpus callosotomy, or hemispherectomy, to placement of a vagal nerve stimulator. These procedures are typically performed in the supine position (rarely prone), often utilizing the horseshoe headrest (Fig. 16.5). However, it should be noted that these procedures are usually performed with a neurologist in the operating room during electrocorticography and

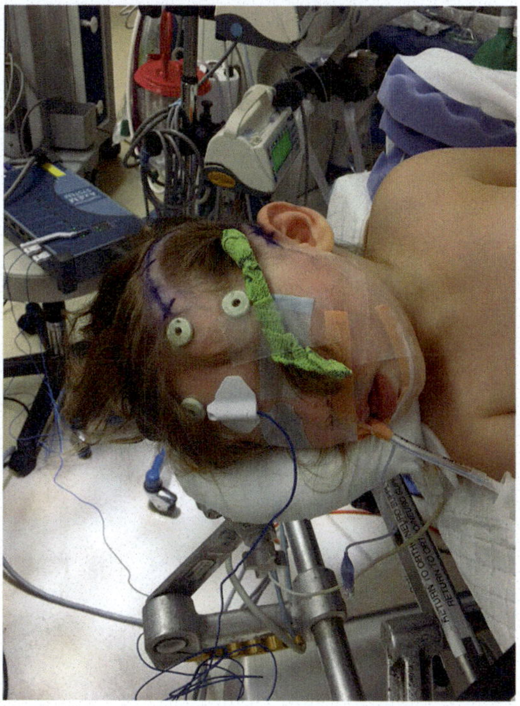

Fig. 16.5 A child positioned supine with padded shoulder roll on horseshoe headrest for resection of an epileptic focus

thus open access to the surgical field by the epilepsy monitoring team is necessary. At our institution, these procedures are typically performed in larger operating rooms to accommodate the increase in personnel.

Trauma

A small child's head is often the point of impact in traumatic injuries and craniotomy for trauma is a common procedure in pediatric neurosurgery. These procedures are typically performed in the supine position, with a padded roll placed under the ipsilateral shoulder to aid in head rotation (achieving a semi-lateral position). The head can be placed on a ring-shaped pad on the operating bed or on the horseshoe headrest. Although cervical fractures are less common in children than in adults, cervical spine immobilization remains essential to avoid secondary injury by manipulation of the patient's neck during positioning or airway during intubation.

Spine Surgery

The most common indication for laminectomy in pediatric patients is spinal dysraphism, and many of these patients have undergone previous myelomeningocele closure followed by several other procedures. Thus, release of a tethered spinal cord will often require electromyographic monitoring (including the anal sphincter) during surgery. The prone position is utilized with appropriate pressure point protection. As a result of increased cervical spine mobility in children, the head may be turned to one side and placed on a ring-pad on the operative bed during the procedure. Urinary catheters are usually placed and continued postoperatively, as these patients typically require bed rest for at least 24 h after surgery. Electromyographic electrodes are placed after the patient is moved into the prone position. A clear surgical drape is often utilized for direct visualization of the lower extremities if nerve root stimulation will be performed during surgery. It is important to discontinue or antagonize muscle relaxants to allow for adequate monitoring.

Conclusion

The positioning of pediatric patients for neurosurgical procedures presents unique challenges to the neurosurgeon, anesthesiologist, and ancillary operating room team. While the prone position is commonly encountered in pediatric neurosurgery, it has several nuances that differ from positioning in adult patients. A thorough understanding of age-dependent variables (such as thermal regulation) and proper positioning practices is essential for minimizing perioperative morbidity.

References

1. Williams K, Thomson D, Seto I, Contopoulos-Ioannidis DG, Ioannidis JP, Curtis S, et al. Standard 6: age groups for pediatric trials. Pediatrics. 2012;129(Suppl 3):S153–60.
2. Triffterer L, Marhofer P, Sulyok I, Keplinger M, Mair S, Steinberger M, et al. Forced-air warming during

pediatric surgery: a randomized comparison of a compressible with a noncompressible warming system. Anesth Analg. 2016;122(1):219–25.

3. Berry C, Sandberg DI, Hoh DJ, Krieger MD, McComb JG. Use of cranial fixation pins in pediatric neurosurgery. Neurosurgery. 2008;62(4):913–8. discussion 8-9.
4. Lee M, Rezai AR, Chou J. Depressed skull fractures in children secondary to skull clamp fixation devices. Pediatr Neurosurg. 1994;21(3):174–7; discussion 8.
5. Anegawa S, Shigemori M, Yoshida M, Kojo N, Torigoe R, Shirouzu T, et al. Postoperative tension pneumocephalus—report of 3 cases. No Shinkei Geka. 1986;14(8):1017–22.
6. Pang D. Air embolism associated with wounds from a pin-type head-holder. Case report. J Neurosurg. 1982;57(5):710–3.
7. Zaazoue MA, Bedewy M, Goumnerova LC. Complications of head immobilization devices in children: contact mechanics, and analysis of a single institutional experience. Neurosurgery 2017;1–8. https://doi.org/10.1093/neuros/nyx315.
8. Baerts WD, de Lange JJ, Booij LH, Broere G. Complications of the Mayfield skull clamp. Anesthesiology. 1984;61(4):460–1.
9. Vitali AM, Steinbok P. Depressed skull fracture and epidural hematoma from head fixation with pins for craniotomy in children. Childs Nerv Syst. 2008;24(8):917–23; discussion 25.
10. Sade B, Mohr G. Depressed skull fracture and epidural haematoma: an unusual post-operative complication of pin headrest in an adult. Acta Neurochir. 2005;147(1):101–3.
11. Singh D, Rath GP, Dash HH, Bithal PK. Anesthetic concerns and perioperative complications in repair of myelomeningocele: a retrospective review of 135 cases. J Neurosurg Anesthesiol. 2010;22(1):11–5.

17 Comorbidities and Positioning: Morbid Obesity and Multiple Trauma

Emily P. Sieg and Shelly D. Timmons

The Polytrauma Patient

Case 1 Illustration

A 29-year-old male arrives as a level 1 trauma activation after prolonged extrication at the site of a multi-vehicle collision. The patient is intubated, in a cervical collar and on a backboard with a Glasgow coma scale of 7-I on arrival. Initial vital signs show a systolic blood pressure of 75/40 and a pulse of 128 despite aggressive resuscitation with crystalloid. The primary and secondary surveys are completed. A Foley and femoral line are placed. On initial neurosurgical evaluation, the patient does not open eyes, is intubated, his pupils are equal and reactive to light, and the motor examination is asymmetrical with withdrawal of the left upper extremity and both lower extremities, and brisk localization of the right upper extremity. FAST exam shows free fluid in the abdomen. Blood pressure is stabilized after transfusion of packed red blood cells, platelets, and fresh frozen plasma, and the patient is able to be taken to the CT scanner.

Head CT reveals an acute 7 mm thick holohemispheric right-sided subdural hematoma leading to 1.2 cm of midline shift and multiple scattered cerebral contusions. Rapid review of the CT of the cervical spine shows no evidence of fracture or dislocation. Before the remaining trauma scans can be obtained the patient becomes hemodynamically unstable once again with significant hypotension and tachycardia, despite further aggressive resuscitation. Given the CT head findings and the FAST findings, the decision is made to take the patient emergently to the operating room (OR) for a right-sided craniotomy and subdural hematoma evacuation with consideration for leaving the bone flap out depending upon operative findings, and a simultaneous exploratory laparotomy. In order to provide appropriate access for the neurosurgery, trauma surgery, and anesthesia teams, a collaborative approach to patient positioning is required.

Positioning for Simultaneous Surgeries

As illustrated in the case presentation, the hypotensive polytrauma patient harboring multiple severe injuries requires evaluation by trauma surgery, neurosurgery, anesthesiology, and orthopaedic surgery. It is imperative that close and ongoing communication occurs between these surgical teams in order to facilitate prioritization

E. P. Sieg · S. D. Timmons (✉)
Department of Neurosurgery, Milton S. Hershey Medical Center, Penn State University College of Medicine, Hershey, PA, USA
e-mail: esieg@pennstatehealth.psu.edu

A. Arthur et al. (eds.), *Perioperative Considerations and Positioning for Neurosurgical Procedures*,
https://doi.org/10.1007/978-3-319-72679-3_17

of those injuries requiring immediate intervention, and ongoing decision-making and coordination of emergency operations, including timing, resuscitation needs, and positioning. A polytrauma patient may present with a traumatic brain injury (TBI) and intracranial surgical lesion and hypotension and/or hypoxia from extracranial injuries necessitating emergent thoracotomy, laparotomy, or pelvic fixation. They may also have other orthopaedic injuries (fractures of upper or lower extremity long bones or acetabulum) requiring surgical repair and, stable or unstable spine injuries [1].

Cervical spine instability can result from ligamentous injury and/or fractures; subluxation or malalignment can lead to permanent spinal cord injury (SCI) and a range of neurological deficits. Endotracheal intubation of the trauma patient should therefore be performed in a neutral position and hyperextension should be avoided during intubation. Log roll procedures should be used at all times during patient transfers, radiological testing, and operating room positioning, in case of thoracic or lumbar spinal column injuries.

Patients with traumatic brain injury who also have intrathoracic or intra abdominal injuries, long bone, acetabular or pelvic fractures, or SCI, may experience hypotension from blood loss or spinal shock. Preventing secondary brain injury by avoiding hypotension and hypoxia is paramount due to the dramatic impact these events have on outcomes after severe TBI (sTBI) [2]. Major extracranial injuries in patients with sTBI are common; incidence is reported in 20–41% of sTBI patients [1]. The need for the simultaneous surgical treatment of intracranial and extracranial injuries is relatively rare; however, the operating room logistics are complicated and time is of the essence in the setting of trauma, particularly with those *in extremis* [3]. Consideration of how to proceed should be given beforehand and all neurosurgeons and trauma surgeons should be prepared mentally before ever encountering the situation in reality.

The proper positioning of the trauma patient in the operating room requires that each team have appropriate access to the patient. A hypotensive trauma patient with a traumatic brain injury may require a thoracotomy, laparotomy, or pelvic fixation concurrent with a craniotomy [3], all of which can generally be done in the supine position on a standard operating room table [4]. The anesthesia team and machines may be placed to one side of the patient contralateral to the craniotomy side and excluded with sterile draping. This is the most expeditious manner in which to set up the room for simultaneous surgeries. Conversely, the patient may be turned 180° from anesthesia, but in this type of scenario, it can be difficult for them to perform all of the necessary procedures (often done under the drapes) and monitor all of the necessary parameters. See Fig. 17.1 for the recommended room setup for simultaneous trauma surgeries.

In cases requiring concurrent surgery, the anesthesiologist must sometimes secure and always maintain access to the airway. If possible, the endotracheal tube should be taped contralateral to the craniotomy side, and an ETT extender used so that the tubing can be directed away from the operative site and protected from pressure from instruments and the hands of the neurosurgeons as they work. Further, access is required to the neck, groin, and limbs for placement of and monitoring of intravascular venous lines that are necessary for ongoing resuscitation with fluid and blood products, and for obtaining serum samples for multiple laboratory studies that will be required throughout the case (e.g., electrolytes, glucose, blood count, coagulation studies). While preferentially lines will have been obtained in the resuscitation room, the rapidity with which patients are taken to the OR may result in suboptimal placement, dislodgement, occlusion, or other malfunction requiring intraoperative replacement. Access to the wrists and groins for arterial line placement and monitoring must also be maintained, as these are required for continuous blood pressure management and acquisition of arterial blood samples for arterial blood gas measurements. Finally, the Foley catheter and drainage system should be positioned between the legs, secured to the thigh, and hung on the anesthesia side (contralateral to the craniotomy) so that the anesthesia personnel can continuously

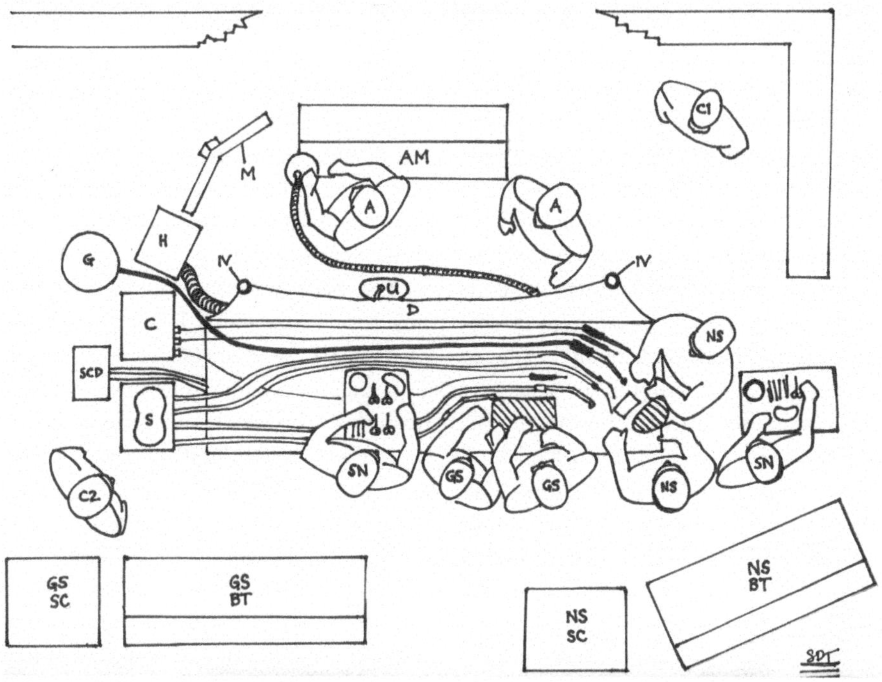

Fig. 17.1 Setup for simultaneous emergency trauma craniotomy and laparotomy. Key: *A* anesthesiologist, *AM* anesthesia machine and cart, *C* cautery unit, *C1* and *C2* circulator 1 and circulator 2, *D* drape, *G* gas cylinder, *GS* general surgeon, *GS BT* general surgery back table, *GS SC* general surgery supply cart, *H* heating blanket unit, *IV* IV pole, *M* monitors, *NS* neurosurgeon, *NS BT* neurosurgery back table, *NS SC* neurosurgery supply cart, *S* suction, *SCD* serial compression device unit, *SN* scrub nurse or technician, *U* urinary catheter collection receptacle

assess the urinary output. Should it drop precipitously, the catheter must be checked for kinking under the drapes, in order to ensure that obstruction is differentiated from hypoperfusion as the etiology of the oliguria. Output must be monitored when mannitol or other diuretics are given to aid with cerebral edema. Finally, the anesthesia team may also need to repeatedly check for blood loss from other injuries under the drapes especially scalp lacerations, facial injuries, compound fractures, and femur/acetabular fractures).

There needs to be ready access to the anesthesia machine and ventilator, as well as adequate space for at least two people to stand in the anesthesia area, due to multiple simultaneous ongoing needs for not only the above intensive monitoring, but also administration of fluids, blood products, and medications. There must be simultaneous ongoing monitoring of the patient's physiology with direct line-of-sight to all displays of vital signs, ventilator settings, respiratory pattern displays, and any implanted neuromonitoring devices such as intracranial pressure read-outs. Finally, the anesthesia team should be placed for ready verbal communication with the surgical teams, circulator, and telephone or voice communication device for rapid communication with the laboratory, the blood bank, and pharmacy. The display monitors should also be positioned so that the surgical teams can quickly, easily, and frequently look up to ascertain the vital signs without resorting to verbal communication, as this can be difficult with multiple ongoing teams talking simultaneously to assistants, technicians, and one another. Noise in the room should be kept to a minimum and conversation should be limited to only that which is essential to the care of the patient.

The neurosurgeon must have access to the head and maintain a sterile field given the high morbidity of intracranial infection. To approach the hemicranium, the patient may be positioned on a gel or foam doughnut headrest with a roll under the ipsilateral shoulder and the neck kept in neutral position with the collar kept in place. The Mayfield head-holder is not required for precision in such an operation and takes additional time that may prove detrimental. Furthermore, placing a patient in fixation pins while multiple teams are working to position, prep, and drape the patient placed the surgeon and assistants as well as the patient at risk for inadvertent lacerations and punctures. The patient should be placed with the vertex of the head slightly overhanging the top of the operating table (2–3 cm) from the very beginning in order to avoid further position changes. This aids in drainage of irrigation fluid downward into the craniotomy drape drainage bag. The contralateral upper extremity is extended on an arm board toward the anesthesia team, and the ipsilateral upper extremity is laid across the upper torso toward anesthesia (for wrist access), but cephalad enough to allow the abdomen to be prepped and accessed by the trauma team. (See "Complications" section below.)

The hair of the entire hemicranium should be quickly clipped to maximize visual inspection for traumatic contusions, hematomas, abrasions, and lacerations around which the incision may need to be planned. Towels are stapled to the cranium to outline a generous exposure to accommodate a large incision and craniotomy. (Alternatively, adhesive paper drapes may be used, but these often become dislodged in rapidly moving emergency cases.) The positioning of the head is done with the slight overhang so that the drainage bag on the adhesive craniotomy drape hangs straight down to properly collect the hemorrhage and irrigation that can be expected to occur in a "crash craniotomy" scenario. If the drainage bag is horizontal and not vertical as it is designed to be placed, spillage of irrigation, bone dust, and blood is difficult to keep clear of the operating field. As a result of fluid pooling, strike-through can occur, or drape separation from the weight of the material pooled on the drapes. Not only does this represent an infectious risk but floor spillage and overflow represents a significant slip risk to surgeons and operating room personnel, especially in a fast-moving crowded scene. Rapidly moving through such a case while maintaining meticulous attention to hemostasis is critical, due to the major blood loss the patient has already experienced and hemodynamic instability. The OR technician or nurse assigned to the neurosurgery team and the back table and Mayo stand for instruments should be positioned at the patient's ipsilateral shoulder.

The neck must be maintained in a neutral position and the collar left in place in the setting of a known or suspected cervical spine injury. This can be challenging in cranial operations involving significant soft tissue injury, especially lacerations and scalp avulsions, that may require non-standard incisions. Heavy scissors may be used to cut out a small portion of the collar to allow sufficient exposure for the inferior limbs of cranial incisions. (This is also an issue when surgery of the posterior fossa is needed, a fortunately unusual event in acute trauma, as this requires the prone position in Mayfield head-holder and fixation pins, and poses a higher risk to the spinal cord during the turning of the patient prone.) See below for further discussion of spinal column injury handling.

The thoracic or trauma surgeons must have access to the chest and abdomen to perform necessary life-saving procedures, including chest tube placement, thoracotomy, and laparotomy. Orthopaedics may also need to have access to the pelvis. All of this can be obtained from the same side as the craniotomy, with the OR technician or nurse and instrument table positioned at the patient's feet.

A thoracotomy may require the lateral position which is also acceptable for a simultaneous craniotomy. The patient should be positioned using standard lateral decubitus techniques, craniotomy side up. He or she may be flexed at the hips but special care to maintain the patient's spine in a neutral position is imperative, so inflatable "bean bag" or gel positioners (placed before the patient is put on the OR table), rolls and pillows, and tape and straps must be strategically placed to maintain neutral spinal alignment throughout the case. The upper arm may be placed on a padded Mayo stand or elevated arm board and will need to be cephalad enough to be

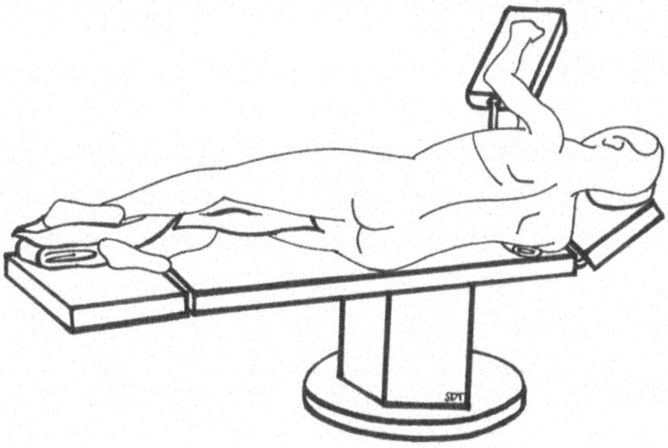

Fig. 17.2 Positioning for simultaneous emergency trauma craniotomy and thoracotomy

out of the way of the thoracic or trauma team, but not over the face and head, so as to allow access for the neurosurgical team (see Fig. 17.2). The anesthesia team may need to repeatedly check position to ensure alignment is maintained through the case, and of course padding needs to be employed as able to avoid pressure points, but this is of secondary consideration for such an extreme emergency and should not delay surgery. (If a thoracotomy is required contralateral to the craniotomy, the position may need to be performed supine, although this is challenging. In this case, the arm is usually elevated to allow improved access to the lateral thorax).

Repair of closed long bone fractures or spinal column fractures without neurological deficit should be delayed, ideally until the patient is hemodynamically stable, surgical intracranial mass lesions have been addressed, and intracranial pressure has been stable within the normal range (typically for at least 24 h). Conversely, pelvic fractures causing exsanguination may require intraoperative fixation with an external compression or pin-fixation device simultaneous to craniotomy to stave blood loss and reverse hypotension. Other exceptions include compound extremity fractures or majorly displaced femur or acetabular fractures. Compound fractures may result in exsanguination or ongoing blood loss (in addition to the infection risk) and can undergo irrigation and application of an external fixation device while other procedures are ongoing or immediately after their completion. They should never be left unattended and unobserved under a drape, but should be rapidly wrapped with sterile gauze and immobilized until such time as this can be performed, with the anesthesia team or other operating room personnel checking under the drapes frequently to assess for ongoing blood loss, about every 15 min until stable if all other events are under control.

Femur and acetabular fractures can also result in massive blood loss into the soft tissue of the thigh. Again, operating room personnel should check for thigh swelling under the drapes frequently. Immobilization of compound fractures and femur or acetabular fractures prevents ongoing tissue trauma and disruption of clotting, and therefore aids in hemostasis. Failure of the patient to respond to ongoing resuscitation efforts should prompt additional re-evaluation of injuries under sterile drapes to assess for ongoing blood loss, especially for those with coagulopathy.

As previously noted, spinal precautions should be maintained as much as possible throughout the initial life-saving emergency surgeries, until a more thorough evaluation of spinal column injury and instability and neurological status may be completed. Spinal cord injury with ongoing cord compression causing a deficit may need to be addressed soon after the initial surgery, but is not typically done in the same setting, unless cervical traction is required (made more difficult by surgical cranial defects). This could be performed under the same anesthetic after any necessary life-saving cranial, thoracic, abdominal, or pelvic surgeries have been completed. However, open surgeries for spinal decompression, stabilization, and fusion are typically done in a subsequent OR setting, and only after hemodynamic stability has been achieved and maintained for a significant length of time.

While modern CT alone is sufficient for experienced and trained interpreters to detect unstable cervical spine injuries in trauma patients, there is frequently no time to adequately review the study prior to emergency craniotomy, beyond a cursory look for major abnormalities (fractures and malalignments). However, should time allow, a thorough review of the CT may allow for removal of the cervical collar and more freedom with operative positioning [5].

Complications

Hernandez et al. [4] found the position described above to be acceptable by 24 of 29 general surgeons (82.76%) and 12 of 12 neurosurgeons (100%). However, the most notable concern, after appropriate access to the patient for all surgical teams and the anesthesia team, is brachial plexus stretch injury due to extension of the ipsilateral arm. While nerve stretch injuries in general occur in less than 1% of surgeries, they may be observed in every body position and may occur as early as 15 min post-positioning [6]. The brachial plexus can be injured by ischemia, compression, or stretch. These lesions are usually not permanent; however, recovery can take up to 18 months or more (leading to muscle atrophy and contracture, sensory loss and skin injury, or atrophic skin changes) so minimizing their occurrence is important. There are several ways to help minimize the chance of brachial plexus injury in the polytrauma hybrid position. First, there must be adequate elevation of the ipsilateral extremity in order to prevent hyperextension and traction on the brachial plexus from the weight of the extremity or arm straps/tape. Additionally, in supine or prone positions, the arm should generally not be abducted at the shoulder above 90° in order to avoid stretch injury (This would be improbable in the supine position for a craniotomy, as higher abduction would impair exposure.). Finally, careful placement of a vacuum "bean bag," gel positioner, and/or tape and safety belts to secure the patient's position and ensure that it does not change from sliding on the operating table if the table is rotated can also help avoid brachial plexus stretch injury [7].

The second concern with this hybrid positioning is that the elevation of the ipsilateral side by the shoulder roll makes the contralateral shoulder and flank dependent, causing potential for extra pressure. As long as the patient is secured to the table appropriately, the operating table can be rotated to bring the contralateral flank, abdomen, and shoulder into better position [4]. However, this may impair cranial access.

In summary, positioning of the polytrauma patient requires cooperation between the anesthesia team, all involved surgical teams, and all OR personnel. Protection of the spine during intubation and positioning as well as avoidance of hypotension and hypoxia in order to prevent secondary brain injury is critical. All teams must carefully and rapidly consider the ramifications to the other teams of positioning required for their operation. Verbal communication amongst all involved should be succinct, clear, and efficient.

The Morbidly Obese Patient

Case 2 Presentation

A 52-year-old female is seen in neurosurgical consultation due to severe back pain radiating into the right leg that started with a "pop" in her back that occurred when she bent over to pick up an object. On physical examination, she has a positive Lasegue's sign (straight leg raise test), and dorsiflexion on the right is weak at 4−/5. An MRI obtained on a special unit shows an L4–5 disc herniation with significant compression of the traversing right L5 nerve root. The patient has tried a Medrol dose pack and rest with no improvement in her symptoms. Her weight is 190 kg, her height is 5 ft. 5 in., and her BMI is 69. Her past medical history includes hypertension, hypercholesterolemia, and poorly controlled diabetes mellitus. Given the failure of medical management, the MRI findings, and the motor weakness on physical examination, surgical intervention is recommended. The patient is referred to the anesthesia clinic for preoperative evaluation. An electrocardiogram, chest X-ray, and laboratory workup are obtained, with no significant abnormalities except hyperglycemia, and a microscopic lumbar discectomy is scheduled.

Positioning of the Morbidly Obese Patient

Morbid obesity is a significant health problem with increasing incidence. A Body Mass Index (BMI) of 25 kg/m^2 and below is considered to be normal, a BMI of 25–30 kg/m^2 is low risk,

30–35 kg/m^2 leads to moderate risk from complications of obesity and a moderate anesthesia risk, 35–40 kg/m^2 is considered high risk, and above 40 kg/m^2 is considered "serious morbid obesity" with very high risk [8]. The patient in the case presentation has a BMI of 69 placing her in the "very high risk" category.

Obese patients have decreased chest wall compliance and inefficient respiratory musculature. With increasing obesity, the work of breathing is increased and with increasing weight, the intra-abdominal pressure is increased, while the total lung capacity and functional residual capacity are decreased [9]. Prone positioning is associated with predictable changes in physiology and also with a number of complications, all of which become more pronounced in the setting of morbid obesity. Thus, preoperative optimization, careful placement into the prone position (or consideration of alternatives), and effective communication between the neurosurgical and OR teams becomes even more crucial [7].

As well as the standard preoperative evaluation, one should consider obtaining an electrocardiogram, and even an echocardiogram as well as a lower extremity duplex to rule out deep vein thrombosis before prone positioning in the morbidly obese patient. Invasive arterial monitoring should be used if cardiopulmonary disease is present, and for those with the inability to gain an accurate cuff pressure due to size discrepancy/poor fit. Central venous catheterization should be considered in those with obesity, cardiopulmonary disease, and poor peripheral venous access [10].

Appropriate selection of operating room equipment must also be considered. Many operating room tables can support patient who weigh up to the 350–500 pound range, and special tables have been designed to support patient who weigh more. However, it must be noted that some OR tables, once articulations in the table begin to be mobilized, may not hold the same amount of weight in certain configurations. Morbidly obese patients have an increased risk of falling off of the operating room table due to weight load shifts and instability. Providing extra support and carefully securing the patient are thus paramount. Adequate padding also becomes more important because the extra weight leads to additional pressure on any areas that come into contact with the operating room table or equipment [11], with the attendant risk of decubitus ulcer formation and nerve compression syndromes, even with relatively short cases. As obese patients are often diabetic, their risk of positioning peripheral neuropathies is cumulatively affected.

Positioning an obese patient in any position, supine, lateral decubitus, "park bench," prone, sitting, or otherwise is challenging and fraught with risk. There is a risk of the patient falling due to personnel being unable to maintain the patient's position while securing him or her, inappropriately sized operating tables and equipment, or partial emergence from anesthesia due to increased drug requirements resulting in patient movement during surgery. Injury to the skin can occur simply from the pressure of straps required to secure patients in place, as they must often be placed under higher tension in the obese patient to be effective. Pooling of prep solutions in the dependent intertriginous areas may result in maceration of tissue, so care must be taken during sterile prep to avoid this. Risk of radiation injury due to increased fluoroscopic requirements for adequate visualization is also higher in obese patients, providing additional challenges to long-term skin integrity. Adjunctive circumferential imaging devices sometimes cannot be used, as they will not fit around the patient, even on a Jackson table. The placement of adjunctive lines, such as IVs, arterial lines, central venous catheters, and urinary catheters may be more difficult. Increased infection risk from diabetes or inability to keep surgical sites adequately cleansed postoperatively are also factors.

The prone position itself has adverse effects on epidural venous pressure and airway pressure in all patients, and these effects are more pronounced in the obese patient [12]. Pressure on the abdominal wall may further accentuate the restrictive nature of the pulmonary disease common in this patient population. The high airway pressures required to ventilate these patients may lead to barotrauma or difficulty with ventilation and cardiopulmonary function. Furthermore, the attendant impaired venous return and cardiac output can lead to decreased spinal cord perfusion and excess surgical blood loss for the neurosurgeon [13, 16].

Palmon et al. compared peak airway pressure, pleural pressure, and mean arterial pressure in patients undergoing posterior spinal surgery in the prone position with a "normal" BMI, a "heavy" BMI, and an "obese" BMI [13]. Obese patients positioned prone on a Wilson frame had an increase in mean arterial pressure and peak airway pressure and a decrease in pulmonary compliance. All patients positioned on chest rolls had an increase in peak airway pressure and a decrease in pulmonary compliance. On the other hand, when using the open Jackson table, there was no change in peak airway pressure or compliance when moving from the supine to the prone position.

All three of these surgical positioners are designed to allow the abdomen to be suspended during prone surgery; however, in the obese patient, the abdominal girth does not allow for its suspension with chest rolls, and even with the Wilson frame in the larger patients. Furthermore, the Wilson frame may tip when expanded high enough to accommodate larger patients and their size and weight may exacerbate this phenomenon. Especially with the Wilson frame, the surgeon and assistant must often be required to stand on step stools to operate at the appropriate height, which can make simultaneous utilization of the microscope, drill, and bipolar cautery more difficult. Reduction of abdominal and thoracic pressures and optimization of respiratory mechanics and venous return thereby improving ventilation, spinal cord perfusion, and surgical blood loss can be achieved by using the Jackson table for obese patients (see Fig. 17.3). In all cases, the table should be placed at the lowest height and even with the bed prior to rolling the patient over to the table into the prone position.

Another option is to adjust the patients positioning based upon obesity status; for example, using the lateral or sitting positions to approach the posterior fossa or the spine instead of the prone position. This is not just an issue related to patient physiology. Depending upon the stature of the surgeon, certain positions may not allow the surgeon to reach the exposed area to operate. It can be especially difficult, even with standing step stools, for surgeons to adequately visualize the depths of exposure of a midline spinal incision in a morbidly obese patient, let along perform the surgical manipulations necessary to carry out the operation safely, effectively making it impossible to position the patient prone.

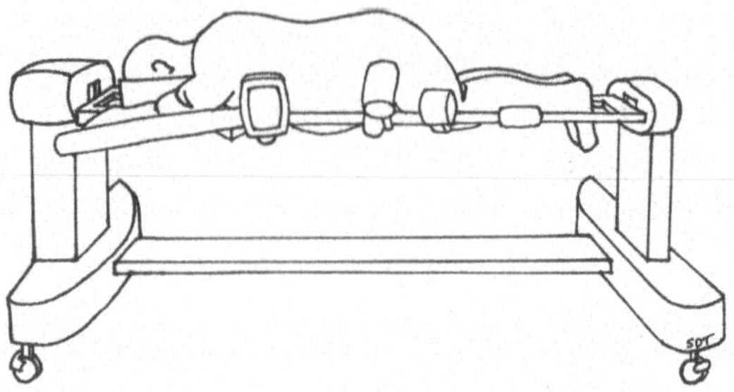

Fig. 17.3 Positioning for the morbidly obese patient

Several studies [14, 15] discuss the use of awake intubation and prone self-positioning as a method for decreasing anesthetic complications and minimizing pressure points during positioning of a morbidly obese patient. In this model, a topical anesthetic and IV sedation are used for awake fiberoptic intubation. The patient is then disconnected from the circuit and allowed to position themselves which minimizes pressure points, skin integrity compromise, and nerve injury. Additionally, spontaneous and adequate oxygenation and ventilation in the prone position can be confirmed before induction of general anesthesia. Patient cooperation and the ability to communicate non-verbally with the operating room team are key for awake intubation and prone self-positioning in the morbidly obese spine patient making patient selection key.

Complications

Morbid obesity is also a risk factor for the development of ischemic optic neuropathy (ION) and subsequent partial or total blindness. While ION may occur in any patient who has been placed prone for surgery, Lee et al. demonstrated in a large multi-institutional study that the odds ratio for ION in the setting of obesity was 2.83 with a confidence interval of 1.52–5.39 [17]. There is no effective treatment for ION so extra vigilance with protective strategies is required.

Positioning should include careful facial padding and support, and visual conformation that the globes are free from pressure. A square foam pad with cut-outs for the face and endotracheal tube is a popular and safe option for use with regular or Jackson flat-top tables. Alternatively, a horseshoe headrest may be used, but these, even when padded, may not appropriately fit the patient's head and face, and therefore risk pressure to the globes. A Mayfield pin-fixation headholder device may also be used, but with very large individuals, the soft tissue may be sufficiently thick that the pins cannot gain adequate penetration of the skull for secure fixation. Furthermore, the face, chin, and neck may be in contact with the metal frame of the Mayfield, rendering it ineffective at avoiding pressure. Finally, cervical fat pads may make it impossible to flex the neck adequately to access the posterior fossa and cervicomedullary junction.

To help avoid ION, the head should be maintained at or above the heart to reduce venous congestion. Minimizing duration in the prone position, maximizing hemostasis, and the use of colloid (and blood products if necessary) to minimize crystalloid administration decrease the risk of ION. However, ION may occur even when all proper precautions are taken and no untoward intraoperative events occur.

In conclusion, positioning for surgery in the morbidly obese patient has a unique set of challenges and pitfalls. Sufficient preoperative workup of cardiac and pulmonary function and glycemic control are important preventive measures to inform the surgeon of the patient's suitability for general anesthesia and surgery in general, and may guide positioning decisions. Placement of arterial lines and central venous catheters should be considered, and the option of awake intubation and self-positioning may be discussed with the patient. Intra-abdominal pressure in the prone position can be minimized by using a Jackson table to improve ventilation, decrease peak airway pressure, improve venous return, and maximize cardiac output. Extra care must be taken when positioning to avoid peripheral nerve injury, decubitus ulcers, and ischemic optic neuropathy.

Conflict of Interest The authors declare no conflict of interest.

References

1. Ecklund JM, Moores LE, editors. Neurotrauma management for the severely injured polytrauma patient. New York: Springer; 2017.
2. Melio FR. Priorities in the multiple trauma patient. Emerg Med Clin North Am. 1998;16:29–43.
3. Wisner DH, Victor NS, Holcroft JW. Priorities in the management of multiple trauma: intracranial versus intra-abdominal injury. J Trauma. 1993;35(2):271–6.
4. Hernandez AM, Roguski M, Qiu RS, Shepard MJ, Riesenburger RI. Surgeons' perspectives on optimal patient positioning during simultaneous cranial procedures and exploratory laparotomy. South Med J. 2013;106(12):679–83. https://doi.org/10.1097/SMJ.0000000000000030.
5. Panczykowski DM, Tomycz ND, Okonkwo DO. Comparative effectiveness of using computed tomography alone to exclude cervical spine injuries in obtunded or intubated patients: meta-analysis of 14,327 patients with blunt trauma. J Neurosurg. 2011;115(3):541–9. https://doi.org/10.3171/2011.4.JNS101672. Epub 2011 May 27.
6. Eggstein S, Franke M, Hofmeister A, Rückauer KD. Postoperative peripheral neuropathies in general surgery. Zentralbl Chir. 2000;125(5):459–63.
7. Agostini J, Goasguen N, Mosnier H. Patient positioning in laparoscopic surgery: tricks and tips. J Visc Surg. 2010;147(4):e227–32. https://doi.org/10.1016/j.jviscsurg.2010.07.010.
8. Bray GA. Pathophysiology of obesity. Am J Clin Nutr. 1992;55(2Suppl):488S–94S.
9. Biring MS, Lewis MI, Liu JT, Mohsenifar Z. Pulmonary physiologic changes of morbid obesity. Am J Med Sci. 1999;318(5):293–7.
10. Maxwell MH, Waks AU, Schroth PC, Karam M, Dornfeld LP. Error in blood-pressure measurement due to incorrect cuff size in obese patients. Lancet. 1982;2:33–6.
11. Ide P, Farber ES, Lautz D. Perioperative nursing care of the bariatric surgical patient. AORN J. 2008;88(1):30–54.
12. Pearce DJ. The role of posture in laminectomy. Proc R Soc Med. 1957;50(2):109–12. PubMed PMID: 13408221; PubMed Central PMCID: PMC1888995.
13. Palmon SC, Kirsch JR, Depper JA, Toung TJ. The effect of the prone position on pulmonary mechanics is frame-dependent. Anesth Analg. 1998;87(5):1175–80.

14. Wu SD, Yilmaz M, Tamul PC, Meeks JJ, Nadler RB. Awake endotracheal intubation and prone patient self-positioning: anesthetic and positioning considerations during percutaneous nephrolithotomy in obese patients. J Endourol. 2009;23(10):1599–602. https://doi.org/10.1089/end.2009.1524.
15. Douglass J, Fraser J, Andrzejowski J. Awake intubation and awake prone positioning of a morbidly obese patient for lumbar spine surgery. Anaesthesia. 2014;69(2):166–9. https://doi.org/10.1111/anae.12387. Epub 2013 Sep 23.
16. Brodsky JB. Positioning the morbidly obese patient for anesthesia. Obes Surg. 2002;12(6):751–8.
17. Postoperative Visual Loss Study Group. Risk factors associated with ischemic optic neuropathy after spinal fusion surgery. Anesthesiology. 2012;116(1):15–24. https://doi.org/10.1097/ALN.0b013e31823d012a.

18 Comorbidities and Positioning: Pregnancy

Thomas Scott Guyton

Maternal Weight Gain

The most obvious change in pregnancy is maternal weight gain. The American Congress of Obstetricians and Gynecologists (ACOG) has made the following recommendations for maternal weight gain [1]. Women with a BMI 18.5–24.9 kg/m^2 should gain 25–35 pounds for a full-term singleton pregnancy. The recommended rate of weight gain in these women is 1 pound per week in the second and third trimester. Even obese mothers (BMI >30 kg/m^2) are recommended to gain 11–20 pounds. Twenty five percent of women are obese at the time of first visit to the obstetrician as defined by a BMI greater than 30 kg/m^2 [2]. Seventy five percent of pregnant women gain more than the recommended amount of weight [2]. While the developing fetus, amniotic fluid, uterus, and increases in circulating blood volume account for increases in maternal weight, fat deposition also occurs. Subcutaneous fat deposits in the thighs account for 16% of fat deposition [3]. Positioning the pregnant woman is complicated by the gravid uterus, an increase in the size of the thighs and hips, and a high rate of obesity.

T. S. Guyton (✉)
Methodist Le Bonheur Healthcare,
Memphis, TN, USA

Physiological Changes During Pregnancy

During pregnancy, cardiac output (CO) increases to a peak at time of delivery and immediately postpartum and returns to pre-pregnant state by 6 weeks postpartum [4]. CO increases by week 5 and reaches a plateau of 45% increase at 24 weeks. Between 24 weeks and term, CO remains the same. During the second stage of labor, CO increases an additional 34% with contractions. Both heart rate and stroke volume increase to account for the increases in CO. After delivery, stroke volume remains elevated for 48 h and then falls dramatically. Heart rate remains up for at least 24 h and then falls dramatically over the next 10 days. After delivery, CO remains at high levels for at least 24 h and then falls to pre-pregnant levels by 2–6 weeks after delivery.

Other circulatory changes include changes in blood pressure, systemic vascular resistance (SVR), pulmonary vascular resistance, and plasma volume [4–6]. Blood pressure falls during pregnancy with a nadir around 20 weeks [4]. Diastolic blood pressure decreases more than systolic. SVR decreases with a decrease of 34% by 20 weeks. Pulmonary changes parallel the changes in CO and SVR with a 44–46% increase in pulmonary artery blood flow and a 17.5%

A. Arthur et al. (eds.), *Perioperative Considerations and Positioning for Neurosurgical Procedures*,
https://doi.org/10.1007/978-3-319-72679-3_18

decrease in pulmonary vascular resistance in the third trimester [5]. Central venous pressure [4] and pulmonary artery pressure [5] do not change with pregnancy. As a compensatory measure for a decreased SVR, plasma volume increases by 1.13 L at term [6]. Plasma volume returns to normal roughly 6 weeks after delivery. Hemoglobin declines in response to hemodilution caused by the increase in plasma volume [5]. Oncotic pressure also declines in response to increased plasma volume [7].

With delivery, normal blood loss for vaginal delivery was approximately 300 mLs [8] and for cesarean section approximately 500 mLs [9]. Uterine contraction after delivery provides an autotransfusion of 300–500 mLs [10].

Respiratory changes in pregnancy include changes in lung volumes, minute ventilation, and oxygen consumption [11, 12]. Functional residual capacity decreases 15–25%. Progesterone stimulates the respiratory center resulting in a 20–45% increase in minute ventilation. Increased minute ventilation is the result of a 30–50% increase in tidal volume. Respiratory rate remains unchanged. The partial pressure of carbon dioxide in the blood is decreased to 27–34 mmHg. Oxygen consumption increases by 18% by the third trimester [12].

Pregnancy causes a host of other changes. Glomerular filtration rate is increased by 40% at term and falls to normal 1 month after delivery [13]. Intra-abdominal pressure increases as the gravid uterus grows. Progesterone induces relaxation of the lower esophageal sphincter tone. Combined these increase the risk of aspiration pneumonitis during intubation [14]. Difficult intubation occurs at a higher frequency during pregnancy [14]. Epistaxis occurs in 20% of pregnant women compared to 6% of controls [15]. Venous thromboembolism is the leading direct cause of maternal mortality in the 2009–2013 Confidential Enquiries into Maternal Deaths [16]. The antenatal pregnant women has a five-fold higher risk than a nonpregnant age matched control [16]. The postpartum women has a 20-fold higher risk [16].

Aortocaval Compression

In 1953, Howard et al. reported two term pregnant women who went into shock when placed supine [17]. One woman would relieve her symptoms by turning on her side, and the symptoms could be elicited again by having her turn back to the supine position. They postulated that this must occur frequently in term pregnant women. They measured the blood pressure in 160 consecutive term pregnant women in the supine and lateral positions and observed that 18 out of the 160 dropped their blood pressure by up to 30 mm mercury (Hg) or to 80 mmHg or less. This hypotension would be relieved by placing the patient on either side or by standing [17]. The hypotension did also not tend to occur during labor where term pregnant women would be supine for long periods of time. They called this supine hypotensive syndrome in late pregnancy [17]. Three to eleven percent of term pregnant patients experience a drop in blood pressure in the supine position sufficient to classify as supine hypotensive syndrome [17–19]. Kerr et al. injected contrast dye into the femoral veins of term pregnant patients just prior to cesarean section and found the inferior vena cava (IVC) to be totally occluded from the bifurcation to above the renal veins in all 12 patients studied [20]. The venous return was by the vertebral plexus of veins and the azygos vein. Return of flow in the vena cava was demonstrated by a second venogram after delivery of the baby [20]. Bieniarz et al. demonstrated displacement of the aorta to the left and diminished flow in the aorta at the level of L4 [21]. The flaccid gravid uterus in the term pregnant woman is recognized to compress the IVC and the aorta in the supine position.

The aortocaval compression has been recently reexamined using magnetic resonance imaging (MRI) and ultrasound. A retrospective study of 56 pregnant patients at a median gestational age of 27 weeks found that 55 out of 56 patients had aortocaval compression on MRI [22]. The compression correlated with the uterine volume on the right side of the spine. The effect of degree of tilt was examined in ten patients using MRI [23]. Increases in IVC size occurred in nine out of ten patients at 30°, but 15° did not have a consistent effect.

For time of onset, McLennan showed a rise in femoral venous pressure with the supine position as early as 13–16 weeks of pregnancy [24]. The earliest report of the supine hypotensive syndrome is at 16 weeks [25]. Twenty weeks gestation is the quoted time where compression of the IVC begins when supine [26]. In support of this statement, cardiovascular MRI of six pregnant women at 20 weeks gestation showed a significant increase in left atrial size, ejection fraction, and stroke volume when turned from supine to the left lateral position indicating an increase in preload with the change in position [27]. The presence of factors other than the size of the uterus may contribute to early onset of aortocaval compression. Obesity, multiple gestation, bicornuate uterus and accompanying ovarian cysts have all been reported as contributing to IVC compression [28–31].

For time of offset, Kerr et al. demonstrated a return of flow in the IVC with delivery [20]. However, the uterus after delivery weighs 1100 g [32]. The uterus will be larger in patients with multiple gestation and those with fibroids [32]. The fundal height of the uterus immediately after delivery averages 16.8 cm with a range between 13 and 22 cm above the symphysis pubis [33]. This corresponds with an average size of 17 weeks gestation with a range from 13 to 22 weeks gestation. The uterus undergoes involution with a decrease in fundal height of 0.8 cm per day for vaginal deliveries [33]. This decrease may be slowed by cesarean section (c-section) [34]. Given the size of the uterus, continued IVC compression can be expected in some patients immediately post delivery.

Importance of Aortocaval Compression

Aortocaval compression results in decreased uterine blood flow. Uterine blood flow is determined by the pressure gradient across the uterine vessels divided by the uterine vasculature resistance. Aortic compression and hypotension from diminished venous return decreases the pressure in the uterine arteries. Forty-seven to seventy percent of patients have a 10% reduction in systolic blood pressure in the supine position [18, 19]. Pressure in the uterine veins as reflected in the femoral veins doubles at term in the supine position from roughly 10 to 20 mmHg [20]. Diminished uterine arterial pressure combined with increased uterine venous pressure results in a decreased gradient across the uterine vessels and reduced uterine blood flow. Even in the patients not demonstrating the supine hypotensive syndrome, the resulting reduction in uterine blood flow may be sufficient to cause fetal distress.

Another important consideration for neurosurgery is that the plexus of veins in the lumbar spine and the azygos vein are the principal collateral vessels for venous return to the heart. The original angiographic studies showed complete occlusion of the IVC in the supine position with the dye returning to the heart via the lumbar plexus of veins [20]. The original angiographic studies also showed partial occlusion of the inferior vena cava in the lateral position but requiring minimal use of collateral venous return [20]. Recent MRI scans have shown increased size of epidural veins and decreased cerebrospinal fluid in the lumbar spinal canal in term pregnant patients in the supine position [35–37]. Positions resulting in the use of lumbar veins as collaterals are important to spine surgery as enlarged epidural veins may make the surgery more difficult. In addition, the enlarged epidural veins will have an adverse effect on intracranial compliance by shifting cerebrospinal fluid (csf) cranially. This effect was seen on MRI imaging of the lumbar spines of supine pregnant women [37]. The effect of fluid in the epidural space on intracranial compliance was demonstrated in two patients recovering from head trauma who had increased intracranial pressures measured after receiving as little as 5–10 mLs of local anesthesia epidurally [38]. The engorged epidural veins are going to occupy space just as the local anesthetic injection did; intracranial compliance will be diminished because csf will be shifted out of the lumbar spine.

How to Reduce Aortocaval Compression in the Supine Position

The key to reducing aortocaval compression in the supine position is to displace the uterus to the left to relieve pressure on the IVC and aorta. One simple method is to tilt the pelvis by placing a 12–15 cm pad underneath the right hip (roughly 15°). In one study, this method achieved increases in brachial blood pressures in 57 out of 57 patients compared to supine and return to control brachial blood pressures in 39 out of 57 patients studied [39]. Manually displacing the uterus to the left also raised brachial blood pressures but was less effective than using a pad to tilt the pelvis [39]. Ultrasound measurements indicate that 76% patients respond to left lateral tilt with a 29% increase in IVC size [40]. Another method to relieve aortocaval compression is to tilt the entire patient. Using MRI in term pregnant women at 0, 15, 30, and 45°, the volume of blood in the IVC between the L1–L2 disk space to the L3–L4 disk space was 3.2, 3.0, 11.5, and 10.9 mLs, respectively [23]. This compares to 21.5 mLs in the nonpregnant patient at 30°. Thus, leftward tilt ≥30° achieved the greatest relief of IVC compression. However, IVC size is still reduced compared to the nonpregnant patient [23]. This finding matches the compression seen on the original venogram in the term pregnant patient in the lateral position [20]. Fifteen degrees or more of leftward tilt appears to normalize arterial blood pressure, and 30° or more is needed to minimize the effects on the IVC in the term pregnant patient.

Recently, the use of the pad under hip has been challenged for use during c-section as not relieving aortocaval compression. The original recommendation was based upon an article by Crawford indicating an improvement in the Apgar scores and pH of the fetus at c-section with the use of pelvic wedge providing 15° leftward tilt [41]. The use of the wedge was not based upon imaging studies of aortocaval compression. Use of the pelvic wedge was shown to help normalize decreased brachial and femoral arterial pressures occurring in the supine position [39]. Fifteen degrees of leftward tilt was shown to offer little benefit over supine in terms of IVC compression at the L1–L4 level in a recent MRI study of ten patients at 37–39 weeks gestation [23]. Both supine and 15° tilt had significant IVC obstruction, and no aortic compression was found in either position. In this study, IVC occlusion occurred in essentially every term pregnant woman in the lumbar region. Not addressed in the MRI study were the effects of tilt during an earlier gestational age and the mechanism of the supine hypotensive syndrome. Contrary to looking at the lumbar IVC, ultrasound of the proximal intrahepatic IVC reflects central venous pressure and includes both flow via the IVC and collateral circulation. Ultrasound of the proximal IVC showed that left lateral tilt resulted in a 29% increase in size of the intrahepatic IVC in 76% of patients between 30 and 42 weeks gestation [40]. A quarter of these women had the largest IVC in the supine position. The majority of women respond to leftward tilt; however, the effect of 15° of leftward tilt on lumbar IVC occlusion is not known during the second trimester.

Fetal Evaluation

ACOG recommends consulting an obstetrician preferably the patient's obstetrician to aid in decision-making [42]. The obstetrician will serve in multiple capacities that effect the patient's position. First, the obstetrician will confirm the gestational age of the fetus. Second, the obstetrician will determine the state of the fetus in utero. Third, the obstetrician will aid in the decision-making on timing of delivery. Fourth, the obstetrician will make decisions regarding inoperative monitoring of the fetus. Last, the obstetrician is going to help manage the patient and the fetus postoperatively particularly in regard to preterm labor.

Estimate of Fetal Gestational Age

Measurement of fundal height can give a crude estimate of gestational age. A tape measure is used to measure from the symphysis pubis to the fundus of the uterus. In general, mean gestational age from 16 to 24 weeks is roughly the fundal height in centimeters. From 25 to 40 weeks, the fundal height is 0.5 to 2 cm greater than the mean gestational age [43]. The reproducibility of this measurement is poor [44], and measurement of fundal height is effected by many variables including obesity [45].

Ultrasound is considered the best method for determining gestational age. From 7 to 12 weeks of gestation, crown-rump length provides the best biometric measure of gestational age [46]. From 12 to 14 weeks, biparietal diameter and crown-rump length are equivalent [46]. Ultrasound performed in the second and third trimesters are less accurate, and multiple other biometric measures such as occipitofrontal diameter, head circumference, abdominal circumference, and femur length are used to improve the accuracy [47, 48]. Measurements of gestational age are accurate to within 5 days of the actual date of conception 95% of the time for ultrasounds done in early gestation [47].

Evaluation of the Fetus In Utero

Ultrasound is the mainstay of evaluating the fetus in utero. Ultrasound can be used to estimate gestational age and fetal weight, detect the presence of more than one fetus, and diagnose placental abnormalities such as abruption or previa. One measurement of fetal well-being in the third trimester is the biophysical profile. Three ultrasound measures of acute fetal well-being: fetal tone, gross body movement, fetal breathing movements, and one chronic measure amniotic fluid volume are combined with the reactivity on the fetal heart rate monitor to comprise the biophysical profile. Each measure is given a score of 0 or 2. Scores of 8 or 10 are considered normal [49]. Lower biophysical profiles will require interpretation by the consulting obstetrician.

Fetal heart rate can be monitored intermittently by fetal Doppler tone measurements as well as by continuous electronic fetal heart rate monitoring. In a low-risk population, continuous fetal heart rate monitoring has no shown benefit in terms of fetal mortality over scheduled intermittent fetal rate monitoring [50]. Continuous fetal heart rate monitoring is most often combined with monitoring of uterine contractions [51]. During the third trimester, the normal fetal heart rate is 120–160. Hypoxia may induce fetal bradycardia or fetal tachycardia. At roughly 24–28 weeks of gestation, the parasympathetic and sympathetic nervous systems mature, and variability in the fetal heart rate starts to occur. The short term or beat to beat variability is the oscillation of the fetal heart rate around baseline. The beat to beat variability has a magnitude of 5–10 beats per minute. A longer term variability of 3–10 cycles per minute with a magnitude of 10–25 beats per minute also occurs. The loss of the short-term variability is thought to be more ominous for fetal hypoxia. Fetal heart rate accelerations in response to uterine contractions, vaginal stimulation, or fetal movement are considered reassuring. Early decelerations are decelerations which occur with the start of a uterine contraction and end with the end of the contraction, and are most commonly caused by fetal head compression by the uterine contraction. Early decelerations are not associated with fetal distress. Late decelerations start at the peak of contraction or after and last past the end of the uterine contraction. Late decelerations are considered a sign of fetal distress [51].

ACOG recommends the decision of what type of monitoring be individualized and guided by an obstetrician [42]. ACOG suggests that in general fetal Doppler heart tone measurements or ultrasound evaluations before and after surgery are sufficient for fetuses prior to gestational age of viability. ACOG suggests that continuous monitoring might be useful for positioning purposes in nonviable fetuses [42]. Continuous fetal heart rate monitoring is recommended for nonobstetric surgeries in which emergent cesarean section is contemplated for fetal distress. Continuous fetal heart monitoring should be performed by someone skilled in its interpretation. When continuous monitoring is used, monitoring should begin prior to surgery to establish a baseline and be continued postoperatively to look for premature labor.

Many problems exist with continuous fetal heart rate monitoring under anesthesia [51]. Premature fetuses have a higher baseline heart rate and lack beat to beat variability because of immaturity of the parasympathetic and sympathetic nervous systems. The fetus has a rest-activity cycle and may have decreased variability during a rest cycle. Parasympathetic and sympathetic agents such as atropine, ritodrine, and terbutaline cross the placenta and alter the resting fetal heart rate and decrease beat to beat variability. Depressant drugs such as opiates, magnesium, and volatile anesthetic agents can all decrease beat to beat variability [51]. An unnecessary emergency cesarean section for decreased beat to beat variability has been reported when continuous fetal rate monitoring was done at 30 weeks gestation for nonobstetric surgery [52]. Continuous fetal heart rate monitoring was not done in several cases in the prone position due to difficulty in performing the monitoring and because of the risk to the mother to stop the surgery to deliver the fetus [53, 54]. Continuous FHR monitoring was not done during a general anesthetic for lumbar laminectomy in the lateral position at 21 weeks because of difficulty performing the monitoring [55] and at 33 weeks because the physicians felt aortocaval compression was unlikely in the left lateral position [56].

Timing of Surgery

Traditionally, surgery that can be delayed has not been performed during the first trimester of pregnancy for fear of possible teratogenicity during the period of organogenesis. Surgery during the second trimester is felt to have a reduced risk of causing preterm contractions and spontaneous abortion compared to the third trimester. ACOG has issued several statements [42]. First, elective surgery should be postponed until after delivery. Second, indicated surgery should never be denied a pregnant woman no matter what the gestational age. Third, no currently existing anesthetic agent given in standard concentrations has shown been to have teratogenic effects in humans. Fourth, ACOG recommends consulting an obstetrician, preferably the patient's obstetrician, to assist in perioperative management.

Nineteen weeks and six days of gestation and less is considered to be previable. Between 20 weeks and 25 weeks and 6 days gestation, the fetus is considered to be periviable. The mortality and morbidity of the infant born between 22 and 26 weeks of gestational age varies greatly depending upon the hospital in which the infant is born [56]. For this reason, consulting a neonatologist to discuss the mortality and morbidity specific to that hospital and to the infant's estimated birth weight and gestational age is best practice. However, for some hospitals, this data is difficult to obtain. Survival and survival with no or mild disability based upon gestational age as seen in Eunice Kennedy Shriver National Institute of Child Health and Human Development Neonatal Research Network in the United States [56], the Neonatal Research Network in Japan [57], and the EPICure studies in England [58] are as follows. Median fetal weight increases weekly from 22 to 26 weeks as follows: 510–540, 586–600, 655–671, 750–799, and 860–879 g, respectively [56, 58]. Percent survival increases weekly from 22 to 26 weeks as follows: 7.3–37.3, 19–64.5, 40–77.7, 66–85.7, and 78–81% respectively [56–58]. Percent survival with no or mild disability from 22 to 26 weeks is as follows: 2.4–12, 5.3–20, 12.2–30.9, 25.7–44.5, and 38.8–58.6% [56–58]. These results for survival percentage and percent survival with mild or no disability exclude neonates receiving comfort care [56]. In weeks 22 and 23, the percentage of neonates receiving comfort care only is 73–78 and 16–28%, respectively [56, 58]. For this reason, these values represent what can be achieved using patient selection. An alternative to using gestational age to predict survival is to use estimated birth weight. Neonatal mortality and morbidity for infants based upon birth weight between 501 and 1500 g is reported for 669 participating North American hospitals from 2000 to 2009 [59]. Mortality for the different groups is reported as 500 to 750 g—36.6%, 751 to 1000 g—11.7%, 1001 to 1250 g—5.7%, and

1251 to 1500 g—3.5% [59]. Major morbidity is reported as 500 to 750 g—82.7%, 751 to 1000 g—57.4%, 1001 to 1250 g—33.1%, and 1251–1500—18.7% [59].

Diagnostic Imaging

ACOG, the American College of Radiology, and the American institute of Ultrasound in Medicine have issued an opinion on the risks of diagnostic imaging [60]. Ultrasonography and MRI are the imaging modalities of choice for pregnant women. No adverse fetal effects have been reported from the use of diagnostic ultrasonography. Highest risk comes from nonobstetric ultrasound system particularly those that do color Doppler. No injuries have been reported to be caused by prenatal MRI during the first trimester using predominantly 1.5 T MRI scanners [61]. The use of gadolinium contrast should be limited only to situations where the benefits of contrast outweigh the risks of teratogenicity. Gadolinium in its free form is teratogenic, and the fetus can accumulate chelated gadolinium in the amniotic fluid so the potential for prolonged exposure to the free form exists [60].

In general, the amount of ionizing radiation from radiography, computed tomography scan, and nuclear medicine imaging is at an acceptable level to the fetus [60]. The goal is to keep the radiation at "As Low As Reasonably Achievable" [60]. The risk to the fetus depends upon both the gestational age and the radiation dose [60]. Before implantation (0–2 weeks), radiation exposure results either in fetal demise or no effect with a threshold of 50–100 mGy. During organogenesis (2–8 weeks), congenital anomalies occur with a threshold around 200 mGy. Between 8 and 15 weeks, severe intellectual disability occurs with a threshold of 60–310 mGy. Between 16 and 25 weeks, severe intellectual disability occurs with a threshold of 250–280 mGy. These doses are typically higher than that associated with a single imaging study. For example, a pelvic CT scan has one of the highest fetal exposure of 10–50 mGy [60]. Of more concern is the risk of carcinogenesis; fetal exposure to 10–20 mGy increases the risk of leukemia by a factor of 1.5–2.0 [60].

Contrast CT scans, nuclear medicine imaging, interventional neuroradiology procedures, and gamma knife procedures have been safely performed on pregnant patients [60]. Oral contrast is not absorbed by the patient, and intravenous contrast crosses the placenta but has not been shown to have adverse effects on the fetus [60]. Nuclear medicine imaging depends upon the isotope. Technetium 99 m has a half-life of 6 h and is a pure gamma ray emitter. Used for ventilation-perfusion studies to detect pulmonary embolus, Technetium 99 m perfusion studies expose the fetus to 5 mGy [60]. Radioactive iodine (iodine 131) has a half-life of 8 days, crosses the placenta, and would not be a safe isotope to use during pregnancy [60]. Interventional neuroradiology procedures have been reported with safe doses of ionizing radiation to lead shielded fetuses. Using lead shielding, a head CT scan and cerebral angiography was reported with a fetal dose of 0.025 mGy [62]. Embolization of an intracranial aneurysm was reported with a fetal exposure between 0.17 and 2.8 mGy [62]. Fetal doses between 32 and 42 mGy were measured during Cyberknife radiosurgery of a maternal brain tumor during the third trimester [63]. Fetal doses of 8.26 mGy were estimated during linear accelerator-based stereotactic radiosurgery of an arteriovenous malformation [64].

Prone Position

One retrospective review of the surgical management of herniated lumbar disks showed that prone position was the most common position used during the first trimester and the early second trimester [65]. The pregnant woman spends essentially no time in the prone position during sleep [66]. The concern is that the weight of the woman pushes the uterus into the inferior vena cava and the aorta. Another potential problem would be compression of the umbilical cord. However, the prone position is used during labor if the uterus and abdomen hang freely. The pregnant woman is placed upon her hands and knees to promote turning of the fetal head from occiput posterior malposition [67] and for fetal distress unrelieved in the lateral positions when aortocaval compression is suspected [68]. The weight of the uterus moves the uterus away from the IVC in the hands and knees position. The lack of compression of the IVC reduces the size of the epidural veins [20].

Multiple open frame prone support systems can be used to allowing the abdomen to hang freely. Typically, these are constructed with two carbon fiber rails with a pair of hip supports and a chest support. Alternatively, blankets placed beneath the anterior superior iliac crest and a thoracic roll placed horizontally across the table can achieve the same effect of the abdomen hanging freely [69]. For craniotomies, special open frame systems such as the Allen four post system attach to the OR table. However, the clearance before the pregnant abdomen hits the table will vary. Recently, a patient at 20 weeks gestation with a cerebellar lesion underwent surgery at my institution. Different positioning aids were tested prior to surgery. Figure 18.1 shows blankets used to support the chest and pelvis in Panel a. The blankets tended to shift and were difficult to adjust; however, the abdomen can be positioned to hang freely as demonstrated in Panel b. Panel a in Fig. 18.2 shows an open frame spinal surgery top from a Mizuho OSI table on two stacked 2 × 4's at the feet and two stacked 2 × 8's at the head bolted to the frame to the operating table. A chest support was created at the head of the table consisting of two stacked 2 × 6's with a 2 in. thick foam pad. The chest support was flush with the head of the table. This solution allowed good stability, ease of adjustment, plenty of room for the gravid uterus, and the ability to use a Mayfield clamp and pins. Panel b in Fig. 18.2 shows a patient positioned using this apparatus.

In general, the prone position is well tolerated. The prone position tends to decrease cardiac output. However, the open frame prone support system has the least effect on cardiac output due largely to the lack of IVC compression [69]. Respiratory function in the prone position tends to be well tolerated because the perfusion is more evenly distributed [70]. Breast enlargement during pregnancy makes position of the chest support more difficult [70]. Ocular injuries have been reported in patients undergoing spine surgery in the prone position [69]. Pregnant women are prone to nosebleeds [15]; in terms of securing the endotracheal tube, taping the endotracheal tube to a suction catheter placed through the nares and brought out through the mouth should be avoided. The biggest complaint is the difficulty in lifting the patient to position [71]. Fetal monitoring is not always done as stopping the surgery to deliver the baby may not be safe for the mother and difficult with placement of the fetal heart rate monitor [53, 54] (see Table 18.1 for overview of the different positions).

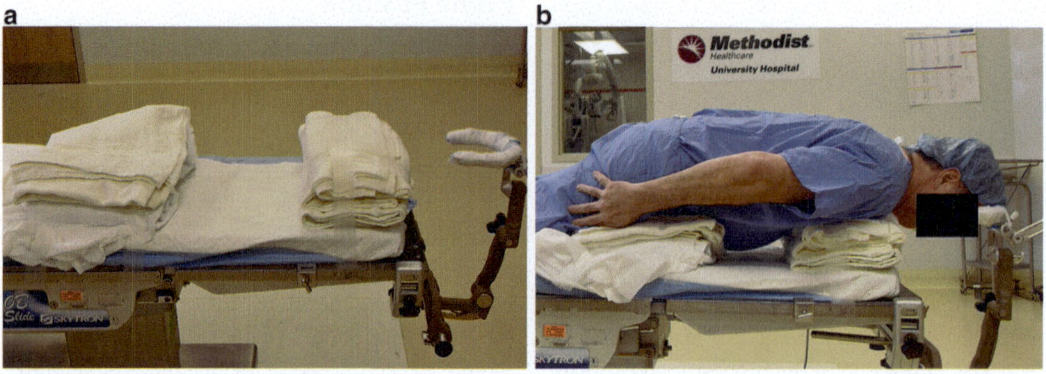

Fig. 18.1 Prone positioning using blankets for craniotomy. Panel **a** shows the blankets on the operating table. Panel **b** shows a model in the prone position for a craniotomy using blankets

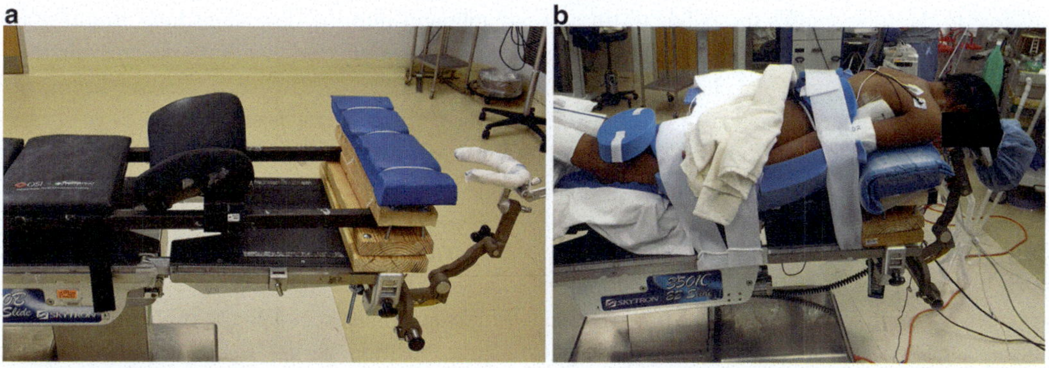

Fig. 18.2 Prone positioning using an open frame system bolted to the operating room table. Panel **a** shows the open frame system bolted to the bed. Panel **b** shows a patient in the prone position for craniotomy using the modified open frame system

Table 18.1 Advantages and disadvantages of different positions

Position	Supine	Prone	Lateral	Sitting
Advantages	1. Familiar position	1. No aortocaval compression 2. Relatively well tolerated	1. Minimal aortocaval compression 2. Works well in obese	1. Good surgical conditions
Disadvantages	1. Aortocaval compression	1. Have to lift patient 2. Obese and third trimester difficult	1. V/Q mismatch 2. Large hips and thighs increase difficulty	1. Venous air embolism 2. Aortocaval compression 3. Need special monitoring 4. Late gestation difficult
Positioning needs	Pad under right hip	Open frame system best	Axillary roll	1. Pad under right hip 2. Leg wraps 3. Frame for headholder
Ease of cesarean section	Easy	Impossible	Difficult	Unlikely
Fetal heart rate monitoring	Easy	Difficult	Easy	Easy

Lateral Position

One study on the surgical management of herniated lumbar disks suggested that the lateral position was the preferred position starting in the late second trimester [65]. The traditional lateral position is left lateral decubitus to minimize aortocaval compression. The original IVC venograms of pregnant women in the lateral position showed partial occlusion [20]. MRI studies showed that the size of the IVC in term pregnant patients in the lateral position is smaller than in nonpregnant women [23].

Positioning the pregnant woman in the lateral position presents a few challenges. First, fat deposition during pregnancy occurs in the hips and thighs. Increasing the height of the pelvis relative to the torso causes the pelvis to tilt and the spine to curve. Extra padding may have to be placed under the abdomen and chest to straighten the spine. Second, one of the goals is to allow the abdomen and gravid uterus to fall away from the IVC. If a bean bag is attempted, the edge will be elevated against the pelvis and thorax and fall away from the abdomen. In many patients, the body habitus does not allow a bean bag to be used. In these patients, flexing the lower leg at the hip and knee and leaving the upper leg straight with pillows between the legs will help stabilize the pelvis. Usually the upper torso is stabilized by securing the arms. The lower arm is most commonly placed on an armboard at roughly 90–120°. Two pillows are placed between the two arms and the upper arm secured. Alternatively, the upper arm is secured using an airplane splint. If the patient's torso is still not secure, folded blankets can be placed on both sides of the chest and secured in place by a Velcro strap over the patient's torso.

Traditionally, the right lateral decubitus position has been felt to place the patient at risk of IVC compression. One author has expressed that right lateral decubitus is contraindicated in the third trimester [72]. This is contradicted by the original description of the supine hypotensive syndrome; relief came when the patient lay on either side [17]. Studies of sleep positions in term pregnant patients indicate 27.3% of the time is spent in the left lateral decubitus position and 27.8% of the time is spent in the right lateral [66]. There are two case reports of the successful use of the right lateral decubitus position during pregnancy. Both are thoracotomies: a diaphragmatic hernia and a tuberculosis infection at T2 [73, 74].

The lateral position is associated with increased CO, decreased SVR, and decreased blood pressure [75]. The most significant problem with the lateral position is ventilation perfusion mismatch [76, 77]. The dependent lung receives greater perfusion. The nondependent lung receives the greatest ventilation. During controlled ventilation with muscle relaxant, the increased intra-abdominal pressure will shift the diaphragm into the dependent lung resulting in decreased ventilation. Arterial oxygen saturation often decreases [77]. C-sections have been performed in the lateral position in cases of severe aortocaval compression [17, 78].

Supine

Pregnant women spend 26.5% of their time in the supine position during sleep [66]. The supine position is used for cesarean section and is associated with aortocaval compression. Typically, a wedge is placed under the right hip to tilt the pelvis roughly 15° to the left. This allows the blood pressure to be maintained, and the fetus to tolerate the procedure. However, the IVC compression does not decrease until the term patient is tilted to the left 30° or more. If the surgical procedure would be bothered by dilated epidural veins or if the intracranial pressure is high, the preterm patient may have to be rotated greater than 30° to the left.

The Sitting Position

A 51 kg woman at 25 weeks gestation underwent a sitting craniotomy for a large cerebellopontine angle meningioma [79]. A pelvic wedge was placed under the right hip to tilt the pelvis to the left. Continuous fetal heart rate monitoring was used. A cardiac echocardiogram was performed to determine whether the atrial septum was intact. Doppler monitoring for air embolism was used and detected a single episode of air embolism. The sitting position provides good surgical exposure, reduces the size of veins in the cranium, reduces the need for retraction, has good pulmonary mechanics, and allows for easy monitoring of the fetus [79, 80].

The principal disadvantage of the sitting position is venous air embolism. In the sitting position, the surgical field is higher than the level of the heart. Pressure in the veins is negative, and entrainment of air into open veins can lead to air embolism [80]. Detection of air embolism involves the use of transthoracic Doppler or transesophageal echocardiography to detect microbubbles, capnography to look for decrease in end tidal CO_2, and end tidal gas monitoring to look decreases in PO_2 [80]. A central venous line is placed with the tip at the junction of the SVC and right atrium to aspirate air in the event of venous air embolism [80]. A patent foramen ovale (PFO) is viewed by some neurosurgeons as an absolute contraindication to the sitting position [80] while others view a PFO as a manageable risk [81, 82]. Autopsy reveals that 27% of people have a patent foramen ovale [83]. These individuals have a risk of paradoxical air embolism. Detection of a PFO by transesophageal echocardiography under propofol requires seeing the atrial septum bulging into the left atrium and good opacification of the right atrium. Improper technique will lead to a false negative roughly 50% of the time [84]. One study of 200 consecutive patients undergoing a sitting craniotomy had 52 patients with a PFO (26%) [81]. Only one patient had a significant venous air embolism as defined by a decrease in end tidal CO_2 >3 mmHg combined with ≥20% decrease of mean arterial blood pressure or increase in heart rate ≥40%. None of the 52 patients with a PFO had a neurological injury [81]. Another study of 600 patients had an incidence of significant venous air embolism of 3.3 and 0.5% of termination of surgery for venous air embolism [82]. There were 24 cases with a confirmed PFO with no evidence of paradoxical air embolism [82].

Hypotension and resulting decreased cerebral perfusion is another problem with the sitting position. The arterial line should be referenced at the level of the mastoid process. Changing from the supine to the sitting position decreases preload and CO and increases SVR [85]. To minimize the decrease in preload, the legs are often wrapped. A pregnant woman with aortocaval compression may be at increased risk for poor venous return particularly an obese patient or one of advanced gestational age. In the case reported, a pelvic wedge was utilized to decrease aortocaval compression [79]. This patient was only 51 kg [79]. A larger individual may have more difficulty with hypotension.

Antibiotic Prophylaxis

Piperacillin, cefazolin, and clindamycin have little overall risk to the fetus. Intravenous vancomycin is felt to be generally safe in pregnancy [86]. All four are used for prophylaxis of group B Streptococcus infections [87]. However, vancomycin is typically reserved for situations where the benefits outweigh the risks [87]. Vancomycin was given to ten pregnant women with methicillin-resistant Staphylococcus aureus infections, and the subsequent children had no hearing loss or nephrotoxicity attributed to the vancomycin [88]. Cefazolin is the first choice for antibiotic prophylaxis for craniotomy during pregnancy [89]. Piperacillin and clindamycin are potential alternatives [87, 89]. Vancomycin can be used typically in the second and third trimester after other alternatives have been considered [87, 89].

Seizure Prophylaxis

Lamotrigine and levetiracetam are considered first-line drugs for women of childbearing age for generalized seizures and focal seizures [90]. In comparison to valproate, phenytoin, and phenobarb, lamotrigine and levetiracetam are not associated with increased risk of congenital anomalies [90]. Valproate usage during pregnancy is associated with increased risk of congenital anomalies and reduced intellectual development [91]. Following the offspring of mothers on valproate monotherapy, the offspring have a reduction in intellectual development that persists at 6 years of age compared to the offspring of mothers on carbamazepine, phenytoin, or lamotrigine monotherapy [92].

Treatment of Intracranial Pressure

The treatment of intracranial pressure can involve the use of external ventricular drainage, spinal drains, hyperventilation, mannitol, lasix, and hypertonic saline solutions. The use of ventricular shunts and external ventricular drainage is well documented in the literature with no adverse effects [93, 94]. Spinal drainage of cerebrospinal fluid is also without adverse effects being used extensively in patients with idiopathic intracranial hypertension [95]. Hyperventilation is typically limited to a PCO_2 of 25–30 mmHg [96] because hyperventilation has been shown to decrease uterine blood flow [97]. Mannitol has been shown to transfer of water from the fetus to the mother. For concern of fetal dehydration, mannitol is recommended to be limited to 0.25–0.5 mg/kg [96]. Lasix has been used with monitoring of urinary output without ill effect [98]. The use of hypertonic saline in humans has not been reported. In the pregnant ewe, prolonged fluid restriction simulating drought conditions has been done with a rise in maternal sodium levels from 147 to 156 mEq/L. Although there does not appear to be fetal demise to chronic elevation, the hypothalamic-pituitary arginine vasopressin regulatory system is altered with the concern of increased risk of hypertension [99].

Tocolysis

Tocolytics are only given if needed. Nifedipine has fewer side effects but may cause hypotension [100]. Betamimetics such as terbutaline are limited by maternal side effects [90]. Indomethacin is limited by fetal side effects [101]. Magnesium sulfate is no longer considered efficacious [102]. Atosiban, an oxytocin receptor antagonist, has a good maternal side effect profile but is not approved in the United States [103].

Neurosurgery with Fetus In Utero

Aspiration pneumonitis prophylaxis such as an histamine-2 receptor blocker and reglan should be given 1 h preoperatively [104]. Pneumocompression devices should be used as the patient should have to be considered hypercoagulable [16]. A pad 12–15 cm high should be placed under the right hip to tilt the pelvis. This pad may be combined with tilting the operating table an additional 15° to relieve aortocaval compression in most patients [23]. The table can be placed in 20° reverse Trendelenburg to decrease ICP and aid in preventing regurgitation and passive aspiration of stomach contents. The pregnant woman has a decreased functional residual capacity [11] and should be preoxygenated to help prevent desaturation. Cricoid pressure can be held to decrease the risk of aspiration. To avoid the increase in intracranial pressure reported with succinylcholine [105], rapid sequence induction using a defasciculating dose of a nondepolarizing muscle and succinylcholine can be used. Alternatively, a small risk of aspiration can be accepted. A nondepolarizing muscle relaxant can be used, and the patient can be gently ventilated holding cricoid pressure. An attempt should be made to blunt the hypertensive response to laryngoscopy.

Intraoperatively, the patient is positioned according to the needs of the surgery. Specifically for craniotomies (see Table 18.2 for considerations for craniotomies), recommendations are to limit hyperventilation to a $PaCO_2$ of 25–30 mmHg [96]. Mannitol is recommended to be limited to 0.25–0.5 mg/kg [96]. Dexamethasone can be safely given to reduce peritumor edema as betamethasone has long been given for fetal lung

Table 18.2 Considerations for craniotomy with intrauterine pregnancy

- Preoperative assessment considers maternal risk and fetal viability
- Team approach recommended
- Obstetrician to determine appropriate fetal heart rate monitoring
- Aspiration prophylaxis/cricoid pressure
- Pelvic tilt to help relieve aortocaval compression during induction
- Antibiotic prophylaxis—Cefazolin [89]
- Phenylephrine—first-line drug for treatment of low blood pressure [96]
- Patient positioned according to patient condition and surgical needs
- Mild hyperventilation to $PaCO_2$ of 25–30 mmHg [96]
- Mannitol 0.25–0.5 mg/kg intravenously [96]
- Decadron as needed
- Seizure prophylaxis with Lamotrigine or Levetiracetam [90]
- Tocolysis given only if needed

maturation [96]. Phenylephrine is now recognized as the first-line drug for maintaining blood pressure not ephedrine [96]. Some anesthesiologists prefer an inhalational anesthesia with narcotics, and others prefer a total intravenous anesthetic [96]. The goals of the anesthetic are: (1) maintain the maternal blood pressure in the patient's normal range, (2) maintain good maternal oxygenation, (3) maintain a relatively normal acid-base status, and (4) use as little phenylephrine as possible.

To illustrate, a patient at 20 weeks gestation underwent a resection of a cerebellar hemangioblastoma in the prone position. The patient was given aspiration prophylaxis and had pneumocompression devices applied. The patient was placed in 20° reverse Trendelenburg with a pad under her right hip at time of induction. After preoxygenation, she was induced with propofol, remifentanil, and zemuron while maintaining cricoid pressure. She was placed in the prone position using the apparatus shown in Figure 18.2b. She was maintained with desflurane and remifentanil. Cefazolin was given for antibiotic prophylaxis. For exposure, only mild hyperventilation was required. Preoperative and postoperative fetal ultrasounds were performed. No intraoperative fetal heart rate monitoring was performed as the fetus would be best resuscitated in utero rather than delivered. No seizure prophylaxis or tocolysis was given.

Neurosurgery with Cesarean Section

Induction of anesthesia begins in the same manner as described above. Rarely, neurosurgery begins at the same time as the cesarean section [106]. More commonly, the c-section is performed first, and the patient is repositioned for neurosurgery [96]. In positioning, the uterus is still of a size to cause aortocaval compression [33]. CO and plasma volume are at the highest levels [4, 6]. Blood loss from c-section is offset by autotransfusion from contraction of the uterus [9, 10]. After c-section, postpartum hemorrhage is treated by lowering the dose of the volatile anesthetic and giving oxytocin derivatives [96]. Ergot derivatives should be avoided as they can cause cerebral vasoconstriction [104].

If neurosurgery can be delayed, the uterus should return to the pelvis at the end of 2 weeks, and aortocaval compression is less likely. CO will have decreased, and increases in plasma volume will have diminished [4, 6]. However, 6 weeks is considered the time that most of the physiologic changes have returned to baseline [4, 6, 13, 33].

Conclusions

Positioning of the pregnant patient must be individualized to meet the needs of the patient, the fetus, and the surgeon. The goals of positioning and anesthesia are to avoid aortocaval compression, compression of the uterus, and to maintain as normal maternal state as possible.

References

1. American College of Obstetricians and Gynecologists Committee Opinion No. 548. Weight gain during pregnancy. Obstet Gynecol. 2013;121(1):210–2.
2. Johnson J, Clifton RG, Roberts JM, Myatt L, Hauth JC, Spong CY, et al. Pregnancy outcomes with weight gain above or below the 2009 Institute of Medicine guidelines. Obstet Gynecol. 2013;121(5):969–75.
3. Sohlström A, Forsum E. Changes in adipose tissue volume and distribution during reproduction in Swedish women as assessed by magnetic resonance imaging. Am J Clin Nutr. 1995;61(2):287–95.
4. Hunter S, Robson SC. Adaptation of the maternal heart in pregnancy. Br Heart J. 1992;68(6):540–3.
5. Sharma R, Kumar A, Aneja GK. Serial changes in pulmonary hemodynamics during pregnancy: a non-invasive study using Doppler echocardiography. Cardiol Res. 2016;7(1):25–31.
6. de Haas S, Ghossein-Doha C, van Kuijk SM, van Drongelen J, Spaanderman ME. Physiological adaptation of maternal plasma volume during pregnancy: a systematic review and meta-analysis. Ultrasound Obstet Gynecol. 2017;49(2):177–87.
7. Clark SL, Cotton DB, Lee W, Bishop C, Hill T, Southwick J, et al. Central hemodynamic assessment of normal term pregnancy. Am J Obstet Gynecol. 1989;161(6 Pt 1):1439–42.
8. Güngördük K, Asicioğlu O, Yildirim G, Gungorduk OC, Besimoglu B, Ark CI. Post-partum oxygen inhalation useful for reducing vaginal blood loss during

the third and fourth stages of labour? A randomised controlled study. Aust N Z J Obstet Gynaecol. 2011;51(5):441–5.
9. Lakshmi SD, Abraham R. Role of prophylactic tranexamic acid in reducing blood loss during elective caesarean section: a randomized controlled study. J Clin Diagn Res. 2016;10(12):QC17–21.
10. Rosseland LA, Hauge TH, Grindheim G, Stubhaug A, Langesæter E. Changes in blood pressure and cardiac output during cesarean delivery: the effects of oxytocin and carbetocin compared with placebo. Anesthesiology. 2013;119(3):541–51.
11. Bhatia PK, Biyani G, Mohammed S, Sethi P, Bihani P. Acute respiratory failure and mechanical ventilation in pregnant patient: a narrative review of literature. J Anaesthesiol Clin Pharmacol. 2016;32(4):431–9.
12. Shinagawa S, Suzuki S, Chihara H, Otsubo Y, Takeshita T, Araki T. Maternal basal metabolic rate in twin pregnancy. Gynecol Obstet Investig. 2005;60(3):145–8.
13. Hussein W, Lafayette RA. Renal function in normal and disordered pregnancy. Curr Opin Nephrol Hypertens. 2014;23(1):46–53.
14. Mushambi MC, Kinsella SM, Popat M, Swales H, Ramaswamy KK, Winton AL, et al. Obstetric Anaesthetists' Association and Difficult Airway Society guidelines for the management of difficult and failed tracheal intubation in obstetrics. Anaesthesia. 2015;70(11):1286–306.
15. Crunkhorn RE, Mitchell-Innes A, Muzaffar J. Torrential epistaxis in the third trimester: a management conundrum. BMJ Case Rep. 2014.; pii:bcr2014203892.
16. Collins J, Bowles L, MacCallum PK. Prevention and management of venous thromboembolism in pregnancy. Br J Hosp Med (Lond). 2016;77(12):C194–200.
17. Howard BK, Goodson JH, Mengert WF. Supine hypotensive syndrome in late pregnancy. Obstet Gynecol. 1953;1(4):371–7.
18. Wright L. Postural hypotension in late pregnancy. "The supine hypotensive syndrome". Br Med J. 1962; 1(5280):760–2.
19. Holmes F. The supine hypotensive syndrome: its importance to the anaesthetist. Anaesthesia. 1960;15:298–306.
20. Kerr MG, Scott DB, Samuel E. Studies of the inferior vena cava in late pregnancy. Br Med J. 1964; 1(5382):532–3.
21. Bieniarz J, Crottogini JJ, Curuchet E, Romero-Salinas G, Yoshida T, Poseiro JJ, et al. Aorto-caval compression by the uterus in late human pregnancy. II. An arteriographic study. Am J Obstet Gynecol. 1968;100:203–17.
22. Kienzl D, Berger-Kulemann V, Kasprian G, Brugger PC, Weber M, Bettelheim D, et al. Risk of inferior vena cava compression syndrome during fetal MRI in the supine position—a retrospective analysis. J Perinat Med. 2014;42(3):301–6.
23. Higuchi H, Takagi S, Zhang K, Furui I, Ozaki M. Effect of lateral tilt angle on the volume of the abdominal aorta and inferior vena cava in pregnant and nonpregnant women determined by magnetic resonance imaging. Anesthesiology. 2015; 122(2):286–93.
24. McLennan CE. Antecubital and femoral venous pressures in normal and toxemic pregnancy. Am J Obstet Gynecol. 1943;45(4):568–91.
25. Kiefer RT, Ploppa A, Dieterich HJ. Aortocaval compression syndrome. Anaesthesist. 2003;52(11): 1073–83.
26. Jeejeebhoy FM, Zelop CM, Lipman S, Carvalho B, Joglar J, Mhyre JM, et al. Cardiac arrest in pregnancy: a scientific statement from the American Heart Association. Circulation. 2015;132(18):1747–73.
27. Rossi A, Cornette J, Johnson MR, Karamermer Y, Springeling T, Opic P, et al. Quantitative cardiovascular magnetic resonance in pregnant women: cross-sectional analysis of physiological parameters throughout pregnancy and the impact of the supine position. J Cardiovasc Magn Reson. 2011;13(1):31.
28. Gaiser R. Anesthetic considerations in the obese parturient. Clin Obstet Gynecol. 2016;59(1): 193–203.
29. Kim YI, Chandra P, Marx GF. Successful management of severe aortocaval compression in twin pregnancy. Obstet Gynecol. 1975;46(3):362–4.
30. Magee DA. Bicornuate uterus and aortocaval compression. Anaesthesia. 1983;38(4):352–4.
31. Kucur SK, Acar C, Temizkan O, Ozagari A, Gozukara I, Akyol A. A huge ovarian mucinous cystadenoma causing virilization, preterm labor, and persistent supine hypotensive syndrome during pregnancy. Autops Case Rep. 2016;6(2):39–43.
32. Hsu KF, Pan HA, Hsu YY, Wu CM, Chung WJ, Huan SC. Enhanced myometrial autophagy in postpartum uterine involution. Taiwan J Obstet Gynecol. 2014;53(3):293–302.
33. Sangestani G, Bashirian S. A normal pattern of uterine involution using s-fd in primiparous women and the prevalence of uterine subinvolution. J Med Sci (Faisalabad, Pak). 2006;6:1011–4.
34. Negishi H, Kishida T, Yamada H, Hirayama E, Mikuni M, Fujimoto S. Changes in uterine size after vaginal delivery and cesarean section determined by vaginal sonography in the puerperium. Arch Gynecol Obstet. 1999;263(1–2):13–6.
35. Xu F, Liu Y, Wei Y, Zhao Y, Yuan H, Guo X. Differences in lumbar dural sac dimension in supine and lateral positions in late pregnancy: a magnetic resonance imaging study. Int J Obstet Anesth. 2016;26:19–23.
36. Takiguchi T, Yamaguchi S, Tezuka M, Furukawa N, Kitajima T. Compression of the subarachnoid space by the engorged epidural venous plexus in pregnant women. Anesthesiology. 2006;105(4):848–51.
37. Hirabayashi Y, Shimizu R, Fukuda H, Saitoh K, Igarashi T. Effects of the pregnant uterus on the extradural venous plexus in the supine and lateral

positions, as determined by magnetic resonance imaging. Br J Anaesth. 1997;78(3):317–9.
38. Hilt H, Gramm HJ, Link J. Changes in intracranial pressure associated with extradural anaesthesia. Br J Anaesth. 1986;58(6):676–80.
39. Eckstein KL, Marx GF. Aortocaval compression and uterine displacement. Anesthesiology. 1974;40(1):92–6.
40. Fields JM, Catallo K, Au AK, Rotte M, Leventhal D, Weiner S, et al. Resuscitation of the pregnant patient: what is the effect of patient positioning on inferior vena cava diameter? Resuscitation. 2013;84(3):304–8.
41. Crawford JS, Burton M, Davies P. Time and lateral tilt at caesarean section. Br J Anaesth. 1972; 44(5):477–84.
42. ACOG Committee on Obstetric Practice Committee opinion no. 474. Nonobstetric surgery during pregnancy. Obstet Gynecol. 2011;117(2 Pt 1):420–1.
43. Papageorghiou AT, Ohuma EO, Gravett MG, Hirst J, da Silveira MF, Lambert A, et al. International standards for symphysis-fundal height based on serial measurements from the fetal growth longitudinal study of the INTERGROWTH-21st Project: prospective cohort study in eight countries. BMJ. 2016;355:i5662.
44. Calvert JP, Crean EE, Newcombe RG, Pearson JF. Antenatal screening by measurement of symphysis-fundus height. Br Med J (Clin Res Ed). 1982;285(6345):846–9.
45. Haragan AF, Hulsey TC, Hawk AF, Newman RB, Chang EY. Diagnostic accuracy of fundal height and handheld ultrasound-measured abdominal circumference to screen for fetal growth abnormalities. Am J Obstet Gynecol. 2015;212(6):820.e1–8.
46. Moore KA, Simpson JA, Thomas KH, Rijken MJ, White LJ, Dwell LM, et al. Estimating gestational age in late presenters to antenatal care in a resource-limited setting on the Thai-Myanmar border. PLoS One. 2015;10(6):e0131025.
47. Ohuma EO, Papageorghiou AT, Villar J, Altman DG. Estimation of gestational age in early pregnancy from crown-rump length when gestational age range is truncated: the case study of the INTERGROWTH-21st project. BMC Med Res Methodol. 2013;13:151.
48. Buscicchio G, Milite V, D'Emidio L, Giorlandino M, Cavaliere A, Padula F, et al. (2008). Analysis of fetal biometric measurements in the last 30 years. J Prenat Med. 2008;2(1):11–3.
49. Czeresnia JM, Araujo Júnior E, Cordioli E, Martins WP, Nardozza LMM, Moron AF. Applicability of the rapid biophysical profile in antepartum fetal well-being assessment in high-risk pregnancies from a university hospital in São Paulo, Brazil: preliminary results. ISRN Obstet Gynecol. 2013;2013:329542.
50. Committee opinion no. 687: approaches to limit intervention during labor and birth. Obstet Gynecol. 2017;129(2):e20–8.
51. Sweha A, Hacker TW, Nuovo J. Interpretation of the electronic fetal heart rate during labor. Am Fam Physician. 1999;59(9):2487–500.
52. Jacob J, Alexander A, Philip S, Thomas A. Prone position craniotomy in pregnancy without fetal heart rate monitoring. J Clin Anesth. 2016;33:119–22.
53. Martel CG, Volpi-Abadie J, Ural K. Anesthetic management of the parturient for lumbar disc surgery in the prone position. Ochsner J. 2015;15(3):259–61.
54. Lee JM, Han IH, Moon SH, Choi BK. Surgery for recurrent lumbar disc herniation during pregnancy: a case report. Korean J Spine. 2011;8(4):304–6.
55. Kathirgamanathan A, Jardine AD, Levy DM, Grevitt MP. Lumbar disc surgery in the third trimester—with the fetus in utero. Int J Obstet Anesth. 2006;15(2):181–2.
56. Rysavy MA, Li L, Bell EF, Das A, Hintz SR, Stoll BJ, et al. Between-hospital variation in treatment and outcomes in extremely preterm infants. N Engl J Med. 2015;372(19):1801–11.
57. Ishii N, Kono Y, Yonemoto N, Kusuda S, Fujimura M. Outcomes of infants born at 22 and 23 weeks' gestation. Neonatal Research Network, Japan. Pediatrics. 2013;132:62–71.
58. Costeloe KL, Hennessy EM, Haider S, Stacey F, Marlow N, Draper ES. Short term outcomes after extreme preterm birth in England: comparison of two birth cohorts in1995 and 2006 (the EPICure studies). BMJ. 2012;345:e7976.
59. Horbar JD, Carpenter JH, Badger GJ, Kenny MJ, Soll RF, Morrow KA, et al. Mortality and neonatal morbidity among infants 501 to 1500 grams from 2000 to 2009. Pediatrics. 2012;129(6):1019–26.
60. American College of Obstetricians and Gynecologists' Committee on Obstetric Practice. Committee opinion no. 656: Guidelines for diagnostic imaging during pregnancy and lactation. Obstet Gynecol. 2016;127(2):e75–80.
61. Ray JG, Vermeulen MJ, Bharatha A, Montanera WJ, Park AL. Association between MRI exposure during pregnancy and fetal and childhood outcomes. JAMA. 2016;316(9):952–61.
62. Lv X, Liu P, Li Y. The clinical characteristics and treatment of cerebral avm in pregnancy. Neuroradiol J. 2015;28(3):234–7.
63. Pantelis E, Antypas C, Frassanito MC, Sideri L, Salvara K, Lekas L, et al. Radiation dose to the fetus during CyberKnife radiosurgery for a brain tumor in pregnancy. Phys Med. 2016;32(1):237–41.
64. Nagayama K, Kurita H, Tonari A, Takayama M, Shiokawa Y. Radiosurgery for cerebral arteriovenous malformation during pregnancy: a case report focusing on fetal exposure to radiation. Asian J Neurosurg. 2010;5(2):73–7.
65. Ardaillon H, Laviv Y, Arle JE, Kasper EM. Lumbar disk herniation during pregnancy: a review on general management and timing of surgery. Acta Neurochir (Wien) [Internet]. 2017; [cited 2017 Jan 31]; Epub 2017 Jan 31. Available from Acta Neurochirurica.

https://link.springer.com/article/10.1007/s00701-017-3098-z.
66. O'Brien LM, Warland J. Typical sleep positions in pregnant women. Early Hum Dev. 2014;90(6):315–7.
67. Hunter S, Hofmeyr GJ, Kulier R. Hands and knees posture in late pregnancy or labour for fetal malposition (lateral or posterior). Cochrane Database Syst Rev. 2007;17(4):CD001063.
68. Thurlow JA, Kinsella SM. Intrauterine resuscitation: active management of fetal distress. Int J Obstet Anesth. 2002;11(2):105–16.
69. Feix B, Sturgess J. Anaesthesia in the prone position. Contin Educ Anaesth Crit Care Pain. 2014;14(6):291–7.
70. Edgcombe H, Carter K, Yarrow S. Anaesthesia in the prone position. Br J Anaesth. 2008;100(2):165–83.
71. Acheson S, Davies M. Safe lifting of anaesthetised patients. Anaesthesia. 2014;69(4):398.
72. Hakan T. Lumbar disk herniation presented with cauda equina syndrome in a pregnant woman. J Neurosci in Rural Pract. 2012;3(2):197–9.
73. Kaul R, Chhabra HS, Kanagaraju V, Mahajan R, Tandon V, Nanda A, et al. Antepartum surgical management of Pott's paraplegia along with maintenance of pregnancy during second trimester. Eur Spine J. 2016;25(4):1064–9.
74. Julien F, Drolet S, Lévesque I, Bouchard A. The right lateral position for laparoscopic diaphragmatic hernia repair in pregnancy: technique and review of the literature. J Laparoendosc Adv Surg Tech A. 2011;21(1):67–70.
75. Fujise K, Shingu K, Matsumoto S, Nagata A, Mikami O, Matsuda T. The effects of the lateral position on cardiopulmonary function during laparoscopic urological surgery. Anesth Analg. 1998;87(4):925–30.
76. Klingstedt C, Hedenstierna G, Baehrendtz S, Lundqvist H, Strandberg A, Tokics L, et al. Ventilation-perfusion relationships and atelectasis formation in the supine and lateral positions during conventional mechanical and differential ventilation. Acta Anaesthesiol Scand. 1990;34(6):421–9.
77. Joo J, Kim YH, Lee J, Choi JH. Difference in the value of arterial and end-tidal carbon dioxide tension according to different surgical positions: does it reliably reflect ventilation-perfusion mismatch? Korean J Anesthesiol. 2012;63(3):216–20.
78. Coffman JC, Legg RL, Coffman CF, Moran KR. Lateral position for cesarean delivery because of severe aortocaval compression in a patient with Marfan syndrome: a case report. A A Case Rep. 2017;8(5):93–5.
79. Giannini A, Bricchi M. Posterior fossa surgery in the sitting position in a pregnant patient with cerebellopontine angle meningioma. Br J Anaesth. 1999;82(6):941–4.
80. Porter JM, Pidgeon C, Cunningham AJ. The sitting position in neurosurgery: a critical appraisal. Br J Anaesth. 1999;82(1):117–28.
81. Feigl GC, Decker K, Wurms M, Krischek B, Ritz R, Unertl K, et al. Neurosurgical procedures in the semi-sitting position: evaluation of the risk of paradoxical venous air embolism in patients with a patent foramen ovale. World Neurosurg. 2014;81(1):159–64.
82. Ganslandt O, Merkel A, Schmitt H, Tzabazis A, Buchfelder M, Eyupoglu I, et al. The sitting position in neurosurgery: indications, complications and results. A single institution experience of 600 cases. Acta Neurochir. 2013;155(10):1887–93.
83. Hagen PT, Scholz DG, Edwards WD. Incidence and size of patent foramen ovale during the first 10 decades of life: an autopsy study of 965 normal hearts. Mayo Clin Proc. 1984;59:17–20.
84. Johansson MC, Eriksson P, Guron CW, Dellborg M. Pitfalls in diagnosing PFO: characteristics of false-negative contrast injections during transesophageal echocardiography in patients with patent foramen ovales. J Am Soc Echocardiogr. 2010;23(11):1136–42.
85. Dalrymple DG, Macgowan SW, Macleod GF. Cardiorespiratory effects of the sitting position in neurosurgery. Br J Anaesth. 1979;51:1079–82.
86. Bookstaver PB, Bland CM, Griffin B, Stover KR, Eiland LS, McLaughlin MA. Review of antibiotic use in pregnancy. Pharmacotherapy. 2015;35(11):1052–62.
87. Apgar BS, Greenberg G, Yen G. Prevention of group B streptococcal disease in the newborn. Am Fam Physician. 2005;75(5):903–10.
88. Reyes MP, Ostrea EM Jr, Cabinian AE, Schmitt C, Rintelmann W. Vancomycin during pregnancy: does it cause hearing loss or nephrotoxicity in the infant? Am J Obstet Gynecol. 1989;161(4):977–81.
89. Bratzler DW, Dellinger EP, Olsen KM, Perl TM, Auwaerter PG, Bolon MK, et al. Clinical practice guidelines for antimicrobial prophylaxis in surgery. Am J Health Syst Pharm. 2013;70(3):195–283.
90. Weston J, Bromley R, Jackson CF, Adab N, Clayton-Simth J, Greenhalgh J, et al. Monotherapy treatment of epilepsy in pregnancy: congenital malformation outcomes in the child. Cochrane Database Syst Rev. 2016;11:CD010224.
91. Tomson T, Marson A, Boon P, Canevini MP, Covanis A, Gaily E, et al. Valproate in the treatment of epilepsy in girls and women of childbearing potential. Epilepsia. 2015;56(7):1006–19.
92. Meador KJ, Baker GA, Browning N, Cohen MJ, Bromley RL, Clayton-Smith J, et al. Fetal antiepileptic drug exposure and cognitive outcomes at age 6 years (NEAD study): a prospective observational study. Lancet Neurol. 2013;12(3):244–52.
93. Hernández-Durán S, Sánchez-Jiménez E, Pérez-Berríos J. Hemangiopericytoma of the foramen magnum in a pregnant patient: a case report and literature review. Surg Neurol Int. 2014;5:13.
94. Jung YJ, Kim MA, Kwon JY, Lee HR, Cho HY, Park YW, et al. Pregnancy outcomes in women with moyamoya disease: experiences at a single center in korea. Yonsei Med J. 2015;56(3):793–7.
95. Bagga R, Jain V, Gupta KR, Gopalan S, Malhotra S, Das CP. Choice of therapy and mode of delivery

in idiopathic intracranial hypertension during pregnancy. MedGenMed. 2005;7(4):42.
96. Wang LP, Paech MJ. Neuroanesthesia for the pregnant woman. Anesth Analg. 2008;107(1):193–200.
97. Levinson G, Shnider SM, deLorimier AA, Steffenson JL. Effects of maternal hyperventilation on uterine blood flow and fetal oxygenation and acid-base status. Anesthesiology. 1974;40(4):340–7.
98. Kazemi P, Villar G, Flexman A. Anesthetic management of neurosurgical procedures during pregnancy: a case series. J Neurosurg Anesthesiol. 2014; 26(3):234–40.
99. Ramirez BA, Wang S, Kallichanda N, Ross MG. Chronic in utero plasma hyperosmolality alters hypothalamic arginine vasopressin synthesis and pituitary arginine vasopressin content in newborn lambs. Am J Obstet Gynecol. 2002;187(1):191–6.
100. Padovani TR, Guyatt G, Lopes LC. Nifedipine *versus* terbutaline, tocolytic effectiveness and maternal and neonatal adverse effects: a randomized, controlled pilot trial. Basic Clin Pharmacol Toxicol. 2015;116:244–50.
101. Hammers AL, Sanchez-Ramos L, Kaunitz AM. Antenatal exposure to indomethacin increases the risk of severe intraventricular hemorrhage, necrotizing enterocolitis, and periventricular leukomalacia: a systematic review with metaanalysis. Am J Obstet Gynecol. 2015;212(4):505.e1–13.
102. Wolf HT, Huusom L, Weber T, Piedvache A, Schmidt S, Norman M, et al. Use of magnesium sulfate before 32 weeks of gestation: a European population-based cohort study. BMJ Open. 2017;7(1):e013952.
103. van Vliet EO, Nijman TA, Schuit E, Heida KY, Opmeer BC, Kok M, et al. Nifedipine versus atosiban for threatened preterm birth (APOSTEL III): a multicentre, randomised controlled trial. Lancet. 2016;387(10033):2117–24.
104. Tawfik MM, Badran BA, Eisa AA, Barakat RI. Simultaneous cesarean delivery and craniotomy in a term pregnant patient with traumatic brain injury. Saudi J Anaesth. 2015;9(2):207–10.
105. Clancy M, Halford S, Walls R, Murphy M. In patients with head injuries who undergo rapid sequence intubation using succinylcholine, does pretreatment with a competitive neuromuscular blocking agent improve outcome? A literature review. Emerg Med J. 2001;18(5):373–5.
106. Wouters B, Sanford DB. Anesthetic management of a simultaneous emergency craniotomy and cesarean delivery. AANA J. 2013;81(5):394–8.

Postoperative Positioning in the Neurointensive Care Unit

19

Abhi Pandhi and Lucas Elijovich

Introduction

Positioning of patients in the operating room (OR) is extremely important to the success of neurosurgical procedures. Patient outcomes are also influenced by positioning outside of the OR including during transport and while in the intensive care unit. Neurosurgeons and critical care providers need to be well versed in the proper positioning in each of their respective settings in order to optimize patient outcomes. Positioning varies based on comorbidities, type of pathology, timing of injury, and type of surgical intervention. The fundamentals of proper positioning are rooted in an understanding of the interaction of neurosurgical pathology with basic principles of neurophysiology, cardiovascular hemodynamics, and respiratory physiology. There are multiple goals when considering proper positioning in intensive care unit. These include minimizing postoperative pain and prevention of delayed complications and mitigating any intraoperative complications. In addition, positioning should optimize the postoperative physiologic conditions for liberation from mechanical ventilation and invasive monitors to shorten the overall ICU length of stay. This chapter will provide a review on basic concepts of ICU positioning with a specific review of postoperative positioning considerations in the neurocritical care unit using a framework based on type of neurosurgical procedure performed.

A. Pandhi · L. Elijovich (✉)
Department of Neurology, University of Tennessee Health Sciences Center, Memphis, TN, USA

Semmes-Murphey Neurologic Institute, University of Tennessee Health Sciences Center, Memphis, TN, USA
e-mail: apandhi@uthsc.edu; lelijovich@semmes-murphey.com

Review of Basic Positions and General Principles

The overwhelming majority of patients in the neurocritical care unit are supine in the immediate postoperative period with varying levels of reverse and standard Trendelenburg positioning. Other less commonly utilized positions include prone and more rarely prolonged or frequent lateral positioning. Independent of the position some of the common concerns for patients in a prolonged immobile state is development of compression neuropathy, deep venous thrombosis, and skin breakdown/pressure ulcers. These are rarely encountered in elective surgical patients with short ICU stays but are of major concern in acutely ill patients, like those with aneurysmal subarachnoid hemorrhage or severe spinal cord injuries, who often have prolonged intensive care units stays [1].

A. Arthur et al. (eds.), *Perioperative Considerations and Positioning for Neurosurgical Procedures*,
https://doi.org/10.1007/978-3-319-72679-3_19

In the supine position, the shoulders, elbow, wrist, and gluteal area need to be sufficiently padded to prevent compression neuropathy. Padding in the ICU is generally accomplished with foam blocks of various shapes and sizes. Towel rolls are also employed and can be placed under the knees with feet suspended by padding under calves to minimize venous restriction to prevent deep venous thrombosis. Air mattresses are the standard equipment to reduce pressure phenomenon on peripheral nerves and venous structures. In addition, the lower extremities should be positioned at the level of the heart to maintain venous return whenever the patient is not upright or actively being mobilized. This will maintain both cardiac output and prevent venous thromboembolism [2, 3]. Patients in the neurocritical care unit are one of the highest risk groups of any ICU patient population for deep venous thrombosis due to the immobility of one or multiple extremities that may accompany critical illness. It is important to emphasize that in addition to positioning use of pharmacologic venous thromboembolism prophylaxis is proven to be efficacious and safe in the immediate perioperative period for all neurosurgical pathologies including aneurysmal subarachnoid hemorrhage, traumatic brain injury, and brain tumors [4–9].

Common positions have predictable physiologic effects that are important to consider in concert with the completed surgery and patient comorbid conditions when recovering in the ICU. In the supine and Trendelenburg positions, there is cranial displacement of the diaphragm and abdominal compartment leading to reduced functional capacity. Atelectasis is also promoted and also worsens ventilation perfusion matching [10, 11]. Trendelenburg positioning with the head down is rarely employed in the NICU due to the deleterious effects of raised intracranial pressure. It has similar effects on pulmonary and cardiovascular physiology to supine positioning but are more pronounced in terms of increased venous return, mean arterial pressure, and cardiac output. Head down positioning can also precipitate airway edema if prolonged and is an important postoperative consideration for spine surgery that will be discussed further below [12, 13].

Prone positioning in the intensive care unit is employed almost exclusively for mechanically ventilated patients with severe hypoxia due to adult respiratory distress syndrome (ARDS). The most common preventable injuries in prone patients are disorders of peripheral nerve compression. Radial and ulnar neuropathies can be prevented by keeping arms in slightly flexed position which prevents excessive traction in either direction. Brachial plexus injuries can occur with rostral or caudal traction on shoulders. Another injury from inadequate padding is due to pressure on anterior superior iliac crest, which can lead to lateral femoral cutaneous neuropathy. Rarely vascular compression of external iliac artery can be seen as well due to prolonged compression in inguinal region. Ideally the face and head should be gently suspended without any site of compression and shoulders overhanging the chest rolls. Careful examination of male genitalia should be done to avoid any compression between thighs or gluteal folds [14].

Patients with ARDS may also require beds that continuously rotate from prone to supine positioning. There are multiple commercially available rotational beds that provide the above described whole body padding including the careful pelvic and cranial suspension. Rotational beds improve oxygenation in ARDS via recruitment of atelectatic lung segments and promote better ventilation perfusion matching and also increase the functional residual capacity. Although ARDS is rare in the neurosurgical population as a whole, it is not uncommon in patients who have poly-trauma including traumatic brain injury (TBI) or spinal cord injury (SCI) [15, 16]. Patients with these types of neurologic injuries who are prone require special attention to intracranial pressure and cerebral and spinal cord perfusion pressure due to disturbed autoregulation which can make cerebral blood flow pressure passive. Prone positioning may precipitate crisis of ICP and or cerebral perfusion if the patient is not properly positioned. The abdomen should be kept suspended to prevent venous compression which can lead to significant epidural venous hypertension which impairs blood flow to the spinal cord via retrograde venous hypertension. Additionally, abdominal compression may compress the vena cava and reducing blood return from the lower extremities impairing preload and as a result reducing the cardiac output. This reduction in cardiac output will in turn impair cerebral and spinal perfusion pressure, particularly when autoregulation is compromised [17].

Prone or rotational positioning poses additional challenge in the neurocritical care unit due to the increased sedation needs of these patients which in conjunction with pharmacologic paralysis severely limits the neurologic exam. For these reasons, prior to being placed in a prone position for ARDS the neurosurgeon and critical care provider must decide whether prophylactic procedures must be performed to minimize the risk of secondary neurologic injury. Predicting individual patient's tolerance for prone positioning must be done on a case by case basis. Generally, this is a last resort for patients who have exhausted all attempts at acceptable oxygenation. A simple trial of lying the patient flat may help indicate tolerability of prone positioning in terms of ICP but the hemodynamic effects of prone positioning are unique and unpredictable. Therefore, in the case of severe TBI maximal efforts like decompressive hemicraniectomy and pharmacologic paralysis with pentobarbital coma should be considered prior to prone positioning.

Transfer of Critically Ill Neurosurgical Patients

One of the first considerations with any operative procedure is the disposition of the patient at the completion of the case. This is institutionally dependent and protocols are useful regarding routine recovery either in the post-anesthesia care unit (PACU) or directly in the intensive care unit. Recovery directly in the NICU has the advantage of direct and fewer transports and improved bed flow. Another important advantage is that the NICU nursing staff is more familiar with early postoperative neurologic complications. However, this is balanced by less experience with managing the normal physiologic response to emergence from anesthesia and potential immediate post-anesthetic complications. Therefore, we feel that transfer directly to the NICU should only occur when a neurointensivist or advanced practice nurse is immediately available upon the patient's arrival to receive a complete handoff from the anesthesia provider. Delayed emergence is the most concerning post-anesthetic complication. This may be due to a number of factors including incomplete clearance of anesthetic, paralytics, opioids, or due to the presence of cholinesterase deficiency, or pre-existing or new neurologic injury [18, 19].

Once admitted to the ICU, transport for imaging or other diagnostic testing outside of the unit after the surgery is often necessary but should not be viewed as a risk-free endeavor. Transport from the ICU requires supine positioning with all of its attendant potential complications in regard to ICP, cardiovascular hemodynamics, and respiratory mechanics. Although routine postoperative CTs are commonly ordered by many neurosurgeons, this practice has not been demonstrated to improve outcomes or significantly reduce complications [20, 21]. On the contrary, several studies demonstrate that the more intrahospital transports a patient experiences the risk of invasive device failure, nosocomial infection, or severe physiologic derangements are increased [22]. Therefore, every diagnostic test should be performed in the ICU when possible and any other tests requiring travel should be minimized if not absolutely necessary.

Neurosurgical Procedures and Intensive Care Unit Positioning

Positioning of the patient post neurological surgery depends largely on the degree and type of pathology and the specific operative intervention performed. Given the large number and wide variety of neurosurgical procedures, it is beyond the scope of this chapter to discuss every surgery and the best postoperative strategy. Therefore, we will discuss positioning as it relates to some of the most common cerebrovascular, cranial, and spine surgeries as a framework to illustrate the key pathophysiologic principles that are common to all neurosurgical procedures with a focus on complication avoidance and management.

Neuroendovascular Surgery

The explosive growth of neuroendovascular surgery in the last 30 years has fundamentally changed the practice of neurosurgery and neurocritical care. It has provided a method of treatment for patients with acute ischemic stroke, improved aneurysmal subarachnoid hemorrhage outcomes, and provided adjunctive multimodality treatments for arteriovenous malformations and brain tumors [23–27]. Despite the minimally invasive nature of these procedures, the postoperative course must be managed with the same care and attention to detail as open neurosurgical procedures. The arterial access point for neuroendovascular surgery is almost always the femoral site and usually ranges from a 4 to 9 French size arteriotomy [28]. Positioning of the leg should remain straight for a period of 4–6 h post procedure after sheath removal. The neurointensivists and nursing staff should note the manner of hemostasis (manual compression or closure device). Regardless of the mode of hemostasis, flexion at the hip or knee or sitting the patient up prematurely may precipitate bleeding from the access site. The sheath may also be sewn in place at the end of the procedure and placed on a pressure bag for blood pressure monitoring. Flexion at the hip may lead to dislodging of the sheath, kinking resulting in thrombosis and inaccurate blood pressures, or force it against the arterial wall which may cause dissection of the femoral artery with repetitive movement.

Mechanical Thrombectomy (MT): Autoregulation and Cerebral Blood Flow

Mechanical thrombectomy (MT) is the standard of care treatment in addition to IV tPA for acute ischemic stroke (AIS) caused emergent large vessel occlusion (ELVO) . Multiple randomized controlled trails (RCTs) and meta-analysis have shown absolute benefit of MT for selected ELVO patients [29–34]. It is rapidly becoming the most common neuroendovascular surgery seen in most NICUs. Post-MT positioning should be focused on optimizing the physiologic conditions for brain perfusion. Autoregulation is disturbed with cerebral blood flow becoming pressure passive in many AIS patients. Therefore, supine positioning is often advocated for these patients [35]. This is particularly important in cases of incomplete recanalization of the occluded artery where cerebral blood flow to vulnerable ischemic tissue is most affected by the pressure passive state. In this situation, it may be preferred to keep the patient supine to augment cerebral blood flow via collateral channels. However, completely supine positioning may be limited by other comorbidities common to the stroke patient such as congestive heart failure or chronic obstructive pulmonary disease [36, 37]. In patients who can't be supine immediately post procedure, reverse Trendelenburg positioning with the access site leg straight is often necessary. The systolic blood pressure from the femoral arterial sheath should be expected to be approximately 20 mmHg higher routinely and as the heart is elevated further above the femoral artery this discrepancy should increase [38].

Endovascular Aneurysm Coiling and Microsurgical Clipping in Subarachnoid Hemorrhage, Positioning for Optimizing Cerebral Blood Flow and Intracranial Pressure

Aneurysmal subarachnoid hemorrhage (aSAH) patients often have prolonged courses in the NICU with severe pathophysiologic derangements in multiple organ systems simultaneously. These include electrolyte and volume status disorders with cerebral salt wasting and SIADH, respiratory failure requiring mechanical ventilation, cardiovascular and cerebrovascular hemodynamic disorders with neurocardiogenic heart failure and cerebral vasospasm, as well ICP crisis. This makes positioning of the patient during the ICU stay crucial to optimal outcome.

All patients with aSAH should be head up to a minimum of 30° to mitigate ICP elevation. The neurointensivist or nurse should also maintain a neutral head position to minimize compromising venous return from the cranium which may raise

ICP. It is common to have anatomic variation with congenitally hypoplastic or absent transverse, sigmoid, and jugular system on one side which can lead to compromised venous return if the head is positioned unfavorably [39]. The disposition of the venous system may be obtained from the angiographer or from review on noninvasive cross-sectional imaging. Additionally, when an ICP monitor is available, the optimum head position can be easily determined by observing the variations of the ICP waveform and pressure with head positioning. The knowledge of a hypoplastic unilateral venous system guides not only the head position but also the site of placement of central venous lines. We prefer to place a subclavian catheter contralateral to the dominant venous drainage of the brain.

If cerebral vasospasm is suspected or confirmed, the standard medical therapy of "triple H," hemodilution, hypervolemia, and induced hypertension is the standard medical treatment. Modern understanding of triple H is that the goal is truly to augment cardiac output while maintaining euvolemia. Hemodilution with hemoglobin levels of approximately 10 g/dL is almost universal with serial phlebotomy required for monitoring in the ICU. In poor grade aSAH, HHG > 3, there is increasing data to support higher CPP goals [40]. Positioning can have important effects on cardiac output, blood pressure and therefore the efficacy of induced hypertension. Preload is maintained by having the lower extremities at the level or above the heart. Like ischemic stroke patients autoregulation may be disturbed in patients with aSAH. However, supine positioning is not recommended because of the concern of increasing ICP and thus reducing the cerebral perfusion pressure.

Craniectomy for Ischemic Stroke, Intracranial Hemorrhage, and Traumatic Brain Injury: Positioning Considerations for Intracranial Pressure Management

Large volume ischemic strokes, cerebellar strokes, intracranial hemorrhage, and traumatic brain injury with resultant edema can all result in lethal elevations of intracranial pressure despite maximal medical management. Randomized clinical trials of decompressive hemicraniectomy of supratentorial ischemic stroke have demonstrated reduced mortality compared to medically managed and improved neurologic outcome for patients less than 60 years of age [41–44]. Similarly, for large cerebellar ischemic and hemorrhagic strokes (>3 cm volume) suboccipital craniectomies are established to be first-line lifesaving procedures that should be performed prior to neurologic deterioration [45, 46].

Positioning after hemicraniectomy should maintain a neutral posture of the head to avoid venous outflow restriction and ICP elevation. Additionally, the head should be positioned to avoid compression of the craniectomy site as this will limit the beneficial effects of the craniectomy on ICP and may damage the brain due to direct pressure. Mechanical compression of the craniectomy site may also result in impaired perfusion in the peri-infarct tissue with expansion of ischemic infarct. Patients requiring craniectomy must also be maintained in an upright (30–45°) posture. After suboccipital decompression, head up positioning is also recommended.

In the subacute period, cerebrospinal fluid (CSF) leakage and pseudomeningocele are both well-known complication of posterior fossa surgery. Both CSF leaking and expanding pseudomeningocele (by virtue of wound breakdown) are risk factors for nosocomial meningitis and should be promptly identified and corrected. Both of these complications may happen spontaneously or be precipitated by attempts at clamping and weaning a ventriculostomy. In these situations, the ventriculostomy should be reopened and if the patient's ICP is able to tolerate supine positioning, a trial of this maneuver is often helpful to help the wound closure and avoid surgical revision of the wound.

Complex Spine Surgery: Positioning Considerations for Postoperative Airway Management and Cerebrospinal Fluid Leakage

Spinal surgery compromises the majority of elective neurosurgical practice. The increasing age and comorbidities of neurosurgical patients and the complexity of spinal instrumentation procedures have made admission to the intensive care unit a routine occurrence. Although the ICU stay is generally short, there are important considerations in regard to positioning for these patients. Morbidity and mortality after spinal fusion is not trivial and has been reported to approach 23 and 0.5%, respectively, and up to 10% of lumbar spine fusions will require care in an ICU [47]. Factors independently associated with increased morbidity after spine surgery include advanced age, male gender, and increased comorbidity burden. Patients who undergo long prone surgery (>4 h) may have extubation delayed due to facial and airway edema. Additionally, anterior-posterior surgeries, prone cases with large blood loss (>1 L), and cervical surgery near the airway should all be considered for delayed extubation due to increased risk of airway edema. At the conclusion of surgery and after flipping to the supine position with the head of bed elevated in the OR if edema is significant then the patient is maintained intubated. In the ICU, the patient should continue to be positioned with the head of bed elevated in reverse Trendelenburg. Most patients who remain intubated after spinal surgery will be extubated successfully within 24 h [48].

After any cervical surgery, careful monitoring for development of a hematoma is a basic part of the postoperative care. Proper positioning is crucial to help mitigate compromise of the airway if a hematoma develops. Supine positioning should be avoided particularly if a hematoma develops as immediate airway obstruction may occur from a rapidly expanding neck hematoma. If the patient is in distress, the difficult airway cart should be brought to the bedside and the surgical site opened immediately prior to lying the patient supine to attempt intubation.

Cerebrospinal fluid leakage occurs due to incidental durotomy in approximately 6.8% of spinal surgeries. Fortunately, the rate of spontaneous resolution of CSF leaks is high with rates reported ranging from 80 to 95% [49]. A persistent leak implies a pressure imbalance between the subarachnoid and epidural compartments. Surgical revision is always an option but has its own intrinsic failure rate of approximately 5–9% [50]. An epidural blood patch will increase the pressure over the closure and can lead to cessation of CSF leaking. The subarachnoid compartment can be addressed by giving medications to reduce CSF production (i.e., acetazolamide), CSF diversion by using drains, or by altering the patient's positioning. The basic principles of fluid dynamics inform positioning. The dural tear site should be elevated to further reduce subarachnoid pressure. Animal studies have demonstrated a 29% reduction in cervical subarachnoid pressure with change of positioning from 0 to 90° [51]. Therefore, after cervical and high thoracic procedures reverse Trendelenburg is preferred in contrast to lumbar or lower thoracic surgeries were Trendelenburg, supine, or prone positioning is standard if CSF leak is suspected. This positioning will reduce CSF volume at the site of surgery and thus minimize subarachnoid pressure across the site of dural injury and encourage wound closure [12].

Cranial and Skull Base Surgery Tumor Surgery: Positioning Considerations for Optimizing Intracranial Pressure and Management of Brain Edema

Postoperative elective brain tumor patients spend a short period in the ICU, generally less than 24 h, principally to ensure that emergence from anesthesia is safe and the airway is stable. However, patients with large tumors or those who present with significant mass effect may have prolonged ICU stays. Management of intracranial pressure and edema in this group of brain tumor patients requires careful attention. Brain tumor patients can manifest both vasogenic edema due to increased capillary permeability and also interstitial edema due to obstructive hydrocephalus and trans-ependymal flow of CSF [52, 53]. The guiding principle for the management of brain edema and intracranial pressure is maintaining neutral head up position at a minimum of 30°. Medical therapy with steroids and hyperosmolar therapy (i.e., mannitol and/or hypertonic saline) are often continued and slowly tapered after surgery reduces mass effect. Head up or reverse Trendelenburg positioning is also important in terms of controlling blood pressure within the desired range to avoid postoperative tumor bed hemorrhage. Due to the edema and the pathologic state of the tumor bed vasculature, regional autoregulation is often disturbed and may be pressure passive similar to the hemodynamic situation encountered in acute ischemic stroke patients. Head up positioning in conjunction with blood pressure control is important to maintain hemostasis of the electrosurgically coagulated blood vessels [54].

Large tumor resections, particularly posterior fossa surgery/skull base surgery, invariably generate some degree of pneumocephalus. The efflux of CSF during surgery produces a negative pressure that is filled by the entry of air. The overwhelming majority of intracranial air is asymptomatic and will resolve spontaneously. Rarely, in the presence of a continued CSF leak a ball valve mechanism is created that allows air to enter but is unable to escape resulting in a tension pneumocephalus. These patients will become symptomatic 2–4 days after the operation due to mass effect. These patients should be positioned supine or head up to minimize CSF leaking and the ball valve effect. Additionally, administration of 100% oxygen will promote movement of nitrogen rich intracranial air due to the gradient of partial pressure favoring nitrogen reabsorbtion into the blood stream. This may stabilize the situation until definitive surgical repair is undertaken [55].

An additional concern in regard to medical treatment of pneumocephalus is rapid removal of air which can theoretically promote venous bleeding.

Conclusions

Positioning of patients in the neurocritical care unit is essential to ensuring the best postoperative outcomes. Proper positioning requires neurocritical care providers to have a fundamental understanding of the surgical procedure, pathophysiology of the treated conditions, and potential complications. We hope the discussion in this chapter has illustrated the important physiologic manipulations that can be attained by proper positioning and how these can mitigate and prevent complications.

References

1. Rozet I, Vavilala MS. Risks and benefits of patient positioning during neurosurgical care. Anesthesiol Clin. 2007;25(3):631–53.
2. Baumann SB, Welch WC, Bloom MJ. Intraoperative SSEP detection of ulnar nerve compression or ischemia in an obese patient: a unique complication associated with a specialized spinal retraction system. Arch Phys Med Rehabil. 2000;81(1):130–2.
3. Bertalanffy H, Eggert HR. Complications of anterior cervical discectomy without fusion in 450 consecutive patients. Acta Neurochir. 1989;99(1–2):41–50.
4. Geerts WH, Bergqvist D, Pineo GF, Heit JA, Samama CM, Lassen MR, et al. Prevention of venous thromboembolism: American College of Chest Physicians Evidence-Based Clinical Practice Guidelines (8th edition). Chest. 2008;133(6 Suppl):381s–453s.
5. Geerts WH, Pineo GF, Heit JA, Bergqvist D, Lassen MR, Colwell CW, et al. Prevention of venous thromboembolism: the Seventh ACCP Conference on Antithrombotic and Thrombolytic Therapy. Chest. 2004;126(3 Suppl):338s–400s.
6. Cohen AT, Tapson VF, Bergmann JF, Goldhaber SZ, Kakkar AK, Deslandes B, et al. Venous thromboembolism risk and prophylaxis in the acute hospital care setting (ENDORSE study): a multinational cross-sectional study. Lancet. 2008;371(9610):387–94.
7. Marehbian J, Muehlschlegel S, Edlow BL, Hinson HE, Hwang DY. Medical management of the severe traumatic brain injury patient. Neurocrit Care. 2017;27(3):430–46.
8. Zakrison TL, Pereira BM, Marttos AC Jr, Fraga GP, Nascimento B Jr, Rizoli S. Venous thromboembolism prophylaxis in patients with traumatic brain injury. Rev Col Bras Cir. 2012;39(6):553–7.
9. Serrone JC, Wash EM, Hartings JA, Andaluz N, Zuccarello M. Venous thromboembolism in subarachnoid hemorrhage. World Neurosurg. 2013;80(6):859–63.
10. Wahba RW. Perioperative functional residual capacity. Can J Anaesth. 1991;38(3):384–400.
11. Mohrman DE, Heller LJ. Cardiovascular responses to physiological stresses. In: Cardiovascular physiology. McGraw Hill; 2014. p. 193.
12. Bundgaard-Nielsen M, Sørensen H, Dalsgaard M, Rasmussen P, Secher NH. Relationship between stroke volume, cardiac output and filling of the heart during tilt. Acta Anaesthesiol Scand. 2009;53(10):1324–8.
13. Harms MP, van Lieshout JJ, Jenstrup M, Pott F, Secher NH. Postural effects on cardiac output and

mixed venous oxygen saturation in humans. Exp Physiol. 2003;88(5):611–6.
14. Carey TW, Shaw KA, Weber ML, DeVine JG. Effect of the degree of reverse Trendelenburg position on intraocular pressure during prone spine surgery: a randomized controlled trial. Spine J. 2014;14(9):2118–26.
15. Reinprecht A, Greher M, Wolfsberger S, Dietrich W, Illievich UM, Gruber A. Prone position in subarachnoid hemorrhage patients with acute respiratory distress syndrome: effects on cerebral tissue oxygenation and intracranial pressure. Crit Care Med. 2003;31(6):1831–8.
16. Petridis AK, Doukas A, Kienke S, Maslehaty H, Mahvash M, Barth H, et al. The effect of lung-protective permissive hypercapnia in intracerebral pressure in patients with subarachnoid haemorrhage and ARDS. A retrospective study. Acta Neurochir. 2010;152(12):2143–5.
17. Backofen JE, Backofen SJ. Changes with prone positioning during general anesthesia. Anesth Analg. 1985;64:194.
18. Sharma MU, Ganjoo P, Singh D, Tandon MS, Agarwal J, Sharma DP, et al. Perioperative complications in endovascular neurosurgery: anesthesiologist's perspective. Asian J Neurosurg. 2017;12(1):6–12.
19. Bruder N, Ravussin P. Recovery from anesthesia and postoperative extubation of neurosurgical patients: a review. J Neurosurg Anesthesiol. 1999;11(4):282–93.
20. Schar RT, Fiechter M, Z'Graggen WJ, Söll N, Krejci V, Wiest R, et al. No routine postoperative head CT following elective craniotomy—a paradigm shift? PLoS One. 2016;11(4):e0153499.
21. Haider AA, Rhee P, Orouji T, Kulvatunyou N, Hassanzadeh T, Tang A, et al. A second look at the utility of serial routine repeat computed tomographic scans in patients with traumatic brain injury. Am J Surg. 2015;210(6):1088–93. discussion 1093-4.
22. Diringer MN, Bleck TP, Hemphill JC III, Menon D, Shutter L, Vespa P, et al. Critical care management of patients following aneurysmal subarachnoid hemorrhage: recommendations from the Neurocritical Care Society's Multidisciplinary Consensus Conference. Neurocrit Care. 2011;15(2):211–40.
23. Molyneux AJ, Kerr R, Stratton I, Sandercock P, Clarke M, Shrimpton J, et al. International subarachnoid aneurysm trial (ISAT) of neurosurgical clipping versus endovascular coiling in 2143 patients with ruptured intracranial aneurysms: a randomised comparison of effects on survival, dependency, seizures, rebleeding, subgroups, and aneurysm occlusion. Lancet. 2005;366(9488):809–17.
24. Molyneux AJ, Kerr RS, Birks J, Ramzi N, Yarnold J, Sneade M, et al. Risk of recurrent subarachnoid haemorrhage, death, or dependence and standardised mortality ratios after clipping or coiling of an intracranial aneurysm in the International Subarachnoid Aneurysm Trial (ISAT): long-term follow-up. Lancet Neurol. 2009;8(5):427–33.
25. Mohr JP, Overbey JR, von Kummer R, Stefani MA, Libman R, Stapf C, et al. The ARUBA trial: current status, future hopes. Stroke. 2010;41(8):e537–40.
26. Lazzaro MA, Badruddin A, Zaidat OO, Darkhabani Z, Pandya DJ, Lynch JR. Endovascular embolization of head and neck tumors. Front Neurol. 2011;2:64.
27. Duffis EJ, Gandhi CD, Prestigiacomo CJ, Abruzzo T, Albuquerque F, Bulsara KR, et al. Head, neck, and brain tumor embolization guidelines. J Neurointerv Surg. 2012;4(4):251–5.
28. Osborne A. Techniques of cerebral angiography. In: Diagnostic cerebral angiography. Philadelphia: Lippincott Williams & Wilkins; 1998. p. 77–89.
29. Broderick JP, Palesch YY, Demchuk AM, Yeatts SD, Khatri P, Hill MD, et al. Endovascular therapy after intravenous t-PA versus t-PA alone for stroke. N Engl J Med. 2013;368(10):893–903.
30. Fransen PS, Berkhemer OA, Lingsma HF, Beumer D, van den Berg LA, Yoo AJ, et al. Time to reperfusion and treatment effect for acute ischemic stroke: a randomized clinical trial. JAMA Neurol. 2016;73(2):190–6.
31. Goyal M, Demchuk AM, Menon BK, Eesa M, Rempel JL, Thornton J, et al. Randomized assessment of rapid endovascular treatment of ischemic stroke. N Engl J Med. 2015;372(11):1019–30.
32. Saver JL, Goyal M, Bonafe A, Diener HC, Levy EI, Pereira VM, et al. Stent-retriever thrombectomy after intravenous t-PA vs. t-PA alone in stroke. N Engl J Med. 2015;372(24):2285–95.
33. Campbell BC, Mitchell PJ, Kleinig TJ, Dewey HM, Churilov L, Yassi N, et al. Endovascular therapy for ischemic stroke with perfusion-imaging selection. N Engl J Med. 2015;372(11):1009–18.
34. Jovin TG, Chamorro A, Cobo E, de Miquel MA, Molina CA, Rovira A, et al. Thrombectomy within 8 hours after symptom onset in ischemic stroke. N Engl J Med. 2015;372(24):2296–306.
35. Wojner AW, El-Mitwalli A, Alexandrov AV. Effect of head positioning on intracranial blood flow velocities in acute ischemic stroke: a pilot study. Crit Care Nurs Q. 2002;24(4):57–66.
36. Lazzaro MA, Novakovic RL, Alexandrov AV, Darkhabani Z, Edgell RC, English J, et al. Developing practice recommendations for endovascular revascularization for acute ischemic stroke. Neurology. 2012;79(13 Suppl 1):S243–55.
37. Munoz-Venturelli P, Arima H, Lavados P, Brunser A, Peng B, Cui L, et al. Head Position in Stroke Trial (HeadPoST)—sitting-up vs lying-flat positioning of patients with acute stroke: study protocol for a cluster randomised controlled trial. Trials. 2015;16:256.
38. Marino P. Indwelling vascular catheters. In: The ICU book. Philadelphia: Wolters Kluwer; 2013. p. 42–44.
39. DH P. The cranial venous system in man in reference to development, adult configuration, and relation to the arteries. Am J Anat. 1956;98(3):307.
40. Schmidt JM, Ko SB, Helbok R, Kurtz P, Stuart RM, Presciutti M, et al. Cerebral perfusion pressure thresh-

olds for brain tissue hypoxia and metabolic crisis after poor-grade subarachnoid hemorrhage. Stroke. 2011;42(5):1351–6.
41. Hofmeijer J, Kappelle LJ, Algra A, Amelink GJ, van Gijn J, van der Worp HB, et al. Surgical decompression for space-occupying cerebral infarction (the Hemicraniectomy After Middle Cerebral Artery infarction with Life-threatening Edema Trial [HAMLET]): a multicentre, open, randomised trial. Lancet Neurol. 2009;8(4):326–33.
42. Juttler E, Unterberg A, Woitzik J, Bösel J, Amiri H, Sakowitz OW, et al. Hemicraniectomy in older patients with extensive middle-cerebral-artery stroke. N Engl J Med. 2014;370(12):1091–100.
43. Vahedi K, Vicaut E, Mateo J, Kurtz A, Orabi M, Guichard JP, et al. Sequential-design, multicenter, randomized, controlled trial of early decompressive craniectomy in malignant middle cerebral artery infarction (DECIMAL Trial). Stroke. 2007;38(9):2506–17.
44. Vahedi K, Hofmeijer J, Juettler E, Vicaut E, George B, Algra A, et al. Early decompressive surgery in malignant infarction of the middle cerebral artery: a pooled analysis of three randomised controlled trials. Lancet Neurol. 2007;6(3):215–22.
45. Juttler E, Schweickert S, Ringleb PA, Huttner HB, Köhrmann M, Aschoff A. Long-term outcome after surgical treatment for space-occupying cerebellar infarction: experience in 56 patients. Stroke. 2009;40(9):3060–6.
46. Pfefferkorn T, Eppinger U, Linn J, Birnbaum T, Herzog J, Straube A, et al. Long-term outcome after suboccipital decompressive craniectomy for malignant cerebellar infarction. Stroke. 2009;40(9):3045–50.
47. Memtsoudis SG, Stundner O, Sun X, Chiu Y-L, Ma Y, Fleischut P, et al. Critical care in patients undergoing lumbar spine fusion: a population-based study. J Intensive Care Med. 2014;29(5):275–84.
48. Anastasian ZH, Gaudet JG, Levitt LC, Mergeche JL, Heyer EJ, Berman MF, et al. Factors that correlate with the decision to delay extubation after multilevel prone spine surgery. J Neurosurg Anesthesiol. 2014;26(2):167–71.
49. Cho JY, Chan CK, Lee SH, Choi WC, Maeng DH, Lee HY. Management of cerebrospinal fluid leakage after anterior decompression for ossification of posterior longitudinal ligament in the thoracic spine: the utilization of a volume-controlled pseudomeningocele. J Spinal Disord Tech. 2012;25(4):E93–102.
50. Kim KD, Wright NM. Polyethylene glycol hydrogel spinal sealant (DuraSeal Spinal Sealant) as an adjunct to sutured dural repair in the spine: results of a prospective, multicenter, randomized controlled study. Spine (Phila Pa 1976). 2011;36(23):1906–12.
51. Carlson GD, Oliff HS, Gorden C, Smith J, Anderson PA. Cerebral spinal fluid pressure: effects of body position and lumbar subarachnoid drainage in a canine model. Spine (Phila Pa 1976). 2003;28(2):119–22.
52. Goriely A, Geers MG, Holzapfel GA, Jayamohan J, Jérusalem A, Sivaloganathan S, et al. Mechanics of the brain: perspectives, challenges, and opportunities. Biomech Model Mechanobiol. 2015;14(5):931–65.
53. Wick W, Kuker W. Brain edema in neurooncology: radiological assessment and management. Onkologie. 2004;27(3):261–6.
54. Kaye AH, Laws ER. In: Brain tumors. Toronto, ON: Saunders; 2011. p. 103–106.
55. Layon AJ, Gabrielli A, Friedman WA. In: Textbook of neurointensive care. New York: Springer; 2014. p. 661.

20 Differential Diagnosis, Treatment, and Prognosis of Peripheral Nerve Injuries Associated with Neurosurgical Procedures

Nickalus R. Khan and Michael S. Muhlbauer

Background

Historically, there were two main theories of the causes of perioperative peripheral nerve injuries (PPNI). The initial theory was that PPNI was due to toxicity from anesthetic agents; however, this was not well supported. The second and correct theory was that PPNI was a result of malpositioning in the operating room. This was published in 1894 [1]. Nearly a century has passed since the initial description of PPNI. Unfortunately, these injuries still occur despite tremendous increases in medical knowledge and technological advancement.

A report from Germany in 2008 found that 17.4% of traumatic nerve injuries were iatrogenic [2]. Two American Society of Anesthesiologists Closed Claim analyses nearly a decade apart showed that 15 and 16% of all claims were related to PPNI [3, 4]. Ulnar neuropathies were the most frequent (28%) followed by brachial plexus (20%) and lumbosacral neuropathies (16%). The incidence of PPNI has been quoted to be 0.03% [5]. These injuries are disappointing to surgeons, especially when they often are not related to the surgical pathology of the patient. The consequences of these injuries are a detriment to the patient, the health care provider, and the overall health care system. Patients often experience pain, delay in return to work, and inability to perform their daily activities of life. Neurological and orthopedic surgical procedures have been shown to have a significantly higher risk of PPNI [5]. During neurosurgical procedures, patients are often placed in sustained positions for prolonged periods of time. The neurosurgeon must understand the anatomy and risk factors associated with PPNI in order to avoid complications during these procedures. In this chapter, we review the pathophysiology, surgical anatomy, diagnosis, and management of peripheral nerve injury during positioning for neurosurgical procedures.

Pathophysiology

The neuron is composed of a cell body, dendrites, and an axon. Dendrites carry information to the cell body and axons carry information away from the cell body. The cell body contains the cytoplasm and the nucleus of the neuron. Neuronal conduction occurs from the dendrite to the cell body to the axon. The axon of a neuron synapses with the dendrite of the next neuron using chemical neurotransmitters (Fig. 20.1).

The membrane of the neuron is baseline negatively charged. When cell of the nerve reaches threshold voltage, the sodium channels open

N.R. Khan · M.S. Muhlbauer (✉)
Department of Neurosurgery, University of Tennessee Health Science Center, Memphis, TN, USA

A. Arthur et al. (eds.), *Perioperative Considerations and Positioning for Neurosurgical Procedures*, https://doi.org/10.1007/978-3-319-72679-3_20

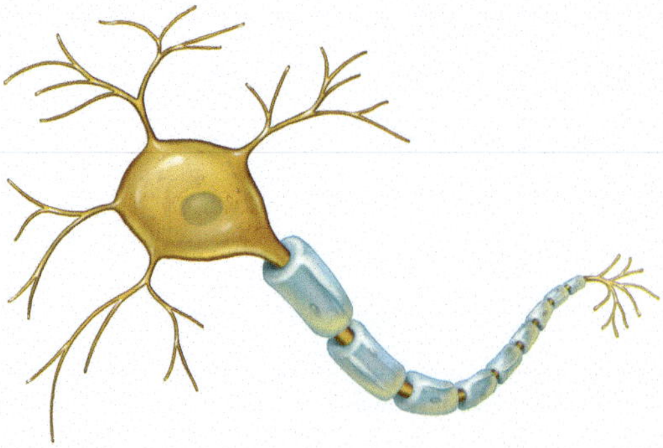

Fig. 20.1 Neuron structure [87] (Image courtesy of AxoGen Corporation)

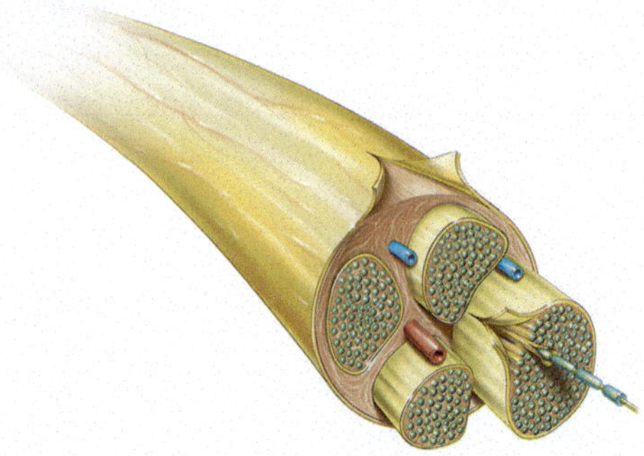

Fig. 20.2 Cross section anatomical diagram of peripheral nerve [87] (Reprinted with permission from AxoGen) (Image courtesy of AxoGen Corporation)

leading to further depolarization of the membrane. This creates a wave of depolarization along the nerve fiber known as an action potential. The peripheral nerve is composed of nerve fibers (axons) bundled together. These bundles are known as nerve fascicles. The endoneurium is a connective sheath that contains the vasa nervorum (blood supply to the nerve) and surrounds the nerve. The nerve fascicles are bundled together in a fibrous tissue known as the perineurium. The epineurium is the fibrous sheath that surrounds the entire nerve. The blood vessels on the epineurium penetrate the perineurium to anastomose with the blood vessels located in the vasa nervorum [6]. The cross section of a peripheral nerve is shown in Fig. 20.2.

There are several distinct but related ways that can damage the peripheral nerve during positioning. At the microscopic level, the final common pathway of nerve injury is ischemia [7–10]. Ischemia can be caused by any mechanism that impedes blood flow to the neuron [11, 12]. This can be caused by direct compression of the nerve or stretch of a nerve [13]. These mechanisms increase intraneural and extraneural pressures which leads to reduced perfusion pressure and nerve ischemia. Nerve ischemia can lead to a focal conduction block in mild injury and demyelination or degeneration in more severe injury. Nerve regeneration is slow and varies from 1 to 4 mm per day and is slower across scar tissue [14]. Remyelination lags behind regeneration by 9–20 days and also proceeds in a proximal to distal direction [15]. If no regeneration occurs within 1–1.5 years, the Schwann cells have likely been replaced by fibrous tissue and the prognosis is poor [16].

Table 20.1 lists these mechanisms of injury and clinical examples of how they could lead to PPNI.

The first major way in which a nerve can be damaged is by stretch. Appendages that are positioned outside the normal physiologic range of motion are subject to stretching the neurovascular structures present within them. This can lead to ischemia, necrosis, and in some cases even tearing of the connective tissue that composes the structure of the nerve. The second major way in which a nerve can be damaged is by compression. Inadvertent positioning that does not utilize adequate padding and care to avoid nerve injury can result in prolonged periods of time of neural compression. Associated risk factors for com-

Table 20.1 Mechanisms of PPNI with specific examples

Mechanisms of injury	Examples
Stretch	Poor positioning of appendages outside normal range of motion
Compression	Poor padding of areas at risk for nerve compression
Direct transection or laceration	Needle trauma from injection for from direct intraoperative damage
Ischemia	Prolonged immobility, local anesthetic agents, tourniquets
Toxicity of injected solutions	Highly concentrated local anesthetic agents

Table 20.2 Classification of nerve injuries [21]

Seddon [19]	Sunderland [20]	Description
Neuropraxia	Type 1	Conduction block • Local myelin damage with nerve still intact
Axonotmesis	Type 2	Axonal injury • Continuity of axons is lost.
	Type 3	Type 2 + Endoneurium injury
	Type 4	Type 2 + Perineurium injury
Neurotmesis	Type 5	Type 4 + Epineurium injury • Complete physiological disruption of entire nerve trunk

pression and stretch injury are as follows: hypothermia, hypotension, hypoxia, and electrolyte disturbances [14, 17]. The final way in which a nerve could be damaged intraoperatively is direct laceration or transection or, in some cases, injection of toxic solutions such as highly concentrated anesthetic agents.

Preoperative History and Physical Assessment

The American Society of Anesthesiologists (ASA) has issued a practice advisory based on evidence consensus that body habitus, pre-existing neurological symptoms, diabetes, peripheral vascular disease, alcohol dependency, gender, and arthritis are important components of a preoperative history and physical assessment to identify those at risk for iatrogenic peripheral neuropathies. This is of utmost importance because when these risk factors are combined with general anesthesia and muscle relaxants the patient becomes at very high risk for iatrogenic nerve injury. The advisory also states that it would be helpful, when appropriate, to ascertain that patients can comfortably tolerate the anticipated operative position [18].

Classification of PPNI

The majority of what we know about peripheral nerve injury and their classification comes from World War I. During this time, the number of traumatic nerve divisions was abundant. The observations from these injuries led to the classification system of Seddon [19] and Sunderland [20]. These classification schemes are listed in Table 20.2.

Specific Nerve Considerations

Upper Extremity

Ulnar Nerve

The ulnar nerve is the most common site of PPNI (28%) according to the ASA closed claims report [4] (Fig. 20.3). The incidence of ulnar nerve injury has been reported to be 0.037% [21]. It is usually injured from compression at the elbow or flexion of the elbow during prolonged surgical procedures. This is reported to effect as many as 1 in 200 adult surgical patients [22] and men may be more susceptible than women [23]. Men have been reported to have a larger tubercle and less adipose tissue protecting the nerve [21]. There are reports of this nerve being damaged in orthopedic surgical pin placement [24], elbow arthroscopy [25], transposition of the nerve for treatment of cubital tunnel syndrome [26, 27], or during radial artery grafting for coronary artery bypass procedures [28]. The authors have also experienced injuries to the ulnar nerve due to oxygen saturation monitors and other monitoring devices that are near the course of the ulnar nerve during surgical procedures.

The ulnar nerve is the longest unprotected nerve in the human body. It originates from the medial cord of the brachial plexus and travels down the humerus to pass behind the medial epicondyle in the "cubital tunnel." This is a common site for direct compression and stretch during surgical procedures. It then enters the

Fig. 20.3 Ulnar nerve

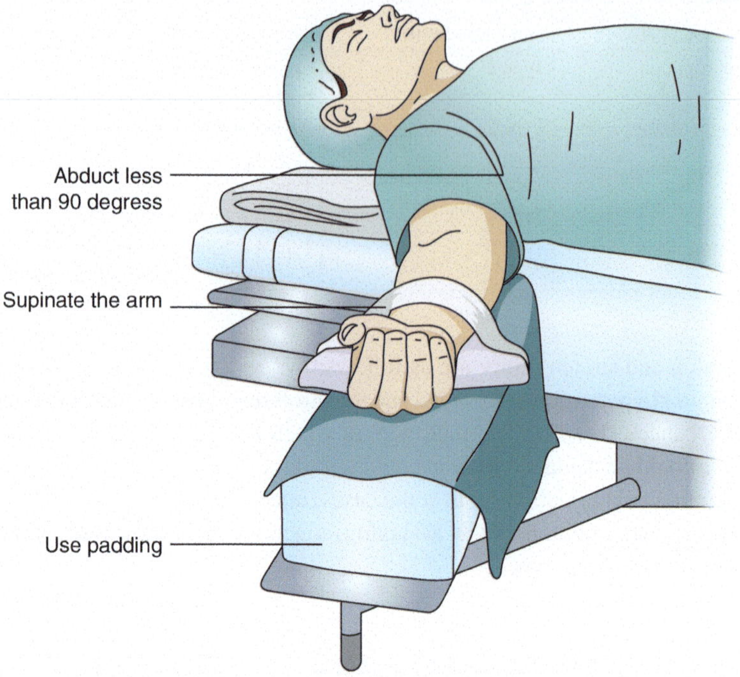

flexor compartment of the forearm and travels distal to supply sensation and motor to the forearm and hand.

The syndrome of compression at the elbow would result in a sensation loss in the palmar and dorsal aspects of fifth digit and the medial portion of the fourth digit. The motor loss would include the intrinsic hand musculature and portions of the flexor forearm musculature (1/2 of flexor digitorum profundus and flexor carpi ulnaris). The loss of the use of these muscles results in weakness of hand flexion (flexor carpi ulnaris), loss of flexion of ulnar half of digits (flexor digitorum profundus) and in severe cases may produce a hand that looks like a "claw hand" at rest.

A study performed in 1999 evaluated the relationship between forearm position and direct pressure on the elbow. This study showed that when the arm was supinated there was dramatically lower pressure over the ulnar nerve (2 mmHg) position compared to the neutral (69 mmHg) and pronated (95 mmHg) positions [29]. The mean area of the cubital tunnel has been shown to considerably decrease when the elbow is in flexion compared to extension [30]. Additionally, flexion of the elbow has been shown to cause up to an 18% elongation of the ulnar nerve [31].

When positioning patients the arm should be abducted less than 90°, slightly supinated, and generous padding should be applied to avoid compression or stretch of the ulnar nerve throughout its course. Figure 20.4 shows an example in the lateral position of generous padding being applied to avoid compression or stretch of the ulnar nerve throughout its course. Figure 20.5 shows improper positioning with too much abduction and arm pronation.

The ASA practice advisory states that the forearm should be placed in the neutral position to avoid elbow flexion. The author's opinion is that the arm should also be slightly supinated in the neutral position and to avoid abduction of the arm. The postcondylar (ulnar) groove of the humerus should be given special attention to avoid compression [18]. A common neurosurgical position that puts the ulnar nerve at risk is the prone "superman" position. In this position, great care should be taken to avoid over-flexion of the elbow and to provide adequate padding of the medial epicondyle area if using armboards.

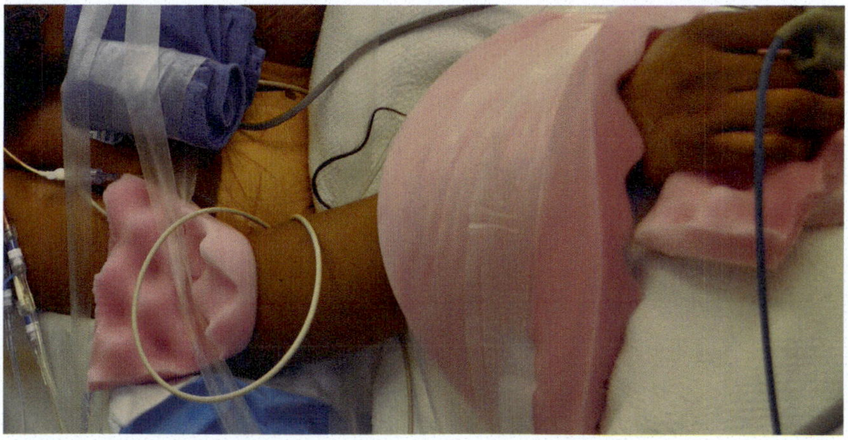

Fig. 20.4 Example in the lateral position of generous padding being applied to avoid compression or stretch of the ulnar nerve throughout its course

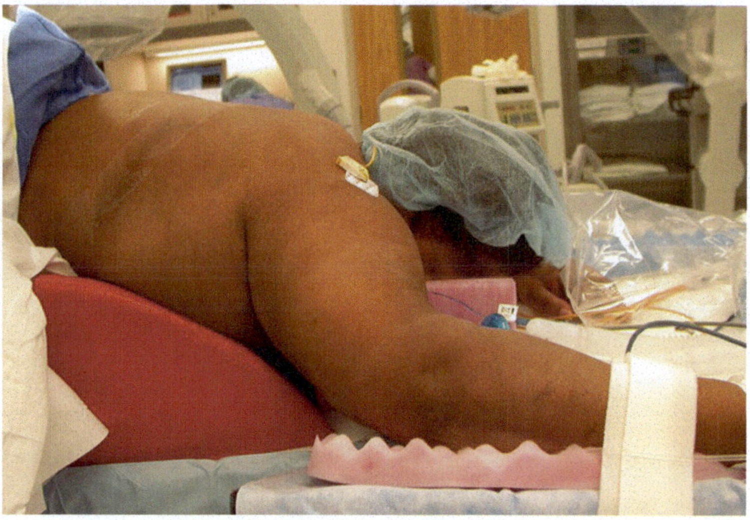

Fig. 20.5 Prone position with patient who has too much arm abduction and pronation putting the ulnar nerve and brachial plexus at risk for injury

Brachial Plexus

The brachial plexus is the second most common site of PPNI according to the ASA closed claims report [4] (Fig. 20.6). The brachial plexus comprises the nerve roots from C5, C6, C7, C8, and T1. It lies between the cervical spinal cord and the axilla and courses over the first rib and behind the clavicle. It supplies somatosensory function to the majority of the upper extremity. The brachial plexus has a superficial and long course and is susceptible to injury at its firm points of attachment: the axillary fascia and the proximal bony vertebra in the neck. During surgical procedures when the muscular tone of a patient is diminished there is risk for brachial plexus injury by stretch or compression if careful detail is not given to positioning techniques. Brachial plexus injuries have been described in the prone position (both surgical and nonsurgical [32]), during obstetrical surgery [33], cardiac surgery [34], urologic surgery [35], and general surgery [36]. There are cases in the literature of patients who had SSEP traced to the brachial plexus during positioning for craniotomy procedures. These changes were concluded to be due to head extension and rotation [37]. The authors have experienced brachial plexus injuries due to excessive taping of the shoulders and stretch on the head during neurosurgical operations.

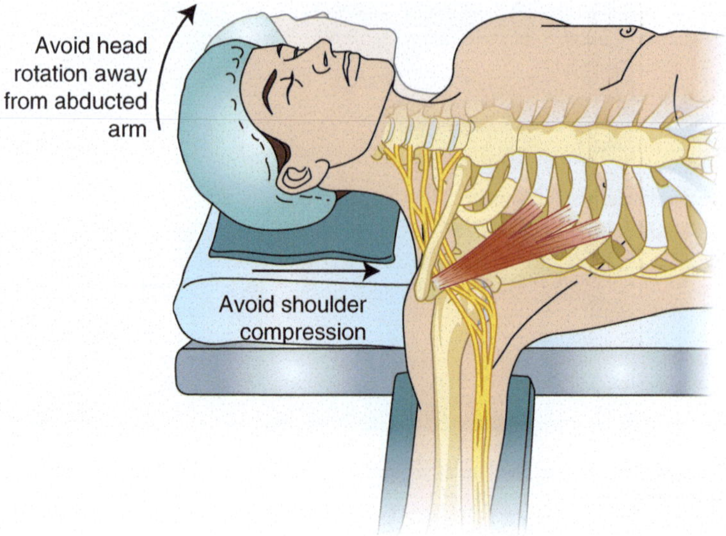

Fig. 20.6 Brachial plexus

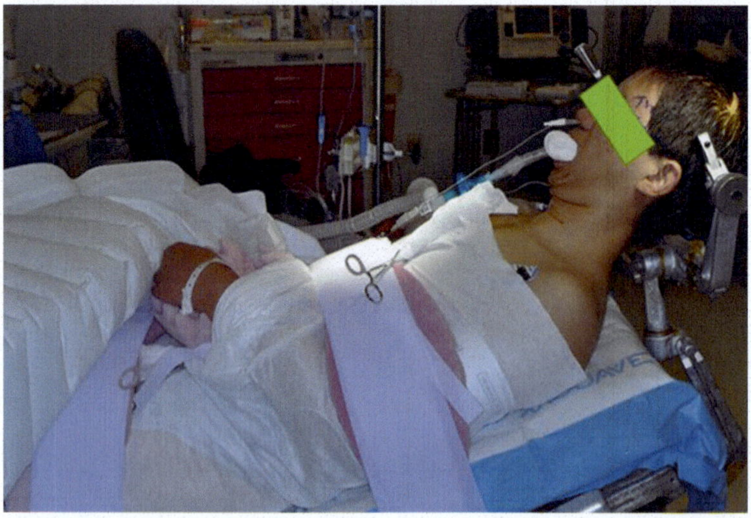

Fig. 20.7 Patient whose shoulders are rotated forward placing strain on the brachial plexus due to improper rigid positioning of the arms at the side

A review article recently found that when the arms are abducted greater than 90 degrees there is a frequent association of brachial plexus injury in the prone position [38]. The brachial plexus injuries described in this chapter improved with extensive rehabilitation within weeks to months [38]. Additionally, extension and external rotation of the abducted arm, lateral neck rotation, and shoulder braces have been associated with brachial plexus injury [39]. The prognosis following brachial plexus injury has been good with most deficits resolving at 3 months and only a small number having permanent neurological deficits [38]. The prevention of brachial plexus injury should lie in avoiding stretch on the neck, over-rotation of the arm, and over-abduction of the arm. Figure 20.7 shows an example of a patient whose shoulders are rotating forward and placing strain on the brachial plexus due to improper rigid positioning of the arms at the side. Figure 20.8 shows an example of external rotation of the arm in the supine position placing stretch on the brachial plexus.

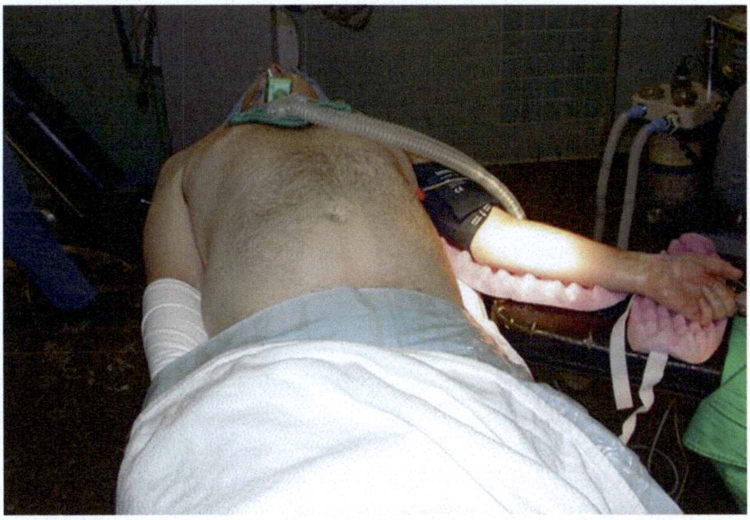

Fig. 20.8 Example of external rotation of the arm in the supine position placing stretch on the brachial plexus

Additionally, the use of adjunct neuromonitoring in the prone position has been shown to potentially help in the prevention of brachial plexus injuries [40]. The ASA practice advisory states that in the supine and prone positions limiting arm abduction to less than 90° may decrease the risk of brachial plexus neuropathy [18]. This advisory also recommends supination of the forearm instead of pronation to prevent rotation of the humerus and stretch on the brachial plexus [18]. A common neurosurgical position that puts the brachial plexus at risk is the prone "superman" position. In this position, great care should be taken to prevent the arm from being abducted greater than 90° to avoid stretch on the brachial plexus. Another common neurosurgical position is the lateral decubitus position. The brachial plexus is compressed between the humeral head and thorax in this position [14]. Placement of an axillary roll underneath the chest has been shown to decrease the pressure over the brachial plexus. The surgeon must make sure not to place the chest roll in the axilla, which would increase the pressure on the brachial plexus and potentially place the patient at higher risk for injury. The authors have also experienced brachial plexus injuries due to overaggressive shoulder taping during anterior cervical spinal procedures.

Median Nerve

The median nerve arises from the median and lateral cords of the brachial plexus. It travels through the arm alongside the brachial artery and eventually passes through the cubital fossa. The nerve exits the cubital fossa between the two heads of the pronator teres where it provides innervation for the superficial flexor musculature of the forearm. The median nerve then gives off two branches: the anterior interosseous nerve and the palmar cutaneous branch. The anterior interosseous nerve supplies the deep musculature of the forearm. The palmar cutaneous branch supplies sensation to the lateral aspect of the palm. The median nerve is the only nerve that passes through the carpal tunnel into the hand where it gives off the recurrent median nerve branch and the common palmar digital branch. The recurrent median nerve innervates the opponens pollicis, flexor pollicis brevis, and abductor pollicis brevis. The median nerve then gives its final innervation to the first and second digit lumbricals. The clinical syndromes associated with injury to the median nerve at the level of the arm include loss of sensation to the radial 3½ digits, loss of the radial half of hand flexion, and loss of pronation. Injury in the forearm could include "anterior interosseous syndrome" which is a pure motor loss of flexion of the radial 3½ digits and pronation without an accompanying sensory loss. An injury to the median nerve at the wrist could present as the familiar "carpal tunnel syndrome."

There is a paucity of literature on the injury of the median nerve during perioperative positioning [41, 42]. This finding is due to the median nerve being anatomically protected by superficial musculature throughout most of its course. However, there are reports of the median n. being injured during radial artery cannulation for hemodynamic monitoring [43, 44]. A task force comprising anesthesiologists found a consensus among expert opinion that "extension of the elbow beyond its normal range of comfortable extension in the perioperative assessment may increase risk of damage to the median nerve" [18].

Axillary Nerve

The axillary nerve provides motor innervation to give the arm abduction from 30 to 90° and sensation to the lateral arm. Injury to the axillary nerve most commonly is seen in shoulder dislocations given its proximity to the neck of the humerus. It can also be damaged in fractures of the surgical neck of the humerus.

There are rare reports of axillary nerve injury from perioperative positioning. An article from 1997 examining 7150 hip replacements identified only 1 axillary nerve injury [45]. There is a single report from 1988 describing both motor and sensory loss of the axillary nerve following a lumbar spine procedure [46]. It is the author's opinion that this rare but known complication can be avoided by limiting the degree of abduction and extension at the shoulder joint.

Radial Nerve

The radial nerve is damaged infrequently during surgical positioning [47]. The incidence of radial nerve injury following general anesthesia has been reported to be 3% [3]. There have been reports of radial nerve injury in general surgery using a Kent retractor, during coronary artery bypass surgery due to a retractor [48–50], a vertical bar used as an anesthesia screen [51], and even a blood pressure cuff [52]. The authors have experienced two cases of radial nerve injury related to malpositioning of fluoroscopic machinery. These injuries occurred when the C-arm was moved towards the head of the patient causing direct compression along the course of the radial nerve. Both of these injuries improved within 3 months following injury; however, one patient sustained permanent neurological deficit.

The radial nerve arises from the posterior cord of the brachial plexus and travels through the arm and enters the spiral groove of the humerus after innervating the triceps brachii. This is an area that could be compromised in a decubitus position with improper armboard positioning causing compression of the nerve [52, 53]. This could also occur as a stretch injury when the arm is abducted beyond 90° [14]. The ASA has issued a practice advisory stating that prolonged pressure on the radial nerve in the spiral groove of the humerus should be avoided [18].

The syndrome caused by this type of injury would result in loss of forearm extension, wrist drop, and weakness in supination. A sensory deficit in the lateral arm, posterior forearm, radial half of dorsum of hand and dorsal parts of digits 3½ excluding the finger tips which are supplied by the median n. If the nerve injury were located at the mid portion of the humerus, then extension of the forearm (triceps brachii m.) would be preserved. If the nerve injury were below the elbow, supination would be preserved (supinator m.). If the injury is in the distal forearm, there may be only a sensory deficit present.

Long Thoracic Nerve

Interestingly, the first description of injury to the long thoracic nerve in 1926 was thought to be due to intraoperative malpositioning [54]. There have been several instances in the literature of damage to this nerve when there is increased stretch between the neck and the upper extremity [55, 56]. This injury has also been reported in retromastoid craniectomy procedures in the park bench position on the dependent side [57]. There have been several small case series showing benefit for early decompression of the long thoracic nerve in nontraumatic injuries resulting in the common "winged scapula" [58, 59]. The author's opinion is that to prevent stretch upon the long thoracic nerve one must avoid increased stretch and tension between the upper extremity and the neck.

Musculocutaneous Nerve

The musculocutaneous nerve arises from the lateral cord of the brachial plexus and pierces the coracobrachialis muscle to travel between and innervate the biceps brachii m. and the brachialis m. After supplying motor innervation to the anterior compartment of the arm, it continues past the elbow in its "cutaneous" portion as the lateral antebrachial cutaneous nerve.

The musculocutaneous nerve is rarely injured during surgical malposition due to its anatomical protection throughout its course. The clinical syndrome caused by injury to the musculocutaneous nerve is weakness in supination and forearm flexion with a sensory deficit present in the lateral forearm. In general, injury to this nerve appears to be related to arm extension, abduction, and internal rotation [60–62].

Lower Extremity

Common Peroneal Nerve

The common peroneal nerve (fibular nerve) arises from the sciatic nerve and is composed of segments L4-S2 of the lumbosacral plexus. It crosses the lateral portion of the popliteal fossa and runs superficially near the biceps femoris m. along the fibular bone where it becomes palpable to touch and is prone to injury. The nerve branches into a superficial fibular nerve and a deep fibular nerve. The superficial branch innervates the fibularis longus and brevis mm. that are involved with foot eversion and plantar flexion. The deep branch innervates the tibialis anterior and the extensor musculature of the foot that are responsible for foot dorsiflexion and extension. The common peroneal nerve supplies sensation to the dorsum of the foot and lateral aspects of the leg and ankle.

The clinical syndromes involved with injury to this nerve involve what is commonly referred to as "foot drop" which is weakness in dorsiflexion, eversion combined with a variable amount of sensation loss along the dorsum of the foot, lateral leg, and ankle.

Injury to the common peroneal nerve during surgery positioning has been attributed to compressive straps around the knee [42] and when using the lithotomy position [63, 64]. A case series of 198,461 consecutive surgeries in the lithotomy position at the Mayo Clinic found there were 43 injuries to the peroneal nerve even when using adequate padding [65]. They found a thin body habitus, history of smoking, and time spent in the lithotomy position as predictors of nerve injury. There have been reports in the neurosurgical literature describing peroneal nerve injury following craniotomy in the sitting position [66, 67] as well as in the lateral suboccipital approach [68] due to overly flexed hips causing nerve stretch.

A report of a severe common peroneal nerve injury in the right lateral decubitus position in a 23-year-old female from 1952 undergoing a nephrectomy illustrates how injury prone the peroneal nerve is in the region of the fibular head where it becomes superficial and often palpable to touch [69].

The author's opinion is to limit excessive hip flexion and knee extension to prevent "stretch" injuries of the peroneal nerve. Additionally, to prevent "compression" of the nerve adequate padding especially around the area of the fibular head should be performed. Compressive straps and braces in this region should be avoided. While adequate padding is recommended, excessive padding is not recommended. We have experienced incidents causing nerve injury at our institution due to excessive padding causing compression.

Sciatic Nerve

The sciatic nerve is formed from the L4-S3 roots of the lumbosacral plexus. The nerve passes through the greater sciatic foramen in the posterior thigh to the popliteal fossa. At the level of the popliteal fossa, the nerve divides into common peroneal and tibial branches. Injury to this nerve would cause loss of motor function to all muscles supplied by the Tibial and Common Peroneal nn. and sensation loss to nearly the entire lower extremity. Injury to the sciatic nerve is a rare iatrogenic peripheral nerve injury [65].

Hip flexion and knee extension have generally been thought to cause more stretch of the sciatic nerve and predisposition it to injury [70]. The ASA practice advisory states that stretching of the hamstring group of muscles and increased hip flexion may increase the risk of sciatic neuropathy [18]. There have also been reports of sciatic nerve compression against the ischial tuberosity in the lateral decubitus positions [71].

Femoral Nerve

The femoral nerve is formed from the L2–L4 roots of the lumbosacral plexus. It runs underneath the inguinal ligament to supply the upper thigh and leg. The femoral nerve provides innervation to the musculature that extends the knee (quadriceps) and sensation to the upper thigh and inner leg. PPNI of the femoral nerve is rare. There have been reports from the general surgery literature of retraction injury when performing intra-abdominal surgery [72]. A case series of surgically repaired iatrogenic nerve injuries from 1990 to 2012 was composed of 5% of femoral nerve injuries [73]. It has also been reported that 60% of femoral nerve injuries are iatrogenic in nature [74–76]. However, the majority of these iatrogenic injuries are due to complications from various operative procedures in the vicinity of the nerve and not due to positioning [76]. There are rare reports of femoral nerve injury when patients have their legs abducted and externally rotated in the lithotomy positions. This position is thought to produce ischemia to the nerve as it passes underneath the inguinal ligament [77, 78]. The authors recommend limiting abduction and external rotation of the lower extremity to reduce the risk of femoral nerve injury.

Obturator, Saphenous, and Pudendal Nerves

Injuries to the obturator, saphenous, and pudendal nerves have been rarely reported. All of the reports available specify direct compression as the result of these injuries. Specifically, the obturator nerve is at risk when compressed against the pubic rami during lithotomy procedures [69], the saphenous nerve when compressed against the tibial tuberosity medially, and the pudendal nerve when compression is placed on the ischial tuberosities. In order to avoid injury to these nerves, their anatomical courses must be understood and areas where they are susceptible to compression as listed above should be appropriately padded.

Uncommon Nerve Injuries

There are nerves which are rarely injured during positioning but which do deserve mention. The supraorbital nerve has been reported to be injured by a tracheal tube or tight head harness [79]. The facial nerve has been injured by compression against the mandible by the anesthetist when holding the jaw forward for airway control [80]. The hypoglossal and lingual nerve has been reportedly injured with overinflated endotracheal tube cuffs, hyperextension of the head and neck, or from direct laryngoscopy alone [81, 82].

Diagnosis of PPNI

The diagnosis of iatrogenic peripheral nerve injury is usually straightforward if a patient develops a neurological deficit following a procedure in a known anatomical pattern that was not present preoperatively. If an injury is detected, an examination by a neurologist or neurosurgeon experienced in traumatic nerve injuries should be sought. Adjunctive neurophysiologic studies or MRI can be performed to further identify the severity and location of injury. After injury has been identified, one must determine if the nerve has been compressed, transected, or stretched in order to determine the best management of the injury.

Management of PPNI

Iatrogenic nerve injuries often present late, which complicates reconstruction. The reasons for late presentation can be a failure to recognize nerve injury, recognizing the nerve injury but waiting too long for spontaneous improvement, or surgeons failing to acknowledge nerve injuries [73].

If a nerve has been sharply transected, repair within several hours to 1 week will give the greatest potential for recovery [83]. However, in the case of contused or stretched nerves later intervention has been performed up to 4 months [84]. Patients who do not have a complete transection should undergo serial neurological and electrophysiological examinations. Those who do not show improvement after 3–4 months should undergo an exploration to perform neurolysis and possible nerve reconstruction. As the time from injury increases, the potential for recovery following reconstruction diminishes dramatically.

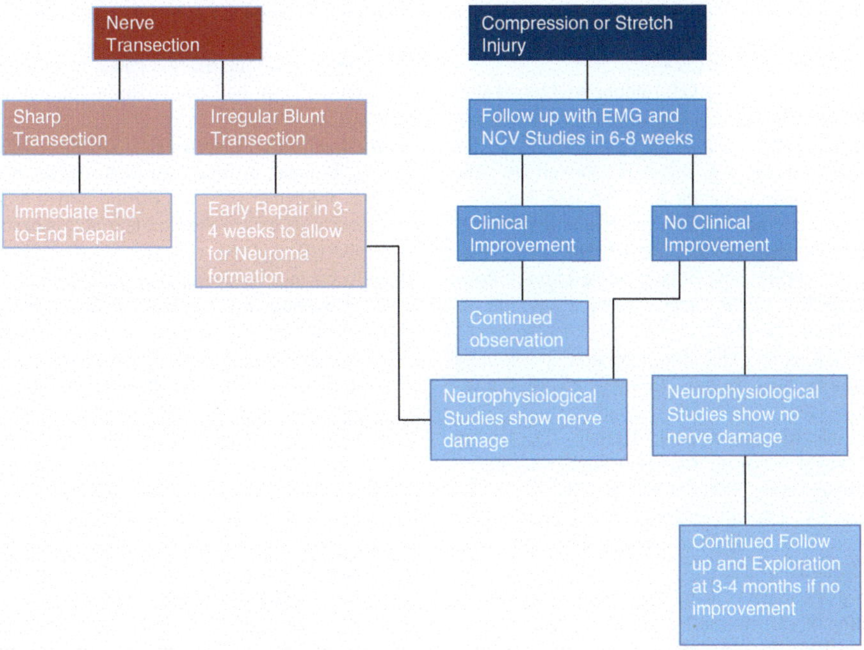

Fig. 20.9 Iatrogenic nerve injury management decision flowchart diagram

The method of reconstruction depends on the pathology of nerve damage. In patients in which a neuroma causes nerve discontinuity, the neuroma should be excised and the two ends of the nerve grafted together [85]. Those nerves in which a neuroma is present but electrostimulation shows that there is continued potential should undergo neurolysis. Those patients who show spontaneous improvement in both clinical and electrophysiological examinations should continue to be followed over time. However, when surgery is performed it should be done under standardized conditions with appropriate surgical instruments and neuromonitoring availability [85].

In conclusion, delay in reconstructive surgery is associated with poor outcomes [83, 86]. A multidisciplinary team performing frequent and thorough examinations to guide the timing and extent of reconstructive surgery is paramount in best management of iatrogenic nerve injuries [85]. The management for iatrogenic nerve injuries at our institution is shown in Fig. 20.9.

References

1. Budinger K. Ueber Lahmungen nach Chloroformnarkosen. Arch Klin Chir. 1894;47:121
2. Kretschmer T, Heinen CW, Antoniadis G, Richter HP, Konig RW. Iatrogenic nerve injuries. Neurosurg Clin N Am. 2009;20(1):73–90. vii
3. Kroll DA, Caplan RA, Posner K, Ward RJ, Cheney FW. Nerve injury associated with anesthesia. Anesthesiology. 1990;73(2):202–7.
4. Cheney FW, Domino KB, Caplan RA, Posner KL. Nerve injury associated with anesthesia: a closed claims analysis. Anesthesiology. 1999;90(4):1062–9.
5. Welch MB, Brummett CM, Welch TD, Tremper KK, Shanks AM, Guglani P, et al. Perioperative peripheral nerve injuries: a retrospective study of 380,680 cases during a 10-year period at a single institution. Anesthesiology. 2009;111(3):490–7.
6. Kamel I, Barnette R. Positioning patients for spine surgery: avoiding uncommon position-related complications. World J Orthop. 2014;5(4):425–43.
7. Swenson JD, Hutchinson DT, Bromberg M, Pace NL. Rapid onset of ulnar nerve dysfunction during transient occlusion of the brachial artery. Anesth Analg. 1998;87(3):677–80.
8. Swenson JD, Bull DA. Postoperative ulnar neuropathy associated with prolonged ischemia in the upper extremity during coronary artery bypass surgery. Anesth Analg. 1997;85(6):1275–7.

9. Yamada T, Muroga T, Kimura J. Tourniquet-induced ischemia and somatosensory evoked potentials. Neurology. 1981;31(12):1524–9.
10. Kozu H, Tamura E, Parry GJ. Endoneurial blood supply to peripheral nerves is not uniform. J Neurol Sci. 1992;111(2):204–8.
11. Myers RR, Yamamoto T, Yaksh TL, Powell HC. The role of focal nerve ischemia and Wallerian degeneration in peripheral nerve injury producing hyperesthesia. Anesthesiology. 1993;78(2):308–16.
12. Bonner SM, Pridie AK. Sciatic nerve palsy following uneventful sciatic nerve block. Anaesthesia. 1997;52(12):1205–7.
13. Winfree CJ, Kline DG. Intraoperative positioning nerve injuries. Surg Neurol. 2005;63(1):5–18. discussion 18
14. Sawyer RJ, Richmond MN, Hickey JD, Jarrratt JA. Peripheral nerve injuries associated with anaesthesia. Anaesthesia. 2000;55(10):980–91.
15. Quilliam TA. Growth changes in sensory nerve fibre aggregates undergoing remyelination. J Anat. 1958;92(3):383–98.
16. Trojaborg W. Early electrophysiologic changes in conduction block. Muscle Nerve. 1978;1(5):400–3.
17. Stoelting RK. Postoperative ulnar nerve palsy—is it a preventable complication? Anesth Analg. 1993;76(1):7–9.
18. American Society of Anesthesiologists Task Force on Prevention of Perioperative Peripheral Neuropathies. Practice advisory for the prevention of perioperative peripheral neuropathies: a report by the American Society of Anesthesiologists Task Force on Prevention of Perioperative Peripheral Neuropathies. Anesthesiology. 2000;92(4):1168–82.
19. Seddon HJ. Three types of nerve injury. Brain J Neurol. 1943;66:237–88.
20. Sunderland S. A classification of peripheral nerve injuries producing loss of function. Brain J Neurol. 1951;74(4):491–516.
21. Lalkhen AG. Perioperative nerve injuries. Revalidation Anaesthetists. 2011;12(1):38–41.
22. Warner MA, Warner DO, Matsumoto JY, Harper CM, Schroeder DR, Maxson PM. Ulnar neuropathy in surgical patients. Anesthesiology. 1999;90(1):54–9.
23. Morell RC, Prielipp RC, Harwood TN, James RL, Butterworth JF. Men are more susceptible than women to direct pressure on unmyelinated ulnar nerve fibers. Anesth Analg. 2003;97(4):1183–8, table of contents.
24. Wind WM, Schwend RM, Armstrong DG. Predicting ulnar nerve location in pinning of supracondylar humerus fractures. J Pediatr Orthop. 2002;22(4):444–7.
25. Rispoli DM, Athwal GS, Morrey BF. Neurolysis of the ulnar nerve for neuropathy following total elbow replacement. J Bone Joint Surg. 2008;90(10):1348–51.
26. Polatsch DB, Bong MR, Rokito AS. Severe ulnar neuropathy after subcutaneous transposition in a collegiate tennis player. Am J Orthop. 2002;31(11):643–6.
27. Kleinman WB. Cubital tunnel syndrome: anterior transposition as a logical approach to complete nerve decompression. J Hand Surg. 1999;24(5):886–97.
28. Ikizler M, Ozkan S, Dernek S, Ozdemir C, Erdinc OO, Sevin B, et al. Does radial artery harvesting for coronary revascularization cause neurological injury in the forearm and hand? Eur J Cardiothorac Surg. 2005;28(3):420–4.
29. Prielipp RC, Morell RC, Walker FO, Santos CC, Bennett J, Butterworth J. Ulnar nerve pressure: influence of arm position and relationship to somatosensory evoked potentials. Anesthesiology. 1999;91(2):345–54.
30. Gelberman RH, Yamaguchi K, Hollstien SB, Winn SS, Heidenreich FP Jr, Bindra RR, et al. Changes in interstitial pressure and cross-sectional area of the cubital tunnel and of the ulnar nerve with flexion of the elbow. An experimental study in human cadavera. J Bone Joint Surg Am. 1998;80(4):492–501.
31. Schuind FA, Goldschmidt D, Bastin C, Burny FA. Biomechanical study of the ulnar nerve at the elbow. J Hand Surg Br. 1995;20(5):623–7.
32. Goettler CE, Pryor JP, Reilly PM. Brachial plexopathy after prone positioning. Crit Care. 2002;6(6):540–2.
33. Raffan AW. Post-operative paralysis of the brachial plexus. Br Med J. 1950;2(4671):149.
34. Po BT, Hansen HR. Iatrogenic brachial plexus injury: a survey of the literature and of pertinent cases. Anesth Analg. 1969;48(6):915–22.
35. Cooper DE, Jenkins RS, Bready L, Rockwood CA Jr. The prevention of injuries of the brachial plexus secondary to malposition of the patient during surgery. Clin Orthop Relat Res. 1988;228:33–41.
36. Brunette KE, Hutchinson DO, Ismail H. Bilateral brachial plexopathy following laparoscopic bariatric surgery. Anaesth Intensive Care. 2005;33(6):812–5.
37. Anastasian ZH, Ramnath B, Komotar RJ, Bruce JN, Sisti MB, Gallo EJ, et al. Evoked potential monitoring identifies possible neurological injury during positioning for craniotomy. Anesth Analg. 2009;109(3):817–21.
38. Uribe JS, Kolla J, Omar H, Dakwar E, Abel N, Mangar D, et al. Brachial plexus injury following spinal surgery. J Neurosurg Spine. 2010;13(4):552–8.
39. Edgcombe H, Carter K, Yarrow S. Anaesthesia in the prone position. Br J Anaesth. 2008;100(2):165–83.
40. Schwartz DM, Drummond DS, Hahn M, Ecker ML, Dormans JP. Prevention of positional brachial plexopathy during surgical correction of scoliosis. J Spinal Disord. 2000;13(2):178–82.
41. Butterworth J, Donofrio PD, Hansen LB. Transient median nerve palsy after general anesthesia: does res ipsa loquitur apply? Anesth Analg. 1994;78(1):163–4.
42. Slocum HC, O'Neal KC, Allen CR. Neurovascular complications from malposition on the operating table. Surg Gynecol Obstet. 1948;86(6):729–34.
43. Cousins TR, O'Donnell JM. Arterial cannulation: a critical review. AANA J. 2004;72(4):267–71.
44. Chowet AL, Lopez JR, Brock-Utne JG, Jaffe RA. Wrist hyperextension leads to median nerve conduction block: implications for intra-arterial catheter placement. Anesthesiology. 2004;100(2):287–91.

45. Posta AG Jr, Allen AA, Nercessian OA. Neurologic injury in the upper extremity after total hip arthroplasty. Clin Orthop Relat Res. 1997;345:181–6.
46. Gwinnutt CL. Injury to the axillary nerve. Anaesthesia. 1988;43(3):205–6.
47. Lee HC, Kim HD, Park WK, Rhee HD, Kim KJ. Radial nerve paralysis due to Kent retractor during upper abdominal operation. Yonsei Med J. 2003;44(6):1106–9.
48. Briffa NP, Price C, Grotte GJ, Keenan DJ. Radial nerve injury in patients undergoing coronary artery bypass grafting. Ann Thorac Surg. 1992;53(6):1149–50.
49. Fernandez de Caleya D, Duarte J, Lozano A, Torrente N. Radial nerve injury caused by external compression during the dissection of the internal mammary artery in coronary surgery. Rev Esp Anestesiol Reanim. 1992;39(6):371–3.
50. Guzman F, Naik S, Weldon OG, Hilton CJ. Transient radial nerve injury related to the use of a self retaining retractor for internal mammary artery dissection. J Cardiovasc Surg. 1989;30(6):1015–6.
51. Britt BA, Gordon RA. Peripheral nerve injuries associated with anaesthesia. Can Anaesth Soc J. 1964; 11:514–36.
52. Lin CC, Jawan B, de Villa MV, Chen FC, Liu PP. Blood pressure cuff compression injury of the radial nerve. J Clin Anesth. 2001;13(4):306–8.
53. Tuncali BE, Tuncali B, Kuvaki B, Cinar O, Dogan A, Elar Z. Radial nerve injury after general anaesthesia in the lateral decubitus position. Anaesthesia. 2005;60(6):602–4.
54. Thorek M. Compression paralysis of the long thoracic nerve following an abdominal opration: report of a case. Am J Surg. 1926;40(26):7.
55. Hubbert CH. Winged scapula associated with epidural anesthesia. Anesth Analg. 1988;67(4):418–9.
56. Lorhan PH. Isolated paralysis of the serratus magnus following surgical procedures; report of a case. Arch Surg. 1947;54(6):656–9.
57. Paluzzi A, Woon K, Bodkin P, Robertson IJ. Scapula alata' as a consequence of park bench position for a retro-mastoid craniectomy. Br J Neurosurg. 2007; 21(5):522–4.
58. Silva JB, Gerhardt S, Pacheco I. Syndrome of fascial incarceration of the long thoracic nerve: winged scapula. Rev Bras Ortop. 2015;50(5):573–7.
59. Nath RK, Melcher SE. Rapid recovery of serratus anterior muscle function after microneurolysis of long thoracic nerve injury. J Brachial Plex Peripher Nerve Inj. 2007;2:4.
60. Ewing MR. Postoperative paralysis in the upper extremity; report of five cases. Lancet. 1950;1(6595): 99–103.
61. Dundore DE, DeLisa JA. Musculocutaneous nerve palsy: an isolated complication of surgery. Arch Phys Med Rehabil. 1979;60(3):130–3.
62. Abbott KM, Nesathurai S. Musculocutaneous nerve palsy following traumatic spinal cord injury. Spinal Cord. 1998;36(8):588–90.
63. Herrera-Ornelas L, Tolls RM, Petrelli NJ, Piver S, Mittelman A. Common peroneal nerve palsy associated with pelvic surgery for cancer. An analysis of 11 cases. Dis Colon Rectum. 1986;29(6):392–7.
64. Hsu KL, Chang CW, Lin CJ, Chang CH, Su WR, Chen SM. The dangers of hemilithotomy positioning on traction tables: case report of a well-leg drop foot after contralateral femoral nailing. Patient Saf Surg. 2015;9:18.
65. Warner MA, Martin JT, Schroeder DR, Offord KP, Chute CG. Lower-extremity motor neuropathy associated with surgery performed on patients in a lithotomy position. Anesthesiology. 1994;81(1):6–12.
66. Keykhah MM, Rosenberg H. Bilateral footdrop after craniotomy in the sitting position. Anesthesiology. 1979;51(2):163–4.
67. Standefer M, Bay JW, Trusso R. The sitting position in neurosurgery: a retrospective analysis of 488 cases. Neurosurgery. 1984;14(6):649–58.
68. Furuno Y, Sasajima H, Goto Y, Taniyama I, Aita K, Owada K, et al. Strategies to prevent positioning-related complications associated with the lateral suboccipital approach. J Neurol Surg B Skull Base. 2014;75(1):35–40.
69. Garland H, Moorhouse D. Compressive lesions of the external popliteal (common peroneal) nerve. Br Med J. 1952;2(4799):1373–8.
70. Burkhart FL, Daly JW. Sciatic and peroneal nerve injury: a complication of vaginal operations. Obstet Gynecol. 1966;28(1):99–102.
71. Lincoln JR, Sawyer HP Jr. Complications related to body positions during surgical procedures. Anesthesiology. 1961;22:800–9.
72. Dillavou ED, Anderson LR, Bernert RA, Mularski RA, Hunter GC, Fiser SM, et al. Lower extremity iatrogenic nerve injury due to compression during intraabdominal surgery. Am J Surg. 1997;173(6):504–8.
73. Antoniadis G, Kretschmer T, Pedro MT, Konig RW, Heinen CP, Richter HP. Iatrogenic nerve injuries: prevalence, diagnosis and treatment. Dtsch Arztebl Int. 2014;111(16):273–9.
74. Kim K, Kim MJ, Ahn S, Bae SY, Kim WS, Yoon J. Frontal Sinus lymphoma presenting as progressive multiple cranial nerve palsy. Yonsei Med J. 2011;52(6):1044–7.
75. Kim DH, Murovic JA, Tiel RL, Kline DG. Intrapelvic and thigh-level femoral nerve lesions: management and outcomes in 119 surgically treated cases. J Neurosurg. 2004;100(6):989–96.
76. Kim DH, Kline DG. Surgical outcome for intra- and extrapelvic femoral nerve lesions. J Neurosurg. 1995;83(5):783–90.
77. Tondare AS, Nadkarni AV, Sathe CH, Dave VB. Femoral neuropathy: a complication of lithotomy position under spinal anaesthesia. Report of three cases. Can Anaesth Soc J. 1983;30(1):84–6.
78. Hopper CL, Baker JB. Bilateral femoral neuropathy complicating vaginal hysterectomy. Analysis of contributing factors in 3 patients. Obstet Gynecol. 1968;32(4):543–7.

79. Barron DW. Supraorbital neuropraxia. Anasthesia. 1955;10:374.
80. Fuller JE, Thomas DV. Facial nerve paralysis after general anesthesia. J Am Med Assoc. 1956;162(7):645.
81. Sommer M, Schuldt M, Runge U, Gielen-Wijffels S, Marcus MA. Bilateral hypoglossal nerve injury following the use of the laryngeal mask without the use of nitrous oxide. Acta Anaesthesiol Scand. 2004;48(3):377–8.
82. Haslam B, Collins S. Unilateral hypoglossal neurapraxia following endotracheal intubation for total shoulder arthroplasty. AANA J. 2013;81(3):233–6.
83. Sunderland S. Nerve injuries and their repair. 2nd ed. Edinburgh: Churchill Livingstone; 1991.
84. Kline DG, Hudson AR, Zager E. Selection and preoperative work-up for peripheral nerve surgery. Clin Neurosurg. 1992;39:8–35.
85. Komurcu F, Zwolak P, Benditte-Klepetko H, Deutinger M. Management strategies for peripheral iatrogenic nerve lesions. Ann Plast Surg. 2005;54(2):135–9. discussion 140-132.
86. Osgaard O, Eskesen V, Rosenorn J. Microsurgical repair of iatrogenic accessory nerve lesions in the posterior triangle of the neck. Acta Chir Scand. 1987;153(3):171–3.
87. Axogenic. About the nervous system. http://www.axogeninc.com/for-patients/about-the-nervous-system. Accessed 29 Jan 2017.

21 Legal Issues in Patient Positioning

Emily Hamm Huseth

Background

Medical malpractice lawsuits have been a feature in American courts for nearly as long as the United States has existed. Cases have been filed with increasing regularity since 1794, the date of the first recorded medical malpractice suit, but it was not until the 1970s that this litigation began to be perceived as a "crisis."[1] Many states have enacted tort reform measures in an effort to combat rising medical malpractice insurance premiums and to maintain physician populations. Yet medical malpractice lawsuits still pervade court dockets.

According to a 2011 study that examined malpractice data from 1991 through 2005 for all physicians covered by a large, national professional liability insurer, 7.4% of physicians annually had a claim, with 1.6% making an indemnity payment.[2] The mean indemnity payment was $274,887, and the median was $111,749.[3] Breaking down this data by specialty revealed substantial variations in risk measures. Neurosurgeons, at 19.1%, had the highest risk of facing a claim annually, while anesthesiologists were slightly below the claim-risk percentage for physicians across all specialties.[4] Claim risk by specialty did not correlate well with the likelihood of indemnity payment; gynecologists had the highest payment rate while being only the 12th highest among specialties for claim risk.[5] Nor did claim risk correlate with the highest average indemnity payments. Though neurosurgeons were the most likely to face a claim, the highest average payment associated with that specialty ($344,811) was lower than that for pathologists ($383,509) and pediatricians ($520,924), two specialties with low claim risk.[6] The study also considered "outlier awards" or those in excess of $1 million. These awards accounted for less than 1% of all payments, and of the 35 total outlier awards included in the data, anesthesiology accounted for seven.[7]

To gain a better understanding of the liability and indemnity payment risk associated with positioning in neurosurgical procedures, I reviewed data obtained from the ASA Closed

[1] Flemma R. Medical malpractice: a dilemma in the search for justice. Marq L Rev. 1985;Winter; 68(2):240–42.

[2] Jena A, Seabury S, Lakdawalla D, Chandra A. Malpractice risk according to physician specialty. N Engl J Med. 2011;365(7):632.

[3] *Ibid.*, 633.

[4] *Ibid.*, 632.

[5] *Ibid.*, 632–33.

[6] *Ibid.*

[7] *Ibid.*, 633.

E. H. Huseth, J.D. (✉)
Harris Shelton Hanover Walsh, PLLC,
Memphis, TN, USA
e-mail: ehuseth@harrisshelton.com

A. Arthur et al. (eds.), *Perioperative Considerations and Positioning for Neurosurgical Procedures*,
https://doi.org/10.1007/978-3-319-72679-3_21

Claims Project (CCP).[8] the CCP recorded 232 neurosurgical claims involving spinal surgery (210) and craniotomies (22) between 2000 and 2016. The CCP categorized these claims into the following outcomes: positioning-related nerve injury (n = 14, 6%); other nerve injury, no evidence of malpositioning (n = 39, 17%); other positioning-related injuries, no nerve injury (n = 22, 9%); postoperative visual loss—ischemic optic neuropathy (n = 28, 12%); and all other neurosurgical claims (n = 129, 56%).

Of the 53 positioning-related and "other" nerve injuries, 47% affected the spinal cord, 21% affected the brachial plexus, and 15% affected the ulnar nerve. These 53 injuries included two deaths, 29 permanent disabling injuries, and 22 temporary or non-disabling injuries. Of the 22 positioning-related injuries where no nerve injury was reported, 10 were skin reactions or pressure sores; seven were eye injuries, including five retinal or vein occlusions, one corneal abrasion, and one claim for ptosis. Liability for each outcome group is summarized in Table 21.1.

Patient positioning thus cannot be overlooked as an area of potential exposure for neurosurgeons, anesthesiologists, and others. The purpose of this chapter is to provide an overview of the law governing medical malpractice and informed consent and to discuss the claims and arguments that have been raised in lawsuits where proper positioning was an issue. However, cases finding no liability on the part of a defendant should not be viewed as a guarantee that the same result will be reached in another court, particularly a court in another state, even under a similar set of facts. Each individual state controls its own tort law, including its own medical practice laws and statutes, and different states impose different requirements on litigants.

Moreover, every case ultimately turns on its own facts. Many of the cases discussed in this chapter may examine only limited aspects of proof because of where the case was procedurally. For example, when a defendant files a motion to dismiss for failure to state a claim (often in the early stages of the case), the court reviewing the motion can consider only what is contained in the pleadings and must presume all of the allegations in the complaint to be true. In other words, the court examines only the legal sufficiency of the complaint, not the strength of the plaintiff's proof or evidence.[9] After engaging in discovery, the defendant may file a motion for summary judgment, which may be granted if "the pleadings, depositions, answers to interrogatories, and admissions on file, together with the affidavits, if any, show that there is no genuine issue as to any material fact and that the moving party is entitled to a judgment as a matter of law."[10] Though a court does consider proof relating to the merits of a claim in evaluating summary judgment motions, it must view the evidence in the light most favorable to the plaintiff.[11] In contrast to both a motion to dismiss and a motion for summary judgment, jury verdicts are made after both sides have presented their proof at trial and the jury has had the opportunity to consider and weigh all of the evidence and to evaluate the credibility of witnesses.

Medical Malpractice

Medical malpractice (or "health care liability" or "medical negligence," depending on the state) is a category of negligence. As a general matter, to make a prima facie case of medical malpractice, a plaintiff must establish the basic elements of negligence: (1) the defendant owed a duty of care to the plaintiff (e.g., the existence of a physician–patient relationship); (2) the defendant breached that duty; (3) the plaintiff suffered an injury; and (4) the defendant's breach of his duty was the actual and proximate cause of the plaintiff's injury. The plaintiff typically has the burden of

[8]The text of this chapter was submitted for prepublication review and approved by the ASA Closed Claims Project Committee.

[9]E.g., *Webb v. Nashville Area Habitat for Humanity, Inc.*, 346 S.W.3d 422, 426 (Tenn. 2011).

[10]E.g., Tenn. R. Civ. P. 56.04 (2016).

[11]E.g., *Amos v. Metro. Gov't of Nashville & Davidson County*, 259 S.W.3d 705, 710 (Tenn. 2008).

Table 21.1 ASA closed claims project liability for outcome groups in neurosurgical claims (Reproduced with permission from the ASA closed claims project committee)

		Positioning-related nerve injury	Other nerve injury (no evidence of malpositioning)	Positioning-related injuries (no nerve injury)	ION	All other neurosurgical claims
Number of cases	Total *N* in each group	14	39	22	28	129
Appropriate anesthetic care	Less than appropriate	1 (8%)	6 (17%)	7 (44%)	5 (24%)	53 (47%)
	Appropriate	11 (92%)	29 (83%)	9 (56%)	16 (76%)	60 (53%)
	Total	12	35	16	21	113
Claim paid? (any payment, including surgeon or hospital)	Yes	4 (29%)	20 (51%)	13 (59%)	17 (61%)	77 (60%)
	No	10 (71%)	19 (49%)	9 (41%)	11 (39%)	51 (40%)
	Total	14	39	22	28	128
Total payment adjusted to 2015 dollars[a]	Median	$120,450	$672,500	$123,300	$438,400	$396,000
	Percentile 25	$38,700	$300,375	$26,800	$268,000	$137,000
	Percentile 75	$635,186	$1,241,500	$330,000	$825,000	$967,500
	# of payments	4	20	13	17	77

[a]Due to small sample size, median and IQ ranges should be interpreted with care. Median and interquartile ranges exclude claims with no payment ($0). Claims with missing data were excluded

proving all of these elements by a preponderance of the evidence.

Standard of Care

The defendant's duty of care to the plaintiff is measured by the "standard of care." In medical malpractice actions, the standard of care is not perfection or even best practice.[12] Instead, it looks to whether a defendant's conduct was "reasonable." But how "reasonableness" is measured varies from state to state.

Tort law in many jurisdictions has, to some degree, mirrored the standardization of training, licensing, and certification requirements for physicians and other medical personnel. A majority of states, including Alabama, California, Florida, Georgia, Mississippi, Missouri, Ohio, Texas, and Wisconsin, apply a national standard of care.[13] One court has described this standard as follows:

> Each physician may with reason and fairness be expected to possess or have reasonable access to such medical knowledge as is commonly possessed or reasonably available to minimally competent physicians in the same specialty or general field of practice throughout the United States, to have a realistic understanding of the limitations on his or her knowledge or competence, and, in general, to exercise minimally adequate medical judgment.[14]

In contrast, a minority of states apply some version of the "locality rule," which looks to the standard of care for the same or similar community in which a defendant practices. Arizona, Virginia, and Washington apply a statewide standard of care; Arkansas, Illinois, Kansas, Maryland, Michigan, Minnesota, Nebraska, North Carolina, North Dakota, Oregon, and Tennessee apply a same or similar community standard; and Colorado, Louisiana, Montana, Pennsylvania, and South Dakota apply a similar community standard for general practitioners and a national standard for specialists.[15]

For example, Tennessee statute requires that a plaintiff prove "[t]he recognized standard of acceptable professional practice in the profession and the specialty thereof, if any, that the defendant practices in the community in which the defendant practices or in a similar community at the time the alleged injury or wrongful action occurred."[16] Any witness who is being offered as an expert on the standard of care must be licensed to practice a profession or specialty "relevant to the issues in the case" in either Tennessee or in a contiguous bordering state, absent a showing that an appropriate expert witness is not available within those geographical restrictions.[17] Experts must also demonstrate familiarity with the medical community in which the defendant practices or a similar community by either firsthand knowledge or by educating themselves on the characteristics of the medical community at issue.[18] Yet, even though Tennessee continues to follow the locality rule, its courts have been influenced by the trend toward national standardization:

> Therefore, expert medical testimony regarding a broader regional standard or a national standard should not be barred, but should be considered as an element of the expert witness' knowledge of the standard of care in the same or similar community. Contrary to statements made in the dissent, this recognition is neither a dilution nor a relaxation nor an invitation of reliance on a national or regional standard of care. It is simply a common sense recognition of the current modern state of medical training, certification, communication, and information sharing technology, as demonstrated in the numerous instances of sworn testimony offered by medical experts in the above-reviewed cases, as well as the thoughtful analysis and discussion by courts in several other jurisdictions, that the consideration of such testimony is justified.[19]

[12] E.g., *Bozarth v. State LSU Med. Ctr./Chabert Med. Ctr.*, 35 So. 3d 316, 324 (La. Ct. App. 2010); *Siirila v. Barrios*, 248 N.W.2d 171, 192 (Mich. 1976).

[13] Lewis MH, Gohagan JK, Merenstein DJ. The locality rule and the physician's dilemma. JAMA. 2007;7(23):2635.

[14] *Hall v. Hilbun*, 466 So. 2d 856, 871 (Miss. 1985).

[15] Lewis et al. *supra* note 13, at 2635.

[16] Tenn. Code Ann. § 29-26-115 (2017).

[17] *Ibid.*

[18] *Shipley v. Williams*, 350 S.W.3d 527, 552-53 (Tenn. 2011).

[19] *Ibid.*, 553 (internal citations omitted).

Plaintiffs have attempted to use internal rules, policies, and protocols of hospitals to establish the standard of care, but many courts have held that these policies, without more, do not conclusively prove the standard of care.[20] This precedent has emerged, in part, to avoid penalizing hospitals that set aspirational policies and procedures.[21] Recommended practices by medical associations also do not, in and of themselves, establish the standard of care. However, like internal hospital policies, such recommendations may be used to support expert testimony.[22]

Congress has recently passed legislation rejecting the notion that federal health care program guidelines, standards, and regulations establish a duty of care or the standard of care in medical malpractice actions. The Medicare Access and CHIP Reauthorization Act of 2015 (MACRA) includes the following provision: "[T]he development, recognition, or implementation of any guideline or other standard under any Federal health care provision shall not be construed to establish the standard of care or duty of care owed by a health care provider to a patient in any medical malpractice or medical product liability action or claim."[23] Therefore, the Patient Protection and Affordable Care Act (PPACA) and Titles XVIII (Medicare) and XIX (Medicaid) of the Social Security Act and their associated standards and regulations (such as quality incentives, conditions of participation, etc.) cannot alone be used to prove the standard of care.[24]

With this background, it is not surprising that case law reflects a variety of expert opinions on standard of care for patient positioning. What is consistent, however, is the suggestion that everyone—from the surgeon to the anesthesiologist to the nursing personnel—may share some role or responsibility in ensuring a patient is properly positioned for surgery.[25]

In *Dierolf v. Doylestown Hospital,* et al. (Pennsylvania), the plaintiff alleged that she suffered a dropped foot following a maxillofacial procedure in the supine position that lasted over six hours. The plaintiff's expert claimed that the defendant anesthesiologist may have placed the straps in an excessively tight manner; that the anesthesiologist should have placed padding under the plaintiff's knee to keep the knees flexed and to avoid compression of the peroneal nerve; and that the plaintiff's leg may have rotated outward during the procedure and exerted pressure on the nerve for an extended period of time. Both the defendant anesthesiologist and her expert witness testified that the use of padding under the knee was contraindicated because the padding itself could cause pressure on the peroneal nerve and create blood pressure issues. The defendant anesthesiologist also testified that, though she could not check the strap during the course of the operation because the surgical drapes needed to remain in place for sterility, she had inspected the straps before the procedure began and saw no indication of excessive tightness. The defendant anesthesiologist also stated that she was "primarily responsible" for avoiding positioning-related nerve injury. The jury found for the defendants.[26]

[20] E.g., *Doe v. St. Francis Hosp. & Med. Ctr.*, 72 A.3d 929, 963–64 (Conn. 2013); *Moyer v. Reynolds*, 780 So. 2d 205, 208 (Fla. Dist. Ct. App. 2001); *Darling v. Charleston Cmty. Mem'l Hosp.*, 211 N.E.2d 253, 257 (Ill. 1965); *Wuest v. McKennan Hosp.*, 619 N.W.2d 682, 689 (S. D. 2000); *Prewitt v. Semmes-Murphey Clinic, P.C.*, No. W2006-00556-COA-R3-CV, 2007 Tenn. App. LEXIS 149, at *47–48 (Tenn. Ct. App. Mar. 23, 2007); *Reed v. Granbury Hosp. Corp.*, 117 S.W.3d 404, 413 (Tex. App. 2003); *Auer v. Baker*, 63 Va. Cir. 596, 600 (Va. Cir. Ct. 2004).

[21] *Wuest*, 619 N.W.2d at 689.

[22] *Estate of Lepage v. Horne*, 809 A.2d 505, 516 (Conn. 2002); *Kipp v. United States*, 880 F. Supp. 691 (D. Neb. 1995); *United States ex rel. Mikes v. Straus*, 84 F. Supp. 2d 427, 432–33 (S.D.N.Y. 1999).

[23] Medicare Access and CHIP Reauthorization Act of 2015, Pub. L. No. 114–10, § 106(d)(1), 129 Stat. 87, 142 (2015).

[24] *Ibid.*, § 106(d)(2); *see Bain v. Colbert County Nw. Ala. Health Care Auth.*, No. 1150764, 2017 Ala. LEXIS 9, at *50 fn.8 (Ala. Feb. 10, 2017).

[25] *Accord* Martin JT. General principles of safe positioning. In: Martin JT, Warner MA, editors. Positioning in anesthesia and surgery. 3rd ed. Philadelphia: W. B. Saunders; 1997. p. 6.

[26] *Dierolf* vs. *Doylestown Hosp.,* et al. Pennsylvania jury verdict review & analysis 1989;7(5).

In *Neidert v. University of Minnesota Medical Center* (Minnesota),[27] the plaintiff alleged that, following an eight-hour heart transplant surgery, he developed compartment syndrome in his left hand due to malpositioning during surgery. In support of his claim, the plaintiff submitted affidavits from his expert witnesses, an anesthesiologist and an orthopedic surgeon, which stated that everyone in the operating room was responsible for proper positioning and padding of the patient and for examining the patient's extremities. On summary judgment, the defendants challenged these experts' affidavits on several grounds, including that the experts' opinions did not differentiate between the different medical personnel present in the operating room (nurses, anesthesia staff, surgeons, etc.) but merely treated them as a group. The court denied the defendants' summary judgment motion,[28] but a jury ultimately returned a defense verdict.[29]

In *Barber v. Dean* (Texas),[30] the plaintiff underwent a CABG procedure that lasted over six hours. Following the harvesting portion of the procedure, the anesthesiologist, aided by several nurses, "tucked" the patient's arm. The plaintiff later complained of pain, burning, numbness, and weakness in his left hand and arm, and he was diagnosed with a left ulnar nerve lesion and ulnar cubital syndrome. The court quoted the opinion of the plaintiff's expert, an anesthesiologist experienced with cardiac surgical procedures, on the standard of care:

> *The applicable reasonable, prudent and accepted standards of care for ... Dr. [Tauriainen] [and] Dr. Dean ... involved a shared responsibility on the part of each of these surgeons, the physician assistant, and nurses to properly position and pad [Malcolm's] left and right upper extremities before the start of the CABG surgical procedure, during the left radial artery harvest, after the left radial [artery] harvest and during the remainder of the surgery in order to prevent peripheral neuropathies to [Malcolm's] upper extremities.*
>
> Of the major nerves in the upper extremities, the ulnar nerve and brachial plexus nerves are and were the most common nerves to be at risk of injury and to become symptomatic and lead to major disability of a patient during and after the perioperative period. Improper surgical patient positioning and padding of upper extremities were well-known causative factors in the development of surgical patients' ulnar neuropathies as of 2004 and such risks had been known by the surgical, physician assistants, hospital, and operating room nursing communities in the United States for many years. As of 2004, reasonably prudent anesthesiologists, cardiovascular and cardiothoracic surgeons, general and traumatic surgeons, physician's professional associations, registered nurses, and physician [] assistants were or should have been aware that surgical patients in supine positions were at risk of developing ulnar nerve injuries and neuropathies during surgery due to external ulnar nerve compression or stretching caused by malpositioning and improper or inadequate padding during surgery. *Prevention of perioperative peripheral neuropathies to [Malcolm], including his left upper extremity, was preventable by proper positioning and padding of his left arm and hand.*
>
> Dr. Moss, with the cooperation of nurses Alexander and Syptak, should have positioned [Malcolm's] right and left upper extremities in a manner to decrease pressure on the postcondylar groove of the humerus or ulnar groove. When his arms were tucked at the side, the neutral forearm position with elbows padded would have been appropriate. When his left upper extremity was abducted on an armboard, that extremity should have been either in supination or a neutral forearm position. His arm should have been extended to less than ninety degrees. They should have applied padding materials such as foam sponges, eggcrate foam, or gel pads, to protect exposed peripheral nerves in [Malcolm's] left arm, particularly at the site of his elbow and left ulnar groove. *Thus, after Drs. [Tauriainen] [and] Dean ... harvested [Malcolm's] left radial artery from his left upper extremity extended on an armboard, they, together with Dr. Moss, and nurses Alexander and Syptak, should have assured that [Malcolm's] left upper extremity was returned to his side in a neutral forearm position and padding of his left elbow and any bony prominences should have been performed to protect his left ulnar nerve and prevent the risk of a left upper extremity neuropathy to the nerve. Also, Drs. [Tauriainen] and Dean ... should have assured and followed procedures so that [Malcom's] left upper extremity was positioned in a neutral forearm position and properly padded to prevent the risk that any of the surgeons or*

[27] *Neidert v. Univ. of Minn. Med. Ctr.*, No. 27-CV-08-11856, 2009 Minn. Dist. LEXIS 112 (Minn. Dist. Ct. July 6, 2009).

[28] *Ibid.*, *2–9 & 39.

[29] *Neidert v. Univ. of Minn. Med. Ctr.*, No. 27-CV-08-11856, 2009 Minn. Dist. LEXIS 105 (Minn. Dist. Ct. Oct. 26, 2009).

[30] *Barber v. Dean*, 303 S.W.3d 819 (Tex. App. 2009).

assistants could come in contact or lean on his left arm during the surgical procedure.[31]

The defendant surgeons filed a motion to dismiss the case, arguing that the plaintiff's expert was not qualified to opine as to the standard of care for cardiovascular and thoracic surgeons and that his report failed to state with specificity the applicable standard of care. Though the trial court granted the defendants' motion to dismiss, the Texas Court of Appeals reversed, finding that the plaintiff's expert was qualified to render opinions as to whether the surgeons had deviated from the standard of care regarding the proper positioning and padding of the plaintiff's arm and that the report specifically stated that all the medical and nursing personnel "owed the same duty to ensure the proper positioning and padding."[32] The case was allowed to proceed.

In *Padilla v. Loweree* (Texas),[33] the plaintiff alleged that she had sustained a brachial plexus injury as a result of improper positioning during a gynecological surgery. In support of her claim, the plaintiff submitted an affidavit by her expert witness, an orthopedic surgeon, that stated that the surgeon was ultimately responsible for the patient's positioning; that the anesthesiologist was responsible for the patient's positioning while the surgeon was operating; and that after the procedure, the surgeon and the anesthesiologist were both responsible for ordering appropriate monitoring and care. The defendants filed a motion to dismiss on the basis that the plaintiff's expert was not qualified to opine as to the standard of care for positioning a patient during gynecological surgery. The trial court denied the defendants' motion, and the Texas Court of Appeals affirmed, noting that "the proper positioning and padding of a patient's arm during the gynecological surgical procedure is not a subject exclusively within the knowledge or experience of a physician specializing in such surgery."[34] This finding appears to be based on the perception that positioning principles are the same in orthopedic and gynecological surgical procedures. The case was allowed to proceed. According to court records, the anesthesiologist was later dismissed on summary judgment, and a nonsuit was taken as to surgeon and surgical center.

[31] *Ibid.*, 830–31 (italics in original).

[32] *Ibid.*, 822, 826–27, 830–31.

[33] *Padilla v. Loweree*, 354 S.W.3d 856 (Tex. App. 2011).

[34] *Ibid.*, 859, 861–64, 866.

Breach of Standard of Care, Causation, and *Res Ipsa Loquitur*

After establishing the standard of care, a plaintiff must show the defendant deviated from it, causing an injury to the plaintiff. These are issues that typically require expert testimony and that may ultimately be determined based on which party's expert the jury finds more credible.

Plaintiffs often seek to apply the doctrine of *res ipsa loquitur* (Latin for "the thing speaks for itself") to establish breach of the standard of care and causation. This approach has been used in cases involving post-anesthesia neuropathies,[35] perhaps because these types of neurological injuries are not always associated with the types of surgeries they follow.[36] As one commentator has noted: "All too often, patients, family members, and consulting or subsequent health care providers make this causation leap of logic without considering alternative causes."[37]

Under *res ipsa*, a jury may infer that a defendant was negligent—even if the plaintiff cannot show what actually happened—if the plaintiff's injury ordinarily would not occur absent negligence.[38] *Res ipsa* does not conclusively establish that the defendant was negligent; it merely allows a jury make this inference from the circumstances. A defendant can rebut this inference by

[35] E.g., *Horner v. N. Pac. Benefit Ass'n Hosps., Inc.*, 382 P.2d 518 (Wash. 1963); *Getch v. Bel-Park Anesthesia Assoc.*, 1998 Ohio App. LEXIS 1920 (Ohio Ct. App. Apr. 15, 1998); *Fitzgerald v. El Camino Hosp.*, No. H032094, 2009 Cal. App. Unpub. LEXIS 7181 (Cal. Ct. App. Sept. 3, 2009).

[36] *See Getch*, 1998 Ohio App. LEXIS 1920, at *1–2.

[37] White KJ. Medicolegal considerations. In: Martin JT, Warner MA, editors. Positioning in anesthesia and surgery. 3rd ed. Philadelphia: W. B. Saunders; 1997. p. 330.

[38] Restatement (Third) of Torts: Liability for Physical and Emotional Harm § 17 cmt. a (2010).

presenting proof that he was not negligent or that the plaintiff's injury was not the result of that defendant's negligence.[39] For example, evidence that the injury at issue is an inherent risk of a surgical procedure may rebut *res ipsa.*[40]

In *Fitzgerald v. El Camino Hospital* (California),[41] a plaintiff alleged that during a thoracoscopic dorsal sympathectomy, her arm fell off an armboard, causing a brachial plexus injury. A jury returned a verdict in favor of the defendants. The plaintiff appealed, claiming that she had established the *res ipsa* conditions and that the defendants had failed to rebut the inference of negligence. The appellate court affirmed the verdict, concluding that there had been conflicting testimony on whether a brachial plexus injury could have occurred during this surgical procedure absent negligence.[42]

In *Seavers v. Methodist Medical Center* (Tennessee),[43] a plaintiff claimed her right ulnar nerve was injured due to negligent positioning while she was being treated for bilateral viral pneumonia in the hospital ICU. The plaintiff's expert neurologist stated that, though he could not offer conclusive proof of causation, the plaintiff's injury was the type that would not have occurred in the absence of negligence by the nursing staff, who were responsible for positioning and turning the plaintiff's body.

The trial court dismissed the plaintiff's claim on summary judgment, concluding that the *res ipsa* theory was not available, and the Court of Appeals affirmed. At that time, Tennessee was one of a minority of states that restricted the use of *res ipsa* in medical malpractice cases to those involving injuries where lay jurors could apply their own common sense to infer negligence, such as where a sponge had been left in a patient's body.[44] If "the subject matter of the alleged malpractice requires a scientific exposition," expert testimony was necessary and the *res ipsa* inference was not permitted.[45] However, the Tennessee Supreme Court reversed, extending the availability of *res ipsa* in medical malpractice cases. The Court concluded that the *res ipsa* conditions could be met even where the injury at issue is outside the jury's common knowledge:

> This is especially true in medical malpractice cases where, as here, a claimant suffers a subtle nerve injury while heavily sedated and under the exclusive care of a hospital nursing staff. Claimants often have no knowledge of what happened during the course of medical treatment, aside from the fact that an injury occurred during that time. In cases where the standard of care or the nature of the injury requires the exposition of expert testimony, such testimony may be as probative of the existence of negligence as the common knowledge of laypersons. The use of expert testimony in that regard serves to bridge the gap between the jury's common knowledge and the complex subject matter that is "common" only to experts in a designated field. With the assistance of expert testimony, jurors can be made to understand the higher level of common knowledge and, after assessing the credibility of both the plaintiff's and defendant's experts, can decide whether to infer negligence from the evidence.[46]

Damages

If a plaintiff establishes the elements of negligence, she must then prove the damages she is seeking to recover. This may include economic and noneconomic damages. Though states may differ somewhat in how they define each category, economic damages are generally described as objectively quantifiable losses, such as medical expenses and lost wages, while noneconomic damages, including pain and suffering and loss of consortium, cannot be objectively quantified. Tennessee's statute differentiates between the two types of damages as follows:

> "Economic damages" means damages, to the extent they are provided by applicable law, for: objectively verifiable pecuniary damages arising

[39] *Ibid.*, § 17 cmt. g.

[40] *Ibid.*, § 17 cmt. e.

[41] *Fitzgerald v. El Camino Hosp.*, No. H032094, 2009 Cal. App. Unpub. LEXIS 7181 (Cal. Ct. App. Sept. 3, 2009).

[42] *Ibid.*, *2–7, 33–44.

[43] *Seavers v. Methodist Med. Ctr.*, 9 S.W.3d 86 (Tenn. 1999).

[44] *Ibid.*, 91–93.

[45] *Ibid.*, 92.

[46] *Ibid.*, 94–95.

> from medical expenses and medical care, rehabilitation services, mental health treatment, custodial care, loss of earnings and earning capacity, loss of income, burial costs, loss of use of property, repair or replacement of property, obtaining substitute domestic services, loss of employment, loss of business or employment opportunities, and other objectively verifiable monetary losses [.]
>
> "Noneconomic damages" means damages, to the extent they are provided by applicable law, for: physical and emotional pain; suffering; inconvenience; physical impairment; disfigurement; mental anguish; emotional distress; loss of society, companionship, and consortium; injury to reputation; humiliation; noneconomic effects of disability, including loss of enjoyment of normal activities, benefits and pleasures of life and loss of mental or physical health, well-being or bodily functions; and all other nonpecuniary losses of any kind or nature.[47]

Though not objectively quantifiable, noneconomic damages awards may be substantial. In *Steele v. Ft. Sanders Anesthesia Group, P.C.* (Tennessee),[48] a plaintiff underwent a decompressive surgical laminectomy to address some mild neurological problems she was experiencing as a result of arthritis-related compression of the spinal cord in her neck. The surgeon elected to perform the surgery in the seated position. When the plaintiff awoke from surgery, she was paralyzed from the neck down.

Prior to the surgery, the anesthesiologist documented a preoperative examination in the plaintiff's chart, but his entry did not mention the plaintiff's diagnosis, the reason for her surgery, her preoperative average blood pressure, what the surgical procedure would be, or that her spinal cord would be under compression. In the preoperative holding area, another anesthesiologist placed a central line and made an entry in the plaintiff's chart, without referring to the plaintiff's diagnosis or that her spinal cord would be under compression. A third anesthesiologist administered anesthesia to the plaintiff in the operating room before turning care over to a CRNA, who, after approximately 15 min, turned the plaintiff's care over to a second CRNA, who administered anesthesia for the remainder of the surgery. Neither CRNA had ever administered anesthesia in a neurosurgical procedure before. The plaintiff's blood pressure dropped during the surgery, and the second CRNA, who administered anesthesia for the majority of the operation, took no action other than to reduce the level of the anesthetic.

The case was first tried in 1992, and the jury found the neurosurgeon who performed the operation not negligent. The jury also found that the anesthesia group, which employed the three anesthesiologists and two CRNAs, had been negligent, but a mistrial was entered when the jury could not agree on causation.

The case was tried again in 1993 as to the liability of the anesthesia group. The proof showed that the anesthesia group deviated from the standard of care by:

> [F]ailing to recognize a special anesthetic risk faced by plaintiff Mrs. Steele; failing to record necessary information regarding the patient's condition on the chart for reference by others as needed in order to recognize and properly evaluate the anesthesia risk by allowing a person with inadequate skill, knowledge, and experience to administer anesthesia to Mrs. Steele; allowing an excessive number of people to participate in Mrs. Steele's care which increased confusion and decreased communication; failing to give adequate fluids during the surgery; and failing to maintain adequate blood pressure, even though the blood pressure could have been easily raised to an acceptable level with prompt treatment.[49]

Expert witnesses for both sides agreed that operating in the seated position presents an increased risk of ischemic injury to the spinal cord and that a person whose spinal cord is under compression would be more susceptible to ischemic injury. The jury awarded the plaintiff $5,600,809.90 as damages and also awarded the plaintiff's husband $2,000,000 for loss of consortium. The trial court suggested a remittitur in the loss of consortium judgment in the amount of $800,000, which reduced the damages award on that claim to $1,200,000. The plaintiff accepted the remittitur under protest.

---

[47] Tenn. Code Ann. § 29-39-101 (2017).

[48] *Steele v. Ft. Sanders Anesthesia Group, P.C.*, 897 S.W.2d 270 (Tenn. Ct. App. 1994).

[49] *Ibid.*, 275.

Both parties appealed. The defendant claimed the jury verdict so exceeded the range of reasonableness that the trial court should have granted a new trial. The plaintiff argued that the remittitur was made in error and that the original jury verdict should be reinstated. The Court of Appeals affirmed the judgment of the trial court in all respects, finding that the proof at trial supported a substantial loss of consortium award and that the award after the remittitur was within the range of reasonableness.[50] Notably, however, this case was decided before Tennessee adopted caps on noneconomic damages awards.

Many states have enacted laws limiting the amount of noneconomic damages a plaintiff can receive in medical malpractice actions and other tort actions.[51] These damages may be capped as low as $250,000 or as high as $1,500,000.[52] For example, in Tennessee, a plaintiff generally cannot recover in excess of $750,000 in noneconomic damages.[53] Where a jury finds there has been a "catastrophic loss"—which includes a spinal cord injury resulting in paraplegia or quadriplegia —noneconomic damages are capped at $1,000,000.[54] However, these caps do not apply to actions where the defendant acted intentionally to harm the plaintiff; the defendant intentionally falsified or destroyed records that contained material evidence; the defendant was under the influence of alcohol or drugs; or the defendant's acts resulted in his being convicted of a felony.[55]

Plaintiffs have brought constitutional challenges to these statutes in various states.[56] Courts in Alaska, California, Indiana, Louisiana, Nebraska, Ohio, West Virginia, and Missouri have upheld their state damages caps.[57] However, damages caps have been invalidated in Florida, Georgia, Illinois, and Wisconsin.[58] Courts in some states, including Tennessee, have, to date, declined to rule on the constitutionality of damages caps on the basis that the issue is not yet ripe; that is, no case involving a plaintiff verdict in excess of the statutory cap has yet been presented for their review.[59]

A plaintiff may also be awarded punitive damages under certain circumstances. The purpose of punitive damages is "not to compensate the plaintiff but to punish the wrongdoer and to deter the wrongdoer and others from committing similar wrongs in the future."[60] The availability of punitive damages varies from state to state. In Tennessee, punitive damages are available only if a plaintiff proves by clear and convincing evidence that the defendant acted "maliciously, intentionally, fraudulently, or recklessly."[61] Tennessee also caps punitive damages awards at the greater of two times the total amount of compensatory damages awarded, or $500,000.00. However, these caps do not apply in cases where a defendant had a specific intent to seriously injure a plaintiff; the defendant intentionally falsified, destroyed, or concealed records containing material evidence to evade liability; the defendant was under the influence of alcohol or drugs; or the defendant's acts resulted in his being convicted of a felony.[62]

Limitations on Medical Malpractice Actions

The time period within which a plaintiff may bring a medical malpractice action is restricted

[50] *Ibid.*, 272–75, 282–84.

[51] *See generally* Avraham, Ronen, Database of State Tort Law Reforms (5th) (May 2014). U of Texas Law and Econ Research Paper No. e555. Available at SSRN: https://ssrn.com/abstract=902711.

[52] See Stein A. Toward a new theory of medical malpractice. Iowa L. Rev. 2012; 97:1253 (citing Cal. Civ. Code § 3333.2(b) (West 2010) and Fla. Stat. Ann. § 766.118(3)(b)).

[53] Tenn. Code Ann. § 29-39-102(a) (2017).

[54] *Ibid.*, § 29-39-102(b).

[55] *Ibid.*, § 29-39-102(h).

[56] Stein, *supra* note 52, at 1254.

[57] *Ibid.*, 1254 n.291; *Dodson v. Ferrara*, 491 S.W.3d 542 (Mo. 2016).

[58] Stein, *supra* note 52, at 1254 n.1291; *N. Broward Hosp. Dist. v. Kalitan*, No. SC15-1858, 2017 Fla. LEXIS 1277 (Fla. June 8, 2017).

[59] *Clark v. Cain*, 479 S.W.3d 830 (Tenn. 2015).

[60] *Hodges v. S.C. Toof & Co.*, 833 S.W.2d 896, 900 (Tenn. 1992) (citation omitted).

[61] Tenn. Code Ann. § 29-39-104(a)(1) (2017).

[62] *Ibid.*, § 29-39-104(a)(5) & (7).

by state statutes of limitations and statutes of repose. A statute of limitations sets the time in which a lawsuit must be filed after a cause of action accrues; if the plaintiff does not file suit within the prescribed time period, she is deemed to have waived her claim.[63] "Thus, the barring of the remedy is caused by a plaintiff's failure to take reasonable steps to assert the cause of action within the time afforded by the statute."[64] Statutes of limitations for medical malpractice cases may range from one[65] to three years.[66]

The date a cause of action accrues is not always the date the medical procedure giving rise to an alleged injury was performed. If the plaintiff reasonably did not discover her injury until some time after the medical procedure, the cause of action is deemed to have accrued on the date of discovery or on the date the injury should have reasonably been discovered. States may also provide for other circumstances that toll, or suspend, the running of the statute of limitations period. One such example is when the plaintiff is a minor or mentally incompetent.[67]

In contrast to statutes of limitations, statutes of repose abolish a cause of action if a plaintiff has not filed suit within a prescribed time after the negligent act occurred, regardless of whether the alleged negligence was discovered or should have reasonably been discovered within that time period. As one court has explained: "Statutes of repose are … not designed, as are statutes of limitations, to necessarily allow a 'reasonable' time in which to file a lawsuit. A statute of repose might theoretically cut off a claim filed within the period allowed by the relevant statute of limitations."[68] Statutes of repose thus serve the purpose of increasing availability of insurance and reducing risk and uncertainty of liability for physicians and other medical practitioners.[69]

[63] E.g., *Lee v. Gaufin*, 867 P.2d 572, 575 (Utah 1993).

[64] *Ibid.*

[65] Tenn. Code Ann. § 29-26-116(a) (2017).

[66] S.C. Code Ann. § 15-3-545 (2016).

[67] E.g., Tenn. Code Ann. § 28-1-106.

[68] *Lee*, 867 P.2d at 576 (citation omitted).

[69] *Ibid.* (citation omitted).

Statutes of repose for medical malpractice actions may range from three[70] to ten years.[71]

As with statutes of limitations, states have made provision for certain exceptions to their statutes of repose. For example, Tennessee permits plaintiffs to bring medical malpractice lawsuits outside the state's three year statute of repose if a defendant has fraudulently concealed evidence of his negligence.[72]

Informed Consent

Medical malpractice claims are often accompanied by claims for lack of informed consent. Informed consent cases typically involve situations in which a patient authorized a procedure but claims that the physician failed to inform her of any or all of the inherent risks.[73]

Though a defendant may not have been negligent in performing the procedure, he may still be found liable for inadequate informed consent if the plaintiff establishes nondisclosure, causation, and injury.[74] What is required to prove these elements differs across states. To determine adequacy of consent, some states inquire whether the undisclosed risks were such that they "could have influenced a reasonable person in making a decision to give or withhold consent."[75] Other states focus on whether "the information provided to the patient deviated from the usual and customary information given to patients to procure consent in similar situations."[76]

With regard to causation, the majority of states apply an objective standard: "If adequate disclosure could reasonably be expected to have caused [a prudent person in the patient's position] to decline the treatment because of the

[70] Tenn. Code Ann. § 29-26-116.

[71] Mo. Rev. Stat. § 516.105 (2017).

[72] Tenn. Code Ann. § 29-26-116.

[73] *Blanchard v. Kellum*, 975 S.W.2d 522, 524 (Tenn. 1998).

[74] *See*, e.g., *Ibid.*, 123; *Foster v. Traul*, 175 P.3d 186, 192 (Idaho 2008).

[75] Tex. Civ. Prac. & Rem. Code § 74.101 (2015).

[76] *Blanchard*, 975 S.W.2d at 524; *see also* Tenn. Code Ann. § 29-26-118.

revelation of the kind of risk or danger that resulted in harm, causation is shown[.]"[77] A minority of states apply a subjective standard, in which causation is established solely by patient testimony that she would not have consented to the procedure had she been advised of the risk in question.[78]

Informed consent has been an issue in a number of cases involving ischemic optic neuropathy following a spinal procedure. In *Foster v. Traul* (Idaho),[79] a plaintiff sought damages against an anesthesiologist, alleging he had experienced bilateral posterior ischemic optic neuropathy (PION) following a back surgery. The plaintiff's medical malpractice claims were dismissed on summary judgment, but he was allowed to proceed with his lack of informed consent claim. The defendant filed a subsequent motion for summary judgment as to this claim, which the trial court granted. However, the Idaho Supreme Court reversed, finding that, based on the affidavits of the parties' respective experts, there was a genuine issue of fact as to whether the plaintiff was injured as a result of the defendant's failure to disclose the risk of PION. The experts agreed that PION occurred in a certain percentage of patients following back surgery, that PION was a risk of the procedure, and that the plaintiff sustained that injury.[80]

In *Nemcik v. United States* (New Jersey),[81] a plaintiff brought suit for medical malpractice and lack of informed consent after being diagnosed with PION following a multilevel spinal fusion surgery. The Court found that, at the time of the surgery, it was not the standard of care for anesthesiologists to inform their patients about the risk of PION:

> The Court finds that while the anesthesiologists who attended to plaintiff were responsible for advising Plaintiff about the risks associated with the anesthetic agents and procedures they would be using throughout the course of the surgery, they were not responsible for informing plaintiff about the risks associated with the surgery itself, such as PION. Moreover, the standard of care for anesthesiologists in 2002 did not mandate that they inform their patients that postoperative vision loss was a risk of spine surgery. Anesthesiologists are generalists in their field and cannot be expected to have knowledge of the risks of each and every kind of surgery. Even [plaintiff's expert anesthesiologist] testified that while it would be prudent to tell a patient of the risk, there was no ASA standard that an anesthesiologist must disclose the risk. Furthermore, the risk factors for PION, such as a lengthy spine surgery in the prone position, are not in the control of the anesthesiologists.[82]

The Court further found that a reasonably prudent person in the plaintiff's position would have undergone the procedure even if he had been informed of the risk of PION. In making this determination, the Court focused on the plaintiff's spinal deterioration and pain levels, the rarity with which PION occurred (between 0.03% and 0.1%), and the fact that the plaintiff testified that had he been told of the risk of PION he would have only "hesitated" about having the surgery. The Court ruled in favor of the defendant on all claims.[83]

In *Dacey v. Huckell* (New York),[84] which was decided in 2015, a plaintiff underwent a lumbar decompression and fusion of levels L1 to S1. When the plaintiff arrived in the operating room, the anesthesiologist secured his airway, anesthetized him, and applied a "Dupaco pillow" to his face before moving him into a prone position on a specialized "Jackson" table. After the six and a half hour procedure was completed, the plaintiff was returned to the supine position, and the pillow was removed from his face. It was then observed that the plaintiff had developed pronounced facial edema. The plaintiff was later diagnosed with transient ischemic optic neuropathy secondary to

[77] *Canterbury v. Spence*, 464 F.2d 772, 791 (D.C. Cir. 1972); *see also Ashe v. Radiation Oncology Assocs.*, 9 S.W.3d 119, 122 fn.1 (Tenn. 1999) (summarizing the states that have adopted the objective standard).

[78] *Ashe*, 9 S.W.3d at 122.

[79] *Foster v. Traul*, 175 P.3d 186, 192 (Idaho 2007).

[80] *Ibid.*, 188 & 192–94.

[81] *Nemcik v. United States*, No. 05-1469, 2008 U.S. Dist. LEXIS 51784 (D. N. J. July 8, 2008).

[82] *Ibid.*, *39–40.

[83] *Ibid.*, *6–7 & 40–42.

[84] *Dacey v. Huckell*, No. 42471, 2015 N. Y. Misc. LEXIS 372 (N. Y. Sup. Ct. Feb. 11, 2015).

hemodynamic compromise. The defendants' expert opined that the incidence of vision loss during non-ophthalmological surgery is so rare that failure to disclose this risk does not constitute a deviation from the standard of care. The plaintiff's expert disagreed. The Court found that there was a genuine issue of fact as to whether the standard of care required disclosure of this risk as well as whether a reasonable patient in the plaintiff's position would have chosen to proceed with the surgery even if this risk had been disclosed. The case was allowed to proceed against the surgeon and the anesthesiologist.[85] According to court records, the suit was settled prior to trial.

Recent Federal Legislative Efforts at Medical Malpractice and Health Care Liability Reform

Though tort reform efforts have generally been concentrated at the state level, federal lawmakers have recently made several efforts to reduce the number of medical malpractice and other health care liability lawsuits or to otherwise limit the possible recovery to plaintiffs in these cases. The latest is the "Protecting Access to Care Act of 2017," which was introduced in the House of Representatives by Rep. Steve King (R-Iowa) on February 24, 2017.[86] In its current form, the bill would apply to any medical malpractice or health care liability action, whether brought in state or federal court, "concerning the provision of goods or services for which coverage was provided in whole or in part via a federal program, subsidy or tax benefit."[87] As such, it would appear to cover suits arising out of "health care products or services paid for at least in part by programs such as Medicare, Medicaid, a subsidy under the Affordable Care Act (ACA), Veterans Administration-provided health care, or the Employee Retirement Income Security Act of 1974."[88]

The bill includes the following provisions:

- The statute of limitations for health care lawsuits would be the *earlier* of one year after the claimant discovers (or reasonably should have discovered) his injury or three years after the date of injury or the date of completion of the health care treatment at issue. No health care lawsuit could be brought after three years had passed from the earlier of the date of injury or the completion of the treatment at issue (except in cases involving fraud, intentional concealment, or leaving a foreign object in a patient). However, this would not preempt any state law that provides for a shorter statute of limitations or that establishes a statute of repose.
- Noneconomic damages would be capped at $250,000. However, these caps would also not preempt any state law setting the amount of damages available in a health care lawsuit.
- Expert witnesses must be licensed to practice in the state where the injury at issue occurred or in a contiguous bordering state and practice a profession or specialty which would make that person's expert testimony "relevant to the issues in the case," thus imposing a version of the locality rule. If a defendant is a board-certified specialist, any expert witness testifying regarding the standard of care for that defendant must also be board-certified in the same specialty. Expert witnesses would also be subject to any state-specific requirements with respect to their qualifications.
- A plaintiff must file with his complaint an affidavit of merit signed by a health care provider stating that the defendant breached the standard of care, what actions should have been taken or omitted by the defendant, and how the defendant's actions caused the plaintiff's injury.[89]

[85] *Ibid.*

[86] All actions H.R.1215—115th Congress (2017–2018) [Internet]. Available from: https://www.congress.gov/bill/115th-congress/house-bill/1215/all-actions-without-amendments?r=1.

[87] Protecting Access to Care Act of 2017, H.R. 1215, 115th Cong., 1st Sess. (2017) (as referred to the Senate).

[88] H.R. Rep. No. 115-55, at 36 (2017) (internal footnotes omitted).

[89] Protecting Access to Care Act of 2017, *supra* note 87.

This bill, as outlined above, passed the House on June 28, 2017, and is now pending in the Senate. However, the likelihood the bill will progress further is low. The bill is opposed by numerous consumer and public interest groups as well as the American Bar Association.[90] Several physicians' groups, including the Association of American Physicians and Surgeons and the American Academy of Family Physicians, have objected to provisions similar to those in the bill that are included in the Trump Administration's proposed budget.[91] Previous bills seeking to impose limits on medical malpractice actions in the states have been unsuccessful.[92]

One piece of failed legislation that sought to go extraordinarily far in standardizing medical malpractice litigation was the Empowering Patients First Act of 2015,[93] which was introduced in the House on May 13, 2015, by Tom Price. The bill proposed that the Secretary of the U.S. Department of Health and Human Services "provide for the selection and issuance of clinical practice guidelines for treatment of medical conditions" with a "physician consensus-building organization" and other physician specialty organizations. If a defendant in a medical malpractice lawsuit established by a preponderance of the evidence that treatment was provided consistent with these clinical practice guidelines, she could not be held liable unless the plaintiff then established the defendant's "liability" by a much higher clear and convincing evidence standard. The bill further provided for grants to states to develop their own "health care tribunals" to resolve malpractice claims through nonjudicial expert review panels and subsequent administrative review process. If, after going through this process, a party was dissatisfied with the outcome, that party could file his claim in a state court, but he would have to forfeit any award he received during the administrative review process. If the expert panel or administrative tribunal previously made a finding in favor of the health care provider on compliance with the clinical practice guidelines or on any other element of a medical malpractice claim, the defendant would be entitled to judgment as a matter of law in the state court unless the plaintiff could produce clear and convincing evidence to the contrary.[94] This bill never made it to a vote.[95]

Acknowledgments The author wishes to thank Douglas Hof, M.D. for providing the ASA Closed Claims Project data referenced herein.

Disclaimer: The views and opinions expressed in this chapter are those of the author and do not necessarily reflect the official policy or position of any agency, organization, employer, or company. Nothing in this chapter is intended to be construed as legal advice and should not be relied upon as such.

[90] H.R. Rep. No. 115-55, at 35.

[91] Dickson V. Providers want trump to stay out of tort reform. Modern Healthcare [Internet]. 2017 May 24 [cited 2017 Jun 18]. Available at: http://www.modernhealthcare.com/article/20170524/NEWS/170529947/providers-want-trump-to-stay-out-of-tort-reform.

[92] *See* Protecting Access to Healthcare Act, H.R. 5, 112th Cong. 2d Sess. (2012); Actions overview H.R.5—112th Congress (2011–2012) [Internet]. Available from https://www.congress.gov/bill/112th-congress/house-bill/5/actions?r=1.

[93] Empowering Patients First Act of 2015, H.R. 2300 §§ 401 *et seq*., 114th Cong., 1st Sess. (2015).

[94] *Ibid.*

[95] All Actions H.R.2300—114th Congress (2015-2016) [Internet]. Available from https://www.congress.gov/bill/114th-congress/house-bill/2300/all-actions?r=1.

Index

A. Arthur et al. (eds.), *Perioperative Considerations and Positioning for Neurosurgical Procedures*,
https://doi.org/10.1007/978-3-319-72679-3

The manufacturer's authorised representative in the EU is Springer Nature Customer Service Centre GmbH, Europaplatz 3, 69115 Heidelberg, Germany. If you have any concerns regarding our products, please contact ProductSafety@springernature.com

Printed and bound by CPI Group (UK) Ltd, Croydon, CR0 4YY
05/10/2026
02228132-0011